# Essentials of Trauma Anesthesia

# Essentials of Trauma Anesthesia

Edited by

**Albert J. Varon**

Professor and Vice Chair for Education, Department of Anesthesiology, University of Miami Miller School of Medicine, and Director of Anesthesiology, Ryder Trauma Center at Jackson Memorial Hospital, Miami, FL, USA

**Charles E. Smith**

Professor at Case Western Reserve University School of Medicine and Director of Cardiothoracic and Trauma Anesthesia, MetroHealth Medical Center, Cleveland, OH, USA

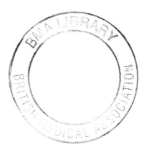

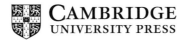
CAMBRIDGE
UNIVERSITY PRESS

CAMBRIDGE UNIVERSITY PRESS
Cambridge, New York, Melbourne, Madrid, Cape Town,
Singapore, São Paulo, Delhi, Mexico City

Cambridge University Press
The Edinburgh Building, Cambridge CB2 8RU, UK

Published in the United States of America
by Cambridge University Press, New York

www.cambridge.org
Information on this title: www.cambridge.org/9781107602564

First published 2012

Printed in the United Kingdom at the University Press, Cambridge

*A catalogue record for this publication is available from the British Library*

*Library of Congress Cataloging-in-Publication Data*

Essentials of trauma anesthesia / edited by Albert J. Varon and Charles E.
Smith.
   p. ; cm.
   ISBN 978-1-107-60256-4 (Paperback)
   I. Varon, Albert J. II. Smith, Charles E.
   [DNLM: 1. Anesthesia.   2. Wounds and Injuries.   3. Critical Care.
4. Perioperative Care.   WO 200]
   617.9′6–dc23

                                                         2011048649

ISBN 978-1-107-60256-4 Paperback

To my wife, Dina, for loving and putting up with me; and to my sons, Michael and Victor, who give me infinite joy.
AJV

To the victims of blunt and penetrating trauma, and to all those who work long and hard to transport, stabilize, diagnose, treat, and rehabilitate them. To my wife Bobby, children Adrienne, Emily, and Rebecca, and parents Thelma and David for their love and support.
CES

# Contents

# Preface

Trauma is the leading cause of death among children, adolescents, and young adults in the United States; it is the second most common single cause of death worldwide.

Those who survive trauma suffer the physical and psychological consequences of injury, which have an enormous impact on patients, their families, and society.

Although few anesthesiologists care exclusively for trauma patients, most will care for trauma patients at one time or another in their clinical practice. These encounters usually occur at the end of the day or in the middle of the night and challenge clinicians to expeditiously manage multi-system derangements despite incomplete patient information.

Active participation of anesthesiologists in the care of severely injured patients provides the best opportunity for improved outcome. We believe participation should not only include involvement in anesthetic management, but also the initial evaluation, resuscitation, and perioperative care of these patients. Unfortunately, current training does not expose trainees to the entire spectrum of trauma care. Although there are a few textbooks that deal with trauma anesthesia, these books are quite extensive, serve mostly as reference books, and are not meant to be read cover-to-cover.

Our intention in creating this text is to provide anesthesiology trainees and practitioners with a concise review of the essential elements in the care of the severely injured patient and to emphasize the role of anesthesiologists in all aspects of trauma care: from time of injury until the patient leaves the critical care areas of the facility. Although a textbook of this size cannot give exhaustive coverage of all issues, we attempt to provide a review of the most important aspects of trauma care from the anesthesiologist's perspective. We also try to identify new trends in surgery and anesthesiology practices that impact on the management of trauma patients.

We present, in three parts, the essential elements of trauma anesthesia care. The first section deals with the core principles of trauma anesthesia including epidemiology, initial evaluation and management, airway management, shock resuscitation and fluid therapy, vascular cannulation, blood component therapy, general and regional anesthesia, monitoring, echocardiography, and postoperative care. A review of chemical and radiological exposure in trauma is also presented. The second section is designed to review anesthetic considerations for traumatic injuries by anatomical area. The third and final section discusses anesthetic management in special trauma populations including burn, pediatric, geriatric, and pregnant patients.

The editors of this book are academic anesthesiologists each with 25 years of experience caring for trauma patients. We were fortunate to recruit expert contributors who are actively engaged in clinical care at leading US and Canadian trauma centers. The chapter contributors were given the task of creating an easily readable and clinically relevant review of current trauma management. As editors we have worked closely with the contributors to attain a consistent style, cover the subject matter in a coherent and logical manner, prevent unnecessary duplication, and provide cross-referencing between chapters. The liberal use of bullet-points and tables facilitated the creation of a portable text that is conducive to the rapid appreciation of the essential elements in trauma care.

We hope this textbook will serve as a useful, practical guide to anesthesiology trainees and practitioners who currently manage or will manage trauma patients. We hope that all anesthesia providers, from the novice to the practitioner, will benefit from this book and more importantly that this will improve their care of trauma patients.

The editors wish to thank the members of the American Society of Anesthesiologists' Committee of Trauma and Emergency Preparedness (COTEP) and our trauma anesthesiology colleagues at MetroHealth Medical Center and the Ryder Trauma Center for helping us select the topics for this book. The editors are also grateful to the chapter authors for contributing to this effort despite their already heavy clinical workload and Eric Scot Shaw who helped edit some of the chapters. Finally, we wish to acknowledge the support of Deborah Russell, Nisha Doshi, Caroline Mowatt, and all the staff at Cambridge University Press in the preparation and timely publication of *Essentials of Trauma Anesthesia*.

*Albert J. Varon, MD, MHPE, FCCM*
*Charles E. Smith, MD, FRCPC*

# Contributors

**Brendan Astley, MD**
Assistant Professor, Case Western Reserve
University School of Medicine
Director, Acute Pain Management
Department of Anesthesia
MetroHealth Medical Center,
Cleveland, OH

**Shawn Banks, MD**
Assistant Professor and Residency
Program Director
Department of Anesthesiology,
University of Miami Miller School
of Medicine
Attending Anesthesiologist
Ryder Trauma Center at
Jackson Memorial Hospital
Miami, FL

**Michael D. Bassett MD**
Assistant Professor,
Case Western Reserve
University School of Medicine
Anesthesiologist,
MetroHealth Medical Center,
Cleveland, OH

**John J. Como, MD, MPH, FACS**
Associate Professor of Surgery
Case Western Reserve University
School of Medicine
Associate Medical Director, Trauma
Services
MetroHealth Medical Center
Cleveland, OH

**Armagan Dagal MD, FRCA**
Assistant Professor, Department of
Anesthesiology & Pain Medicine,
Adjunct Assistant Professor,
Department of Neurological Surgery
Division Head of Spine and Orthopaedic
Anesthesia Services
Harborview Medical Center,

University of Washington
Seattle, WA

**Christian Diez, MD**
Assistant Professor and Associate
Residency Program Director
Department of Anesthesiology,
University of Miami Miller School of
Medicine
Attending Anesthesiologist
Ryder Trauma Center at Jackson
Memorial Hospital
Miami, FL

**Sylvia Y. Dolinski MD**
Associate Professor of Anesthesiology
and Critical Care
Director, Critical Care Fellowship
Medical College of Wisconsin
Milwaukee, WI

**Richard Dutton, MD, MBA**
Professor of Anesthesiology
University of Maryland School
of Medicine
R Adams Cowley Shock Trauma Center
Baltimore, MD

**Ashraf Fayad MD, FRCPC, FFARCSI,
FACC, FASE**
Associate Professor
Director, Perioperative Echocardiography
for Non-cardiac Surgery Program
Department of Anesthesiology
University of Ottawa
Ottawa, Canada

**Yvette Fouche, M.D**
Assitant Professor of Anesthesiology
University of Maryland School
of Medicine
Director, Trauma Anesthesiology Division
R Adams Cowley Shock Trauma Center
Baltimore, MD

**Megan Gatlin, DO**
Resident Physician
Department of Anesthesiology,
Jackson Memorial Hospital
Miami, FL

**Ralf E. Gebhard, MD**
Professor of Anesthesiology and Associate
Professor of Orthopedics and
Rehabilitation
Director, Division of Regional Anesthesia
and Acute Perioperative Pain Management
Department of Anesthesiology,
University of Miami Miller School
of Medicine
Miami, FL

**Suneeta Gollapudy MD,**
Assistant Professor of Anesthesiology
Director, Division of Neuroanesthesia
Director, Division of Post Anesthesia Care
Unit, Department of Anesthesiology
Medical College of
Wisconsin Froedtert Memorial Lutheran
Hospital Milwaukee, WI

**Andreas Grabinsky, MD**
Program Director and Section Head,
Emergency and Trauma Anesthesia
Assistant Professor of Anesthesiology
Harborview Medical Center
Seattle, WA

**Thomas E. Grissom, M.D.**
Associate Professor of Anesthesiology
University of Maryland School of Medicine
R Adams Cowley Shock Trauma Center
Baltimore, MD

**Pertti Hakala, MD**
Assistant Professor
Department of Anesthesiology,
University of Miami Miller School
of Medicine
Attending Anesthesiologist
Ryder Trauma Center at Jackson Memorial
Hospital
Miami, FL

**Olga Kaslow, M.D., Ph.D.**
Director, Trauma Anesthesiology Service,
Associate Professor, Department of
Anesthesiology
Medical College of Wisconsin
Froedtert Memorial Lutheran Hospital
Milwaukee, WI

**Robert Kettler, M.D.**
Associate Professor,
Department of Anesthesiology
Medical College of Wisconsin
Froedtert Memorial Lutheran Hospital
Milwaukee, WI

**Jeb Kucik, MD, DMCC, FCCP**
Lieutenant Commander, Medical Corps,
U.S. Navy
Anesthesia Program Director, Navy
Trauma Training Center
Los Angeles, CA, USA
Assistant Professor of Anesthesiology
University of Southern California Keck
School of Medicine

**Jessica A. Lovich-Sapola MD**
Director, Pre-Surgical Testing
Assistant Professor, Case Western Reserve
University School of Medicine
Anesthesiologist, MetroHealth Medical
Center, Cleveland, OH

**Scott Margraf, DO**
Resident Physician, Department of
Anesthesiology, University of Southern
California
Lieutenant, United States Navy Reserve
Navy Operational Support Center
Los Angeles, CA

**Joseph H. McIsaac, III, MD, MS**
Chief of Trauma Anesthesia,
Hartford Hospital
Hartford, CT, USA
Associate Clinical Professor of Anesthesiology
University of Connecticut School of Medicine
Associate Adjunct Professor of Biomedical
Engineering
University of Connecticut Graduate School

**Richard McNeer, MD, PhD**
Assistant Professor of Anesthesiology and
Biomedical Engineering
University of Miami Miller School of
Medicine
Attending Anesthesiologist
Ryder Trauma Center at Jackson Memorial
Hospital
Miami, FL

**Nicholas Nedeff, MD**
Assistant Professor
Department of Anesthesiology, University
of Miami Miller School of Medicine
Attending Anesthesiologist
Ryder Trauma Center at Jackson Memorial
Hospital
Miami, FL

**Edgar J. Pierre, MD**
Associate Professor
Department of Anesthesiology, University
of Miami Miller School of Medicine
Attending Anesthesiologist
Ryder Trauma Center at Jackson Memorial
Hospital
Miami, FL

**Ramesh Ramaiah, MD, FRCA, FCARCSI**
Assistant Professor
Department of Anesthesiology and Pain
Medicine
University of Washington Harborview
Medical Center
Seattle, WA

**Sripad Rao, MD**
Assistant Professor
Associate Director, Division of Regional
Anesthesia and Acute Perioperative Pain
Management
Department of Anesthesiology, University
of Miami Miller School of Medicine
Attending Anesthesiologist
Ryder Trauma Center at Jackson Memorial
Hospital
Miami, FL

**Sam Sharar**
Professor, University of Washington
Department of Anesthesiology and Pain
Medicine; Pediatric Anesthesia Section Head
Harborview Medical Center
Seattle, WA

**Deepak Sharma MBBS, MD, DM**
Assistant Professor, Department of
Anesthesiology & Pain Medicine
Adjunct Assistant Professor, Department of
Neurological Surgery
Program Director, Neuroanesthesiology
Fellowship
Harborview Neuroanesthesiology
Education Head
Harborview Medical Center,
University of Washington
Seattle, WA

**Roger Shere-Wolfe, M.D.**
Assistant Professor of Anesthesiology
University of Maryland School of Medicine
R Adams Cowley Shock Trauma Center
Baltimore, MD

**Robert Sikorski, MD**
Assistant Professor of Anesthesiology
University of Maryland School of Medicine
R Adams Cowley Shock Trauma Center
Baltimore, MD

**Charles E. Smith MD, FRCPC**
Professor, Case Western Reserve University
School of Medicine
Director, Cardiothoracic and Trauma
Anesthesia
MetroHealth Medical Center, Cleveland, OH

**Michael J. Souter MB, ChB, FRCA**
Professor, Anesthesiology & Pain
Medicine
Adjunct Professor, Neurological Surgery
University of Washington, Seattle, WA
Chief of Anesthesiology, Harborview
Medical Center
Medical Co-Director, Neurocritical Care
Service, HMC

**Christopher Stephens, M.D.,**
Assistant Professor of Anesthesiology
University of Maryland School of Medicine
R Adams Cowley Shock Trauma Center
Baltimore, MD

**Brandon A. Van Noord, MD**
Resident Physician, Department of
Anesthesiology, University of Southern
California
Lieutenant, United States Navy Reserve
Navy Operational Support Center
Los Angeles, CA

**Albert J. Varon, MD, MHPE, FCCM**
Professor and Vice Chair for Education,
Department of Anesthesiology,
University of Miami Miller School of
Medicine
Director of Anesthesiology,
Ryder Trauma Center at

Jackson Memorial Hospital
Miami, FL

**Monica S. Vavilala, MD**
Professor, Anesthesiology & Pain Medicine
and Pediatrics
Professor (Adj), Neurological Surgery and
Radiology
Associate Director, Harborview Injury
Prevention and Research Center
(HIPRC)
University of Washington, Seattle, WA

**Michael Woo MD, CCFP (EM), RDMS**
Director, Emergency Medicine
Ultrasonography Fellowship Program
Director
Associate Professor
Department of Emergency Medicine
University of Ottawa
Ottawa, Canada

# Abbreviations

AANS = American Association of Neurological Surgeons
ABG = Arterial blood gas
ACES = Abdominal cardiac evaluation with sonography in shock
ACLS = Advanced cardiac life support
ACS = American College of Surgeons
AEC = Airway exchange catheter
AI = Aortic insufficiency
AKI = Acute kidney injury
ALI = Acute lung injury
ARDS = Acute respiratory distress syndrome
ARF = Acute renal failure
ASA = American Society of Anesthesiologists
ASD = Atrial septal defect
ASIA = American Spinal Injury Association
ASRA = American Society of Regional Anesthesia and Pain Management
ATLS = Advanced trauma life support
BBB = Blood brain barrier
BIS = Bispectral index
BP = Blood pressure
BSA = Body surface area
BUN = Blood urea nitrogen
BVM = Bag-valve-mask
CAD = Coronary artery disease
CBC = Complete blood count
CBF = Cerebral blood flow
CDC = Centers for Disease Control
CFD = Color flow Doppler
CHEMM = Chemical Hazards Emergency Medical Management
CMAP = Compound muscle action potential
$CMRO_2$ = Cerebral metabolic rate of oxygen
CNS = Central nervous system
CO = Carbon monoxide
CO = Cardiac output
$CO_2$ = Carbon dioxide

COPD = Chronic obstructive pulmonary disease
COT = Committee on Trauma
CP = Cricoid pressure
CPAP = Continuous positive airway pressure
CPB = Cardiopulmonary bypass
CPP = Cerebral perfusion pressure
CPR = Cardiopulmonary resuscitation
CRM = Crisis resource management
C-section = Caesarean section
CSF = Cerebral spinal fluid
$CSF_P$ = Cerebral spinal fluid pressure
C-spine = Cervical spine
CT = Computed tomography
CTA = Computed tomography angiography
CVP = Central venous pressure
CXR = Chest X-ray
DIC = Disseminated intravascular coagulation
DLT = Double lumen tube
DNA = Deoxyribonucleic acid
DPL = Diagnostic peritoneal lavage
DVT = Deep venous thrombosis
ECG = Electrocardiogram
ED = Emergency department
eFAST = Extended focused assessment with sonography for trauma
EMG = Electromyography
EMS = Emergency medical services
ER = Emergency room
ESKD = End-stage kidney disease
$EtCO_2$ = End-tidal carbon dioxide
ETT = Endotracheal tube
Ex fix = External fixation
FAST = Focused assessment with sonography for trauma
$FEV_1$ = Forced expiratory volume in one second
FFP = Fresh frozen plasma
$FiO_2$ = Fraction of inspired oxygen
FOB = Fiberoptic bronchoscope

FRC = Functional residual capacity
GABA = Gamma-aminobutyric acid
GCS = Glasgow Coma Scale
GFR = Glomerular filtration rate
GSW = Gunshot wound
Gy = Grays
$H_2S$ = Hydrogen sulfide
HCN = Hydrogen cyanide
HTS = Hypertonic saline
ICH = Intracranial hypertension
ICP = Intracranial pressure
ICU = Intensive care unit
IDSA = Infectious Disease Society of America
INR = International normalized ratio
IO = Intraosseous
IOP = Intraocular pressure
IR = Interventional radiology
ISS = Injury severity score
IV = Intravenous
IVC = Inferior vena cava
LA = Left atrium
LAX = Long axis
LMA = Laryngeal mask airway
LR = Lactated Ringer's solution
LTA = Laryngeal tube airway
LV = Left ventricle
MAC = Minimum alveolar concentration
MAP = Mean arterial pressure
MEP = Motor evoked potential
MILI = Manual in-line immobilization
MR = Mitral regurgitation
MRI = Magnetic resonance imaging
MV = Motor vehicle
$N_2O$ = Nitrous oxide
NASCIS = National Acute Spinal Cord Injury Study
NG = Nasogastric
NHTSA = National Highway Traffic Safety Administration
NIH = National Institutes of Health
NIOSH = National Institute for Occupational Safety and Health
NMBD = Neuromuscular blocking drug
NMDA = N-methyl-D-aspartate
NS = Normal saline

NSAID = Non-steroidal anti-inflammatory drug
OCR = Oculo-cardiac reflex
OLV = One-lung ventilation
OR = Operating room
ORIF = Open reduction internal fixation
PA = Pulmonary artery
$PaCO_2$ = Arterial carbon dioxide tension
PACU = Postanesthesia care unit
$PaO_2$ = Arterial oxygen tension
PAOP = Pulmonary artery occlusion pressure
PAP = Pulmonary artery pressure
PAPR = Powered air-purifying respirators
PCA = Patient-controlled analgesia
PCC = Prothrombin complex concentrates
PE = Pulmonary emboli
PEEP = Positive end-expiratory pressure
Perc fix = Percutaneous fixation
PFO = Patent foramen ovale
PPE = Personal protective equipment
PPV = Pulse pressure variation
PRBC = Packed red blood cell
PT = Prothrombin time
$P_{\bar{v}}CO_2$ = Mixed venous carbon dioxide tension
$P_{\bar{v}}O_2$ = Mixed venous oxygen tension
RA = Right atrium
rad = Radiation absorbed dose
RBCs = Red blood cells
rem = Roentgen-equivalent man
rFVIIa = Recombinant factor VIIa
RIFLE = Risk, Injury, Failure, Loss, and End-stage kidney disease
RR = Respiratory rate
RSI = Rapid sequence induction
RUL = Right upper lobe
RUSH = Rapid ultrasound for shock and hypotension
RV = Right ventricle
RWMA = Regional wall motion abnormality
SAX = Short axis
SBP = Systolic blood pressure
SCA = Society of Cardiovascular Anesthesiologists

**SCCP** = Spinal cord perfusion pressure
**SCI** = Spinal cord injury
**SCIWORA** = Spinal cord injury without radiographic abnormality
**SCM** = Sternocleidomastoid muscle
**S$_{cv}$O$_2$** = Central venous oxygen saturation
**SIRS** = Systemic inflammatory response syndrome
**SjvO$_2$** = Jugular venous oxygen saturation
**SpO$_2$** = Oxygen saturation measured by pulse oximeter
**SPV** = Systolic pressure variation
**SSEP** = Somatosensory evoked potentials
**START** = Simple triage and rapid assessment
**STASCIS** = Surgical Treatment for Acute Spinal Cord Injury Study
**STE** = Speckle-tracking echocardiography
**Sv** = Sievert

**S$_{\bar{v}}$O$_2$** = Mixed venous oxygen saturation
**SVR** = Systemic vascular resistance
**SVV** = Stroke volume variation
**TBI** = Traumatic brain injury
**TBSA** = Total body surface area
**TEE** = Transesophageal echocardiography
**TIG** = Tetanus immune globulin
**TIVA** = Total intravenous anesthesia
**TOXALS** = Advanced life support for acute toxic injury
**TTE** = Transthoracic echocardiography
**US** = Ultrasound
**VAP** = Ventilator-associated pneumonia
**VATS** = Video-assisted thoracic surgery
**Vfib** = Ventricular fibrillation
**WISER** = Wireless information system for emergency responders
**YPLL** = Years of potential life lost

# Chapter
# 1
# Trauma epidemiology, mechanisms of injury, and prehospital care

John J. Como, Charles E. Smith, and Andreas Grabinsky

## Trauma epidemiology

Trauma is defined as physical damage to the body as a result of mechanical, chemical, thermal, electrical, or other energy that exceeds the tolerance of the body. Although trauma is often thought of as a series of unavoidable accidents, in reality it is a disease with known risk factors. Like other diseases such as cancer and heart disease, trauma risk factors are modifiable and injuries can be avoided before their occurrence. There are three phases of injury:

1. Pre-injury
2. Injury
3. Post-injury

The pre-injury phase includes the events prior to trauma and is impacted by risk factors such as drug and alcohol intoxication, medical and environmental conditions, and behavioral factors. The injury phase is when energy is transferred to the victim's body through a series of mechanisms related to blunt, penetrating, crush, blast, and rotational injury. The post-injury phase commences as soon as transfer of energy is complete. Since approximately 50% of trauma deaths are catastrophic events (massive head injury, upper spinal cord, heart, and great vessel trauma), which occur within moments of the injury, the only way to avoid them is through preventive strategies. An understanding of the basic epidemiology of traumatic injury is thus imperative if we wish to decrease the burden of this disease on society.

The most effective means of reducing mortality from trauma is modification of risk factors and prevention of injuries through education, legislation, and research. Examples of preventive measures for motor vehicle trauma include:

- Legislation concerning alcohol consumption
- Proper child occupant restraint in cars
- Front and rear seatbelts
- Air bags
- Speed limit controls
- Laminated windshields
- Crash resistant fuel systems
- Energy absorbing steering wheels

*Essentials of Trauma Anesthesia*, ed. A. J. Varon and C. E. Smith. Published by Cambridge University Press.
© Cambridge University Press 2012.

## Age Groups

| Rank | <1 | 1–4 | 5–9 | 10–14 | 15–24 | 25–34 | 35–44 | 45–54 | 55–64 | 65+ | Total |
|---|---|---|---|---|---|---|---|---|---|---|---|
| 1 | Congenital Anomalies 5,785 | Unintentional Injury 1,588 | Unintentional Injury 965 | Unintentional Injury 1,229 | Unintentional Injury 15,897 | Unintentional Injury 14,977 | Unintentional Injury 16,931 | Malignant Neoplasms 50,167 | Malignant Neoplasms 103,171 | Heart Disease 496,095 | Heart Disease 616,067 |
| 2 | Short Gestation 4,857 | Congenital Anomalies 546 | Malignant Neoplasms 480 | Malignant Neoplasms 479 | Homicide 5,551 | Suicide 5,278 | Malignant Neoplasms 13,288 | Heart Disease 37,434 | Heart Disease 65,527 | Malignant Neoplasms 389,730 | Malignant Neoplasms 562,875 |
| 3 | SIDS 2,453 | Homicide 398 | Congenital Anomalies 196 | Homicide 213 | Suicide 4,140 | Homicide 4,758 | Heart Disease 11,839 | Unintentional Injury 20,315 | Chronic Low. Respiratory Disease 12,777 | Cerebrovascular 115,961 | Cerebrovascular 135,952 |
| 4 | Maternal Pregnancy Comp. 1,769 | Malignant Neoplasms 364 | Homicide 133 | Suicide 180 | Malignant Neoplasms 1,653 | Malignant Neoplasms 3,463 | Suicide 6,722 | Liver Disease 8,212 | Unintentional Injury 12,193 | Chronic Low. Respiratory Disease 109,562 | Chronic Low. Respiratory Disease 127,924 |
| 5 | Unintentional Injury 1,285 | Heart Disease 173 | Heart Disease 110 | Congenital Anomalies 178 | Heart Disease 1,084 | Heart Disease 3,223 | HIV 3,572 | Suicide 7,778 | Diabetes Mellitus 11,304 | Alzheimer's Disease 73,797 | Unintentional Injury 123,706 |
| 6 | Placenta Cord Membranes 1,135 | Influenza & Pneumonia 109 | Chronic Low. Respiratory Disease 54 | Heart Disease 131 | Congenital Anomalies 402 | HIV 1,091 | Homicide 3,052 | Cerebrovascular 6,385 | Cerebrovascular 10,500 | Diabetes Mellitus 51,528 | Alzheimer's Disease 74,632 |
| 7 | Bacterial Sepsis 820 | Septicemia 78 | Influenza & Pneumonia 48 | Chronic Low. Respiratory Disease 64 | Cerebrovascular 195 | Diabetes Mellitus 610 | Liver Disease 2,570 | Diabetes Mellitus 5,753 | Liver Disease 8,004 | Influenza & Pneumonia 45,941 | Diabetes Mellitus 71,382 |
| 8 | Respiratory Distress 789 | Perinatal Period 70 | Benign Neoplasms 41 | Influenza & Pneumonia 55 | Diabetes Mellitus 168 | Cerebrovascular 505 | Cerebrovascular 2,133 | HIV 4,156 | Suicide 5,069 | Nephritis 38,484 | Influenza & Pneumonia 52,717 |
| 9 | Circulatory System Disease 624 | Benign Neoplasms 59 | Cerebrovascular 38 | Cerebrovascular 45 | Influenza & Pneumonia 163 | Congenital Anomalies 417 | Diabetes Mellitus 1,984 | Chronic Low. Respiratory Disease 4,153 | Nephritis 4,440 | Unintentional Injury 38,292 | Nephritis 46,448 |
| 10 | Neonatal Hemorrhage 597 | Chronic Low. Respiratory Disease 57 | Septicemia 36 | Benign Neoplasms 43 | Three Tied* 160 | Liver Disease 384 | Septicemia 910 | Viral Hepatitis 2,815 | Septicemia 4,231 | Septicemia 26,362 | Septicemia 34,828 |

*The three causes are: Complicated Pregnancy, HIV, Septicemia.
**Source:** National Vital Statistics System, National Center for Health Statistics, CDC.
**Produced by:** Office of Statistics and Programming, National Center for Injury Prevention and Control, CDC.

**Figure 1.1.** Leading causes of death in the United States – 2007.

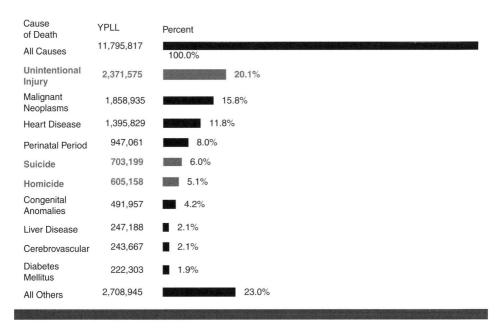

| Cause of Death | YPLL | Percent |
|---|---|---|
| All Causes | 11,795,817 | 100.0% |
| Unintentional Injury | 2,371,575 | 20.1% |
| Malignant Neoplasms | 1,858,935 | 15.8% |
| Heart Disease | 1,395,829 | 11.8% |
| Perinatal Period | 947,061 | 8.0% |
| Suicide | 703,199 | 6.0% |
| Homicide | 605,158 | 5.1% |
| Congenital Anomalies | 491,957 | 4.2% |
| Liver Disease | 247,188 | 2.1% |
| Cerebrovascular | 243,667 | 2.1% |
| Diabetes Mellitus | 222,303 | 1.9% |
| All Others | 2,708,945 | 23.0% |

Produced By: Office of Statistics and Pogramming, National Center for Injury Prevention and Control, CDC
Date Source: National Center for Health Statistics (NCHS) Vital Statistics system.

**Figure 1.2.** Years of potential life lost (YPLL) before age 65, United States – 2007.

The problem of traumatic injury in the United States is enormous. In the United States, trauma (including unintentional injury, homicide, and suicide) was the third leading cause of death in 2007 after heart disease and malignant neoplasms for people of all ages; it was also the leading cause of death in children and in adults up to 44 years of age (see Figure 1.1). In total, about one person will die every three minutes due to injury in the United States. As the majority of fatal injuries occur in the young, trauma is also responsible for more years of potential life lost than any other disease, accounting for 31.2% of years lost from all causes (see Figure 1.2). The two leading causes of injury death are those due to vehicular injuries and those due to firearms, which together account for about half of fatal injuries (see Figure 1.3).

In addition to death, the problem of non-fatal injury is also staggering. In 2009 a total of 29,636,366 people in the United States suffered from non-fatal injuries requiring medical treatment. Of those, 2,161,199 required hospitalization or transfer to another facility. In the same year, an additional 2,003,585 people suffered from non-fatal violence-related injuries requiring medical treatment and 359,281 patients were either hospitalized or transferred. The ten leading causes of non-fatal injuries stratified by age in the United States in 2008 are listed in Figure 1.4. In almost every age group the leading cause of non-fatal trauma admissions is falls.

The costs to society are tremendous and include:

- Emergency medical services (EMS)
- In-hospital medical care
- Rehabilitation
- Wage and productivity loss

# Age Groups

| Rank | <1 | 1–4 | 5–9 | 10–14 | 15–24 | 25–34 | 35–44 | 45–54 | 55–64 | 65+ | Total |
|---|---|---|---|---|---|---|---|---|---|---|---|
| 1 | Unintentional Suffocation 959 | Unintentional Drowning 458 | Unintentional MV Traffic 456 | Unintentional MV Traffic 696 | Unintentional MV Traffic 10,272 | Unintentional MV Traffic 6,842 | Unintentional Poisoning 7,575 | Unintentional Poisoning 9,006 | Unintentional MV Traffic 4,177 | Unintentional Fall 18,334 | Unintentional MV Traffic 42,031 |
| 2 | Homicide Unspecified 174 | Unintentional MV Traffic 428 | Unintentional Fire/Burn 136 | Homicide Firearm 154 | Homicide Firearm 4,669 | Unintentional Poisoning 5,700 | Unintentional MV Traffic 6,135 | Unintentional MV Traffic 6,262 | Unintentional Poisoning 3,120 | Unintentional MV Traffic 6,632 | Unintentional Poisoning 29,846 |
| 3 | Unintentional MV Traffic 122 | Unintentional Fire/Burn 204 | Unintentional Drowning 122 | Suicide Suffocation 119 | Unintentional Poisoning 3,159 | Homicide Firearm 3,751 | Suicide Firearm 2,879 | Suicide Firearm 3,531 | Suicide Firearm 2,786 | Unintentional Unspecified 4,855 | Unintentional Fall 22,631 |
| 4 | Homicide Other Spec., classifiable 86 | Homicide Unspecified 174 | Homicide Firearm 47 | Unintentional Drowning 102 | Suicide Firearm 1,900 | Suicide Firearm 2,306 | Homicide Firearm 2,038 | Suicide Poisoning 2,015 | Unintentional Fall 1,739 | Suicide Firearm 3,895 | Suicide Firearm 17,352 |
| 5 | Unintentional Drowning 57 | Unintentional Suffocation 149 | Unintentional Suffocation 42 | Unintentional Other Land Transport 80 | Suicide Suffocation 1,533 | Suicide Suffocation 1,770 | Suicide Suffocation 1,839 | Suicide Suffocation 1,589 | Suicide Poisoning 1,147 | Unintentional Suffocation 3,209 | Homicide Firearm 12,632 |
| 6 | Unintentional Fire/Burn 39 | Unintentional Pedestrian, Other 124 | Unintentional Other Land Transport 40 | Unintentional Fire/Burn 78 | Unintentional Drowning 630 | Suicide Poisoning 802 | Suicide Poisoning 1,419 | Unintentional Fall 1,304 | Suicide Suffocation 725 | Adverse Effects 1,631 | Suicide Suffocation 8,161 |
| 7 | Undetermined Suffocation 34 | Homicide Other Spec., classifiable 61 | Unintentional Pedestrian, Other 32 | Unintentional Poisoning 69 | Homicide Cut/pierce 444 | Undetermined Poisoning 687 | Undetermined Poisoning 1,020 | Homicide Firearm 1,159 | Unintentional Fire/Burn 505 | Unintentional Fire/Burn 1,179 | Suicide Poisoning 6,358 |
| 8 | Homicide Firearm 30 | Homicide Firearm 48 | Homicide Suffocation 21 | Unintentional Suffocation 60 | Undetermined Poisoning 365 | Homicide Cut/Pierce 466 | Unintentional Fall 593 | Undetermined Poisoning 1,155 | Unintentional Suffocation 484 | Unintentional Poisoning 1,149 | Unintentional Unspecified 6,019 |
| 9 | Undetermined Unspecified 28 | Unintentional Struck by or Against 44 | Unintentional Firearm 20 | Suicide Firearm 53 | Suicide Poisoning 362 | Unintentional Drowning 381 | Unintentional Drowning 417 | Unintentional Fire/Burn 496 | Homicide Firearm 446 | Suicide Poisoning 604 | Unintentional Suffocation 5,997 |
| 10 | Unintentional Fall 24 | Unintentional Fall 36 | Unintentional Struck by or Against 20 | Unintentional Firearm 26 | Unintentional Other Land Transport 310 | Unintentional Fall 334 | Homicide Cut/pierce 409 | Unintentional Drowning 481 | Adverse Effects 398 | Suicide Suffocation 583 | Undetermined Poisoning 3,770 |

**Source:** National Center for Health Statistics (NCHS), National Vital Statistics System.
**Produced by:** Office of Statistics and Programming, National Center for Injury Prevention and Control, CDC.

**Figure 1.3.** Leading causes of injury deaths by age group highlighting unintentional injury deaths, United States – 2007. MV: motor vehicle

## Age Groups

| Rank | <1 | 1–4 | 5–9 | 10–14 | 15–24 | 25–34 | 35–44 | 45–54 | 55–64 | 65+ | Total |
|---|---|---|---|---|---|---|---|---|---|---|---|
| 1 | Unintentional Fall 125,097 | Unintentional Fall 878,612 | Unintentional Fall 639,091 | Unintentional Fall 607,365 | Unintentional Struck By/Against 1,031,192 | Unintentional Fall 813,125 | Unintentional Fall 798,775 | Unintentional Fall 913,341 | Unintentional Fall 742,735 | Unintentional Fall 2,114,113 | Unintentional Fall 8,551,037 |
| 2 | Unintentional Struck By/Against 37,010 | Unintentional Struck By/Against 371,404 | Unintentional Struck By/Against 399,995 | Unintentional Struck By/Against 583,948 | Unintentional Fall 918,574 | Unintentional Overexertion 675,349 | Unintentional Overexertion 584,738 | Unintentional Overexertion 448,656 | Unintentional Struck By/Against 230,874 | Unintentional Struck By/Against 229,304 | Unintentional Struck By/Against 4,492,287 |
| 3 | Unintentional Other Bite/Sting 13,092 | Unintentional Other Bite/Sting 134,920 | Unintentional Cut/Pierce 106,907 | Unintentional Overexertion 283,813 | Unintentional MV Occupant 743,738 | Unintentional Struck By/Against 654,918 | Unintentional Struck By/Against 529,223 | Unintentional Struck By/Against 424,305 | Unintentional Overexertion 213,174 | Unintentional Overexertion 178,344 | Unintentional Overexertion 3,278,300 |
| 4 | Unintentional Foreign Body 11,035 | Unintentional Foreign Body 123,369 | Unintentional Other Bite/Sting 83,107 | Unintentional Cut/Pierce 135,610 | Unintentional Overexertion 735,400 | Unintentional MV Occupant 528,751 | Unintentional MV Occupant 412,047 | Unintentional MV Occupant 350,291 | Unintentional MV Occupant 197,380 | Unintentional MV Occupant 176,571 | Unintentional MV Occupant 2,581,605 |
| 5 | Unintentional Other Specified 8,271 | Unintentional Cut/Pierce 81,571 | Unintentional Pedal Cyclist 80,743 | Unintentional Pedal Cyclist 108,016 | Other Assault* Struck By/Against 475,386 | Unintentional Cut/Pierce 411,514 | Unintentional Cut/Pierce 320,785 | Unintentional Cut/Pierce 289,857 | Unintentional Cut/Pierce 156,046 | Unintentional Cut/Pierce 112,015 | Unintentional Cut/Pierce 2,072,604 |
| 6 | Unintentional Unknown/ Unspecified 6,722 | Unintentional Overexertion 78,018 | Unintentional Overexertion 75,796 | Unintentional Unknown/ Unspecified 100,842 | Unintentional Cut/Pierce 452,297 | Other Assault* Struck By/Against 308,662 | Unintentional Other Specified 228,808 | Unintentional Other Specified 225,469 | Unintentional Other Specified 95,934 | Unintentional Poisoning 74,623 | Other Assault* Struck By/Against 1,297,555 |
| 7 | Unintentional Cut/Pierce 5,916 | Unintentional Other Specified 69,043 | Unintentional MV Occupant 57,236 | Unintentional MV Occupant 75,969 | Unintentional Other Specified 203,484 | Unintentional Other Specified 196,247 | Other Assault* Struck By/Against 198,019 | Unintentional Poisoning 169,088 | Unintentional Poisoning 84,040 | Unintentional Other Bite/Sting 73,062 | Unintentional Other Specified 1,109,782 |
| 8 | Unintentional Cut/Pierce 5,916 | Unintentional Fire/Burn 50,708 | Unintentional Foreign Body 56,624 | Other Assault* Struck By/Against 73,372 | Unintentional Unknown/ Unspecified 191,276 | Unintentional Other Bite/Sting 146,982 | Unintentional Poisoning 132,444 | Other Assault* Struck By/Against 152,308 | Unintentional Other Bite/Sting 72,088 | Unintentional Unknown/ Unspecified 65,524 | Unintentional Other Bite/Sting 993,923 |
| 9 | Unintentional Inhalation/ Suffocation 4,975 | Unintentional Unknown/ Unspecified 45,017 | Unintentional Other Transport 45,158 | Unintentional Other Transport 57,597 | Unintentional Other Bite/Sting 167,310 | Unintentional Unknown/ Unspecified 126,719 | Unintentional Other Bite/Sting 128,813 | Unintentional Other Bite/Sting 122,059 | Other Assault* Struck By/Against 46,004 | Unintentional Other Transport 60,997 | Unintentional Unknown/ Unspecified 806,819 |
| 10 | Unintentional MV Occupant 4,818 | Unintentional Dog Bite 38,214 | Unintentional Unknown/ Unspecified 41,967 | Unintentional Other Bite/Sting 52,489 | Unintentional Other Transport 125,828 | Unintentional Poisoning 103,881 | Unintentional Unknown/ Unspecified 101,767 | Unintentional Unknown/ Unspecified 81,359 | Unintentional Unknown/ Unspecified 45,563 | Unintentional Other Specified 44,520 | Unintentional Poisoning 732,316 |

*The "Other Assault" category includes all assaults that are **not** classified as sexual assault. It represents the majority of assaults.
**Source:** NEISS All Injury Program operated by the Consumer Product Safety Commission (CPSC).
**Produced by:** Office of Statistics and Programming, National Center for Injury Prevention and Control, CDC.

**Figure 1.4.** National estimates of the 10 leading causes of non-fatal injuries treated in hospital emergency departments, United States – 2008. MV: motor vehicle

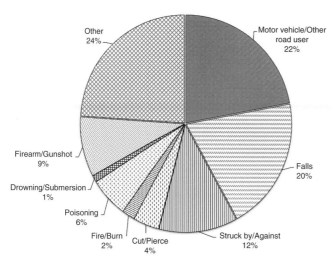

**Figure 1.5.** Percent cost of injury by mechanism.

- Damage to property and goods
- Costs to employers, such as having to train and hire new workers
- Administrative costs
- Private and public health insurance
- Police and legal costs
- Costs arising from fatal and non-fatal trauma

Taking into account both fatal and non-fatal injuries, injury accounts for $406 billion per year if both medical costs and lost productivity are considered. The pie chart in Figure 1.5 illustrates the percentage costs of injury by mechanism.

## Funding for research

While there are well-funded research and prevention programs for chronic diseases like cancer, cardiovascular disease, and HIV/AIDS due to high public awareness, trauma is often viewed as the result of unavoidable accidents, and support for research or prevention programs is comparatively small. In 2010, the National Institutes of Health (NIH) appropriated $372 million for injury research. In the same year $5.8 billion was spent on cancer research, $2.1 billion on research for cardiovascular disease, and $3.1 billion on HIV/AIDS.

## Prevention

Efforts of trauma prevention programs are often hampered by many factors, such as the decisions by motorcyclists and bicycle riders not to use helmets and the reluctance of employers and laborers to invest in safety devices for workplace/machinery safety. Regulations in the form of incentives, laws, or oversight are often required to increase compliance and improve trauma prevention. Unfortunately, special interest groups have commonly opposed seatbelt or helmet laws, as these are viewed as a restriction of freedom and

**Table 1.1.** Reduction in motorcycle fatalities after enacting motorcycle helmet law

| State | Reduction |
|---|---|
| California | 37% |
| Oregon | 33% |
| Nebraska | 32% |
| Texas | 23% |
| Maryland | 20% |
| Washington | 15% |

individual rights. When laws to prevent injuries have been introduced, significant improvements in mortality have often been demonstrated.

As an example, the use of helmets by motorcycle riders reduces the risk of death by 37% and is 67% effective in preventing brain injuries. States with helmet laws have an 86% compliance rate in wearing helmets, while states without such laws have only a 55% rate of helmet use. All states that have introduced helmet laws have experienced significant decreases in motorcycle fatalities (see Table 1.1).

The National Highway Traffic Safety Administration (NHTSA) estimates that three-point safety belts in frontal positions are 45–60% effective in preventing fatalities in frontal collisions and 50–65% effective in preventing moderate-to-critical injuries. Despite this knowledge, the national rate of seatbelt usage is only 82%. States that have enacted primary seatbelt laws have increased seatbelt usage rates by an average of 14% over states without seatbelt laws. According to the NHTSA, nationally 250 additional lives could be saved per year and 6,400 serious injuries prevented for every one percentage-point increase in seatbelt use.

## Mechanisms of injury

Transfer of energy occurs due to blunt and penetrating trauma according to Sir Isaac Newton's first law of motion, which states that "a body in motion will stay in motion unless acted upon by an outside force." Severity of injury is related to three factors:

1. Kinetic energy absorbed by the body ($KE = mass \times velocity^2/2$)
2. Direction the energy travels through the body.
3. Body structure density: solid (water dense) organs are more likely to rupture than hollow (air dense) organs. Bone and cartilage are more rigid and have greater density.

## Falls

In the United States, falls are the most common cause of non-fatal injuries. In 2007, 8,035,635 non-fatal unintentional falls were reported, requiring 746,160 admissions or transfers to other facilities. In the same year, 22,631 patients suffered fatal injuries due to unintentional falls. Falls from a height, such as a ladder or a scaffold, are more common in the working age population. As the patient age increases, falls down stairs and falls from standing become more common. Falls are much more common and are more likely to be lethal in the elderly population. As an example, in those aged 65 and over, the mortality rate for unintentional falls in 2007 was 0.94% compared with 0.08% in those aged 35–44. The incidence of falls has been increasing, and given the widespread use of anticoagulants in the elderly, it is likely that the severity of injuries, even from ground level falls, will increase. Characteristics of the contact surface, position of the person upon landing, and change in velocity determine the injury severity.

- Landing on feet: full force is transmitted up the axial skeleton with injuries to the calcaneus, tibia, femoral neck, and spine. Intra-abdominal organs may be avulsed off their mesenteries or peritoneal attachments.
- Landing on back: energy is transferred over a larger area.
- Landing on head: severe head injury and cervical spine fractures.

## Transportation-related injuries

Motor vehicle collisions are the leading cause of death due to injury (Figure 1.3). In addition, vehicular trauma fatalities rank third in terms of years of life lost (the number of remaining years that the person would be expected to live had they not died) behind only cancer and heart disease. In 2008, almost six million motor vehicle crashes were reported, resulting in over two million injuries. Injuries may occur from frontal or rear impact, from lateral and rotational impact, and due to restraint devices. Each of these impacts is associated with characteristic patterns of injury.

- Frontal impact – down and under: fracture dislocations of the ankle, tibia, knee; fractures of the femur and acetabulum.
- Frontal impact – up and over: rib fractures, sternal fracture, blunt cardiac injury (contusion, valve disruption, rupture), pulmonary trauma, cervical spine fracture, facial fractures, head injury, abdominal trauma.
- Lateral impact: injury of clavicle, ribs, lung, pelvis, and spleen. Other injuries may occur: femur fracture, aortic tear.
- Rear impact: whiplash injuries.
- Sideswipe/rotational: combination of injury patterns as in frontal and lateral impacts.
- Rollover: complicated spectrum of injuries depending on forces, restraints, roof deformation, and ejection.
- Ejection: may result in severe crush or total amputations. Increased risk of death.
- Seatbelt and air bag: restraint devices protect against head, face, chest, abdominal, and extremity trauma. The lap belt when worn above the iliac crest can result in hyperflexion of the torso over the seatbelt with anterior compression fracture of the lumbar spine (Chance fracture). A shoulder restraint may cause trauma to the clavicle. Deployment of the airbag can cause corneal, facial, and neck trauma.

To prevent injuries due to seatbelts, booster seats are recommended for small children. Rollover crashes with ejection of the passenger are considered to have the greatest injury potential, as just about any type of injury can result, due to the multitude of forces involved in this injury pattern.

Most people who die in motor vehicle crashes are the vehicle occupants; less than one-quarter of fatalities caused by motor vehicle crashes involve pedestrians, bicyclists, and motorcycle riders. In 2008, a total of 37,423 people, or just over 100 per day, died in motor vehicle collisions. Motor vehicle crashes were the leading cause of death for every age from 5 through 34 in the United States (Figure 1.3). The fatality rate of these collisions has decreased in the last few decades by the widespread use of better automotive design and the use of seatbelts and airbags, emphasizing the role of preventive strategies in decreasing injury mortality.

With motorcycle and bicycle collisions, the potential for injury is high, because the passenger is frequently ejected and there is very little protection for the passenger. A massive amount of energy is transferred to the cyclist on impact. The main piece of equipment that offers protection is a helmet. Injury patterns are as follows:

- Frontal impact, ejection: any part of the head, chest, or abdomen can hit the handlebars. Blunt abdominal injuries and femur fractures may occur.
- Lateral impact or ejection: open or closed extremity fractures occur on the impacted side. Secondary injury occurs upon landing.
- Laying down the bike: increases the stopping distance for kinetic energy to dissipate. Soft tissue injuries and road burn on the down limb. Injury severity decreased by wearing protective gear.
- Helmets: these are designed to reduce direct force to the head and disperse it over the entire foam padding of the helmet. There is no doubt that helmets reduce the risk of fatal head injury after motorcycle and bicycle collisions.

Pedestrian injuries often affect children, the elderly, and intoxicated persons. The pattern of injury depends on the height of the patient and the type of vehicle.

- Bumper impact: tibia-fibula fractures, knee dislocations, and pelvic injuries.
- Hood and windshield impact: truncal injuries such as rib fractures or splenic trauma. If the victim is thrown into the air, other organ compression injuries may occur.
- Ground impact: this occurs when the patient slides off the car and hits the ground and may result in head and face injuries as well as extremity fractures.

# Penetrating trauma

Gun-related deaths are the second leading injury-related fatality in the United States, second only to motor vehicle collisions. In 2007, there were 17,352 suicides and 12,632 homicides due to firearms. In total, there were 30,335 violence-related firearm deaths in the United States in 2007, while there were 54,165 violence-related non-fatal gunshot injuries, a mortality rate of 35.9%. The problem of homicide due to guns is particularly acute in the young, inner-city, African-American male population. Homicide due to firearms is the second-leading cause of death, only behind unintentional motor vehicle traffic, in those aged 10–14 and 15–24. The firearm death rate has steadily increased over the past few decades, due almost exclusively to the homicide rate in the adolescent and young adult population. Attempting to prevent such inner-city violence has become an important public health effort.

Determinants of tissue damage from a bullet are:

- Amount of energy transferred to the tissues.
- Time it takes for the transfer to occur.
- Surface area over which the energy is transferred.
- Velocity of the bullet (kinetic energy).
- Wound ballistics like cavitation, trajectory, yaw, tumbling, and fragmentation.
- Entry and exit wounds. These are critical determinants of trajectory and path of the missile. The trajectory may not be linear if the bullet ricochets off bony structures.

Another significant mechanism of penetrating trauma is that of stab wounds. Stab wounds produce damage by sharp, cutting edges. Surrounding damage is minimal, and there is no blast effect as seen in gunshot wounds. Mortality, while still present, is generally much lower. In 2007, 2,600 patients died due to violence-related cutting and piercing deaths in the United States. In the same year, a total of 175,482 non-fatal such injuries occurred. The mortality rate due to this mechanism is 1.5%.

## Blasts or explosions

Blasts or explosions cause injury in three distinct manners:

1. Primary: direct effect of high-pressure waves on the tympanic membrane, lung (pulmonary edema, hemorrhage, bullae, or rupture), and bowel. Intraocular hemorrhage and retinal detachment may occur.
2. Secondary: objects rendered mobile by the explosion may cause penetrating and/or blunt trauma.
3. Tertiary: the patient may become mobile from the blast and injuries may be similar to those sustained from a fall or ejection.

# Prehospital care

In order for trauma victims to have the highest chance for a successful outcome, it is essential that they receive optimal care as soon as possible after the injury. In the United States, most trauma victims will first encounter the healthcare system via the EMS system, which is a network of services encompassing rescue operations, prehospital emergency care by specially trained personnel (emergency medical responder, emergency medical technician, advanced emergency medical technician, and paramedic). Each provider has different training requirements and scope of practice. This system is based on the premise of bringing EMS providers to the patients. These trained providers are responsible for the initial assessment and management of the trauma patient in the field. The emphasis is to bring the patient as fast as possible to the hospital after basic rescue techniques such as airway management and intravenous (IV) access are performed at the scene. The emphasis is clearly on rapid transport to the hospital for definitive treatment, since trauma patients who are exsanguinating need to have bleeding addressed as soon as possible to increase their chance of survival. Definitive control of most bleeding cannot be controlled in the field; therefore, transport to the hospital, where a trauma surgeon is available, must proceed as quickly as possible.

In 1966, the paper *Accidental Death and Disability: the Neglected Disease of Modern Society* was published. It was argued that there were no standards in prehospital care. As a response to this, the Department of Transportation published the Emergency Medical Technician – Ambulance (EMT-A) curriculum in 1969, followed by the EMS Systems Act of 1973. The two groups of patients who stood to benefit from this system were the cardiac patient and the trauma patient. It became apparent in the 1980s that definitive care between these two groups of patients is fundamentally different. Since the trauma patient who is exsanguinating needs operative intervention as soon as possible, any delay in reaching a trauma center is detrimental to survival. Therefore, prolonged attempts at stabilization of the trauma patient in the field should be avoided. EMS personnel should limit the field time with such a patient to 10 minutes or less. The patient should be brought to the closest hospital capable of providing care for the patient's injuries. This may involve bypassing a closer hospital in favor of a trauma center which is further away, but will allow admission of the patient to the operating room more expeditiously. The concept of the trauma system is imporatant in this regard, in that EMS providers need to know the capabilities of the hospital(s) in their region.

The basic approach that the EMS provider must follow is similar to that taught in the Advanced Trauma Life Support (ATLS) course, with one significant addition: scene safety. If this is not done, the EMS provider risks putting himself/herself at danger and thus also becoming injured, to the detriment of the provider and the patient. Law enforcement must often work with EMS so that the scene of the injury is as safe as possible. After scene safety is ensured, the primary survey is addressed, and the patient is then transported to the nearest appropriate facility. For the patient with internal bleeding, transport to the nearest center capable of providing surgical control is essential. This should not be delayed for interventions such as IV access.

# Trauma management in the prehospital phase

## Airway and ventilation management

Loss of airway or breathing is the most rapid cause of death, and definitive control of the airway of the severely injured trauma patient should be a consideration. Airway manage-ment in the field is usually more difficult than in the hospital. In the field, airway management is affected by the lack of resources, adverse environment, and uncontrolled patient factors. Rapid sequence intubation by EMS in the field is controversial, as there is a risk of losing a partially patent airway by the administration of a neuromuscular blocking drug. Alternatives such as laryngeal tube airways or laryngeal mask airways may be considered. Whenever management of the airway is attempted in the field, cervical spine injury must be taken into consideration, and in-line cervical immobilization must be performed should there be a risk of cervical spine trauma. Cricothyroidotomy may be performed in the field in the "cannot intubate, cannot ventilate situation."

## Breathing

The EMS provider should administer oxygen in the field and consider assisted ventilation if injury to the chest is suspected. If the patient does not appear to be taking adequate tidal volumes, tracheal intubation may be considered. Tension pneumothorax should be recog-nized clinically and treated with a needle placed into the pleural space via the second intercostal space in the mid-clavicular line. An open pneumothorax is treated in the field by an occlusive dressing taped down on three sides so that a one-way valve is created that allows air to escape from the pleural space into the environment but does allow re-entry.

## Circulation

When considering circulation, the EMS provider has two goals: vital organ perfusion must be maintained, and external bleeding controlled. Perfusion should be assessed by determining the patient's mental status, noting the skin color, and examining the quality of the pulse. A simple assessment of mental status should be done using the mnemonic AVPU, where

- A = Alert and responsive
- V = Responds only to verbal stimulus
- P = Responds only to pain (trapezius pinch, sternal rub)
- U = Unresponsive

**Table 1.2.** National Association of Emergency Medical Services Physicians and American College of Surgeons Committee on Trauma guidelines for withholding or termination of resuscitation in prehospital traumatic cardiopulmonary arrest*

## Criteria

1. Resuscitation efforts may be withheld in any blunt trauma patient who, based on out-of-hospital personnel's thorough primary patient assessment, is found apneic, pulseless, and without organized ECG activity upon the arrival of EMS at the scene.

2. Victims of penetrating trauma found apneic and pulseless by EMS, based on their patient assessment, should be rapidly assessed for the presence of other signs of life, such as pupillary reflexes, spontaneous movement, or organized ECG activity. If any of these signs are present, the patient should have resuscitation performed and be transported to the nearest emergency department or trauma center. If these signs of life are absent, resuscitation efforts may be withheld.

3. Resuscitation efforts should be withheld in victims of penetrating or blunt trauma with injuries obviously incompatible with life, such as decapitation or hemicorporectomy.

4. Resuscitation efforts should be withheld in victims of penetrating or blunt trauma with evidence of significant time lapse since pulselessness, including dependent lividity, rigor mortis, and decomposition.

5. Cardiopulmonary arrest patients in whom the mechanism of injury does not correlate with clinical condition, suggesting a nontraumatic cause of the arrest, should have standard resuscitation initiated.

6. Termination of resuscitation efforts should be considered in trauma patients with EMS-witnessed cardiopulmonary arrest and 15 minutes of unsuccessful resuscitation and cardiopulmonary resuscitation (CPR).

7. Traumatic cardiopulmonary arrest patients with a transport time to an emergency department or a trauma center of more than 15 minutes after the arrest is identified may be considered nonsalvagable, and termination of resuscitation should be considered.

8. Guidelines and protocols for traumatic cardiopulmonary arrest (TCPA) patients who should be transported must be individualized for each EMS system. Consideration should be given to factors such as the average transport time within the system, the scope of practice of the various EMS providers within the system, and the definitive care capabilities (that is, trauma centers) within the system. Airway management and intravenous (IV) line placement should be accomplished during transport when possible.

9. Special consideration must be given to victims of drowning and lightning strike and in situations where significant hypothermia may alter the prognosis.

10. EMS providers should be thoroughly familiar with the guidelines and protocols affecting the decision to withhold or terminate resuscitative efforts.

11. All termination protocols should be developed and implemented under the guidance of the system EMS medical director. On-line medical control may be necessary to determine the appropriateness of termination of resuscitation.

12. Policies and protocols for termination of resuscitation efforts must include notification of the appropriate law enforcement agencies and notification of the medical examiner or coroner for final disposition of the body.

13. Families of the deceased should have access to resources, including clergy, social workers, and other counseling personnel, as needed. EMS providers should have access to resources for debriefing and counseling as needed.

14. Adherence to policies and protocols governing termination of resuscitation should be monitored through a quality review system.

* With permission from: Hopson LR, Hirsh E, Delgado J, et al. Guidelines for withholding or termination of resuscitation in prehospital traumatic cardiopulmonary arrest: joint position statement of the National Association of EMS Physicians and the American College of Surgeons Committee on Trauma. *J Am Coll Surg* 2003;**196**:106–112.

Time should not be wasted attempting to determine the blood pressure as this may delay patient transport. Almost all external bleeding may be controlled with direct pressure. A pressure dressing with gauze may be considered if manpower is low, or tourniquets may be used if direct pressure fails to control the hemorrhage. Time should not be taken in the exsanguinating patient to establish IV access if this is at the expense of getting the patient to a trauma center in the fastest time possible.

Traditionally, fluid resuscitation has been considered the standard of care in the pre-hospital setting despite a lack of evidence supporting this practice. Recent data have demonstrated that IV access should not be performed in the prehospital setting if it delays transport to definitive care. If access is obtained, IV fluid should be withheld until active bleeding has been addressed. This is particularly true for penetrating torso wounds. If fluid is given, it should be given in small (i.e., 250 cc) boluses, titrating to a palpable radial pulse, rather than as a continuous infusion. During transport, fluids should otherwise be run at a "keep vein open" rate.

The situation in which the trauma patient is found in cardiopulmonary arrest in the field deserves special consideration. Most trauma patients who are found in cardiopulmonary arrest in the field have exsanguinated. Advanced Cardiac Life Support (ACLS) algorithms will not help this situation. Futile resuscitative efforts will also place the field healthcare providers at needless risk of exposure to blood and body fluids, and at risk for trauma to themselves at the scene. Accordingly, the National Association of Emergency Medical Services Physicians and the American College of Surgeons Committee on Trauma have published guidelines for withholding or termination of resuscitation in prehospital traumatic arrest (see Table 1.2).

## Disability/Exposure

The EMS provider should make a rapid determination of the patient's Glasgow Coma Scale (GCS) score (see Table 2.3 in Chapter 2) and pupillary response. A gross assessment of extremity motor function should be made. Full spinal immobilization, using a rigid cervical collar and a backboard, should be maintained if there is any suspicion of injury to the spine.

A rapid look at the patient's body should also be undertaken to complete the primary survey. This, however, may not be practical due to environmental conditions. Again, transport to definitive care should not be delayed. If fractures are noted, time should not be taken to splint each fracture at the expense of moving the patient to the trauma center in the shortest time possible.

## Triage

The purpose of triage is to match patients with the resources necessary to most effectively and efficiently deal with their injuries. Triage protocols should be formulated so that patients are brought to the closest and most appropriate facility. When multiple casualty incidents occur, the goal is to do the most good for the most people. A widely used triage categorization is ID-ME based on likelihood of survival and degree of injury.

- I = Immediate. The patient has detectable vital signs but will die if they do not receive immediate care within two hours. Examples are head injury with altered mental status, severe respiratory distress, extensive burns, uncontrolled bleeding, decompensated shock, extensive thoracic, abdominal, or pelvic injuries, and traumatic amputation.
- D = Delayed. The patient has a serious injury and obviously needs medical treatment but will not rapidly deteriorate. Examples are moderate dyspnea, compensated shock,

moderate to severe bleeding that is controlled, penetrating injury without airway compromise, open fractures, severe abdominal pain with stable vital signs, compartment syndrome, and uncomplicated spine injury.
- M = Minimal. The patient has minor injuries but is fully conscious and able to walk. These patients are often referred to as "walking wounded" and can take care of themselves for extended periods of time. Examples are closed fractures or dislocations without shock, minor to moderate bleeding that is controlled, burns involving less than 20% body surface area (BSA) not involving the airway or joints, strains and sprains, and minor head injury.
- E = Expectant. The patient has little or no chance of survival. Examples are cardiac arrest from any cause, severe head injury, burns larger than 70% BSA, irreversible shock, and gunshot wound to the head with GCS score $\leq 5$.

The START triage system (Simple Triage and Rapid Assessment) is commonly used by EMS and military personnel to focus on four specific factors:
1. Ability to ambulate
2. Respirations (respiratory rate, RR)
3. Pulse
4. Mental status

If the patient is able to ambulate, they can be removed from the scene. Non-ambulatory patients are then triaged according to the following:
- Respirations (no respirations = Expectant or Deceased; RR > 30 = Immediate; RR < 30 go to next assessment).
- Pulse (no radial pulse or delayed capillary refill > 2 sec = Expectant).
- Mental status (unable to follow commands or unresponsive = Immediate; able to follow commands = Delayed).

Triage is dynamic and changes may occur based on response to simple maneuvers (e.g., chin lift, jaw thrust), availability of additional or more highly trained personnel, and other factors. The patient should be taken to the trauma center within the system that has the most appropriate resources to care for the specific injuries the patient might have. The goals of the prehospital providers are to prevent further injury, initiate resuscitation, and provide safe and rapid transport of the injured patient.

## Key points
- While much emphasis is understandably focused on the in-hospital care of the injured patient, injury prevention and prehospital care are essential if the burden of trauma on the individual and on society as a whole is to be diminished.
- Traumatic injuries are the third-leading cause of death in the United States, and for many of these injuries, death occurs within minutes of injury, making injury prevention the only way of treating these patients.
- For those who survive the initial insult, efficient prehospital care is essential in bringing the patient to the most appropriate facility.
- Field time should be minimized so that the potentially exsanguinating patient can be brought to a trauma center as soon as possible, where expeditious operative control of bleeding can be accomplished.

# Further reading

1. Centers for Disease Control and Prevention. Injury Prevention and Control. Available at: www.cdc.gov/injury/overview/data.html. Accesssed October 14, 2011.

2. Cotton BA, Jerome R, Collier BR, et al. Guidelines for prehospital fluid resuscitation in the injured patient. *J Trauma* 2009;**67**:389–402.

3. Hopson LR, Hirsh E, Delgado J, et al. Guidelines for withholding or termination of resuscitation in prehospital traumatic cardiopulmonary arrest: joint position statement of the National Association of EMS Physicians and the American College of Surgeons Committee on Trauma. *J Am Coll Surg* 2003;**196**:106–112.

4. MacKenzie EJ, Fowler CJ. Epidemiology. In: Feliciano DV, Mattox KL, Moore EE, eds. *Trauma*, 6th edition. New York, NY: McGraw-Hill; 2008.

5. McNamara ED, Johe DH, Endly DA, eds. *Outdoor Emergency Care*, 5th edition. Upper Saddle River, NJ: Pearson; 2011.

6. National Institutes of Health. Estimates of Funding for Various Research, Condition, and Disease Categories (RCDC). Available at: http://report.nih.gov/rcdc/categories/. Accessed October 13, 2011.

7. National Highway Traffic Safety Administration (NHTSA), United States Department of Transportation. Fatality Analysis Reporting System (FARS) Encyclopedia. Available at: www-fars.nhtsa. dot.gov/Main/index.aspx. Accessed October 13, 2011.

8. Salomone JP, Salomone JA. Prehospital care. In: Feliciano DV, Mattox KL, Moore EE, eds. *Trauma*, 6th edition. New York, NY: McGraw-Hill; 2008.

9. World Health Organization. Violence and Injury Prevention and Disability. Available at: www.who.int/violence_injury_prevention. Accessed October 13, 2011.

10. Yee DA, Devitt JH. Mechanisms of injury. Causes of trauma. *Anesthesiol Clin North Am* 1999;**17**:1–16.

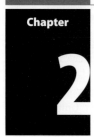

**Chapter**

**2**

# Initial evaluation and management

Thomas E. Grissom, Christopher Stephens, and
Robert Sikorski

## Introduction

Severely injured trauma patients challenge the healthcare system at all levels. Trauma patient care is resource intensive and frequently requires coordination across multiple specialties, especially with multiple injuries and multi-organ system involvement. Although frequently referred to as a "surgical disease," trauma resuscitation benefits from a multi-disciplinary approach. The anesthesiologist's role in the management of these patients can be a significant contributor to improved care – from initial resuscitation to the rehabilitative phase. While anesthesiologists practicing in designated trauma centers are more likely to be involved in the initial care of the trauma patient, an understanding of the early evaluation, management, and resuscitation of these patients will aid in later interactions and provide an understanding of management priorities during the first and subsequent surgical procedures. Successful perioperative care of these patients requires a good understanding of these basics, supplemented by preparation, flexibility, and the ability to react quickly to changing circumstances.

In the United States, very few anesthesiologists consider trauma their primary specialty. However, recommendations for "Level 1" trauma center status, made by the American College of Surgeons (ACS) Committee on Trauma (COT), require the presence of an experienced anesthesiologist and the immediate availability of an open operating room (OR) as core standards for certification. With expanded trauma care being delivered by emergency medicine physicians, US anesthesiologists may not be as readily consulted for early airway management and their initial interaction may not occur until the patient presents to the OR. The European model has taken a different approach, with anesthesiologists frequently working in the prehospital environment or serving as the leader of a hospital's "trauma team." This variable exposure to early trauma evaluation and management creates a need for ongoing education of providers that covers many recent innovations in trauma care. These include technologies for rapid volume resuscitation, "damage control" surgical techniques, and diagnostic modalities such as focused assessment with sonography for trauma (FAST), rapid computed tomography (CT), and angiography.

This chapter provides an overview of important areas of trauma care for the anesthesiologist to utilize during the initial evaluation and management of the injured patient. Recognizing the need to expedite surgical care, without extensive delay for optimizing chronic medical conditions, is one of the primary differences between trauma anesthesia and other anesthesiology specialties. This review will serve as a foundation for subsequent chapters where specific aspects of airway management, vascular access, resuscitation, and anesthetic considerations are discussed.

*Essentials of Trauma Anesthesia*, ed. A. J. Varon and C. E. Smith. Published by Cambridge University Press.
© Cambridge University Press 2012.

# Before the patient arrives

**Prehospital coordination:** Ideally, the receiving hospital should be set up to obtain information from the prehospital system prior to, or during, patient transport from the scene. Advanced notification allows the hospital's trauma team to mobilize and ensure necessary personnel and resources are available and ready in the receiving unit. This should include laboratory, operative suite, and radiology personnel. Patient and scene-specific information, including mechanism and time of injury, events related to the injury, patient history, and prehospital interventions will help the anesthesiologist and other team members prepare for triage and initial treatment.

**Trauma area setup:** The resuscitation or trauma area should be prepared to receive the patient. This should include the following equipment:

- Airway management and ventilation devices:

  - laryngoscope (check bulb brightness and integrity)
  - appropriate blade selection and sizes
  - appropriately sized endotracheal tubes (check cuff integrity) with stylet and 10 cc syringe attached
  - oropharyngeal and nasopharyngeal airways, tracheal tube introducer ("gum elastic bougie"), and other airway adjuncts immediately available
  - bag-valve-mask attached to high-flow oxygen with capnogram adapter attached (preferred if available) or colorimetric end-tidal carbon dioxide ($CO_2$) device
  - wall suction on and functioning, with rigid suction tip (Yankauer) attached
  - drug kit with rapid sequence intubation agents readily available
  - alternative airway devices present and readily available (laryngeal mask airway or other supraglottic airway device, video laryngoscope, cricothyroidotomy kit, scalpel)
  - mechanical ventilator for subsequent ventilatory requirements

- Vascular access:

  - intravenous access supplies including large-bore peripheral intravenous catheters
  - warmed intravenous crystalloid solutions
  - central venous catheter kits (introducer or large-flow double lumen catheter kit)
  - intraosseous needles and device for placement
  - arterial line kits and transducer cables available

- Monitors:

  - electrocardiogram
  - pulse oximeter
  - non-invasive blood pressure
  - temperature
  - continuous waveform capnogram
  - invasive arterial pressure monitoring should be readily available

- Equipment:

  - ultrasound machine readily available for FAST exam and insertion of intravascular catheters
  - surgical trays for chest tube placement, cricothyroidotomy, and vascular access

- Universal (standard) precautions:
  - face mask
  - eye protection
  - water-impervious apron
  - gloves

## Prioritizing trauma care

The ACS COT has developed the Advanced Trauma Life Support (ATLS) course for physicians. This organized system for treating the trauma patient is an excellent guide for those programs that infrequently treat trauma patients and serves as a foundation for trauma care at all levels. It is a concise, well-structured program for trauma centers with a surgeon-based approach to the initial evaluation and management of the trauma patient. Over the past decades this model has gradually begun to shift to a multi-disciplinary approach for the initial evaluation and treatment of those critically ill patients that require immediate, simultaneous interventions. Nonetheless, it provides a basic script for the first minutes of diagnosis and treatment of the trauma patient, including advanced training and planning to ensure a smooth, team-based approach.

With ATLS, the initial focus is on recognizing life-threatening problems following trauma, during which survival rates may be improved with rapid interventions like airway management and control of arterial hemorrhage. Prioritizing care during the first 60 minutes post-injury, often referred to as the "golden hour," is the most important lesson of ATLS. Put simply, better outcomes are more likely to be achieved with faster diagnosis and treatment. Resolution of urgent needs during the primary survey is followed by a meticulous secondary survey and further diagnostic studies designed to reduce the occurrence of missed injuries. Knowing the basic tenets of ATLS is essential for any physician who interacts with trauma patients. A simple representation of the ATLS protocol is shown in Table 2.1.

ATLS emphasizes the ABCDE of the trauma mnemonic: *A*irway, *B*reathing, *C*irculation with hemorrhage control, *D*isability, and *E*xposure/Environmental control. During the initial evaluation, the presence of the anesthesiologist is paramount since he or she can contribute significantly to these objectives. For example, a significant percentage of critically injured patients require early airway intervention because of a low or decreasing Glasgow Coma Scale (GCS) score, hypoxemia, shock, or other elements of airway or respiratory failure (Table 2.2). Management of the trauma airway necessitates advanced training and experience due to the possibility of blood in the airway and anatomical distortion secondary to soft tissue swelling or injury (see Chapter 3). In this patient population, there is often inadequate time for preoxygenation, which contributes to more rapid oxygen desaturation and limits the time available to secure a definitive airway. Because the incidence of mild to moderate hypoxia is common, the presence of a skilled anesthesiologist can benefit the patient. Similarly, many anesthesiologists have experience with resuscitation, rapid establishment of vascular access, and familiarity with the concepts espoused by crisis resource management (CRM) principles. As a member of a "team of experts," the anesthesiologist is ideally suited for a role in the initial evaluation and management of the trauma patient.

**First contact:** Since treatment priorities and initial assessment are based on injuries, vital signs, and injury mechanisms, clinicians should carefully listen to the prehospital provider's field report, as this information can be invaluable in determining the potential for a serious injury.

**Table 2.1.** Simplified assessment and management of the trauma patient (adapted from the Advanced Trauma Life Support curriculum of the American College of Surgeons)

| | Assessment | Action |
|---|---|---|
| **Airway** | • Vocal response<br>• Auscultation | • Chin lift/jaw thrust<br>• Bag-valve-mask assist with 100% $O_2$<br>• Oral and nasopharyngeal airways<br>• Intubation |
| **Breathing** | • Auscultation<br>• Pulse oximetry<br>• Arterial blood gas<br>• Chest X-ray | • Mechanical ventilation<br>• Tube thoracostomy |
| **Circulation** | • Vital signs<br>• Capillary refill<br>• Response to fluid bolus<br>• CBC, coagulation studies<br>• Type and cross-match<br>• FAST exam<br>• Pelvic X-ray | • Adequate intravenous access<br>• Warmed fluid administration<br>• Apply pressure to hemorrhage<br>• Pelvic binder<br>• Warmed uncross-matched blood<br>• Surgery |
| **Neurologic Disability** | • Determination of GCS<br>• Motor and sensory exam<br>• Cervical spine films<br>• Head/neck/spine CT | • Support of oxygenation/ perfusion<br>• Emergent surgery<br>• Intracranial pressure monitoring |
| **Exposure and secondary survey** | • Laboratory studies<br>• ECG<br>• Indicated X-rays and CT scans<br>• Detailed history and physical exam | • Remove all clothes<br>• Further surgical treatment as indicated<br>• Detailed review of lab and radiographic findings<br>• Urinary catheterization<br>• Gastric decompression |

Abbreviations: CBC = complete blood count; ECG = electrocardiogram; GCS = Glasgow Coma Scale score; FAST = focused assessment with sonography for trauma; CT = computed tomography.

**Primary survey:** While the ABCDE approach in the primary survey serves as a model for initial evaluation and management of the trauma patient, there are some caveats that assume primary importance throughout the process. In the setting of visible external hemorrhage, attempts must be made to control the hemorrhage on initial presentation. Placement of tourniquets or initiation of other hemorrhage control devices or methods should proceed if unable to control hemorrhage with direct pressure. If not previously placed in the field, a rigid cervical collar should be applied to patients at risk for cervical spine injury. Throughout the evaluation process, including airway maintenance, the

**Table 2.2.** Causes of airway obstruction or inadequate ventilation in the trauma patient

- Airway obstruction
- Direct injury to the face, mandible, or neck
- Hemorrhage in the nasopharynx, sinuses, mouth, or upper airway
- Diminished consciousness secondary to traumatic brain injury, intoxication, or analgesic medications
- Aspiration of gastric contents or a foreign body (e.g., dentures)
- Misapplication of oral airway or endotracheal tube (esophageal intubation)
- Inadequate ventilation
- Diminished respiratory drive secondary to traumatic brain injury, shock, intoxication, hypothermia, or oversedation
- Direct injury to the trachea or bronchi
- Pneumothorax or hemothorax
- Chest wall injury
- Aspiration
- Pulmonary contusion
- Cervical spine injury
- Bronchospasm secondary to smoke or toxic gas inhalation

patient's head and neck should not be hyperextended, flexed, or rotated, and appropriate attempts should be made to protect the cervical spine.

- Airway (Chapter 3): One of the fastest methods of determining airway patency is asking the patient to speak. If unable to speak, is the patient able to make any sounds at all demonstrating any degree of airway patency? Perform a quick inspection of the mouth, nose, and neck. Is there upper or lower airway obstruction? Are teeth intact? Is there blood or gastric contents in the oropharynx? Suction the mouth and begin assisting ventilations with a bag-valve-mask as needed. Consider transient use of airway adjuncts (oral or nasopharyngeal airways) to facilitate ventilation. If the patient is unable to maintain his or her airway, prepare to intubate.
- Breathing: Perform a rapid chest exam and listen for presence of breath sounds – are they equal bilaterally? How well is the patient ventilating? Are there signs of chest injury (flail chest, contusions, wounds of any type)? Place a pulse oximeter and provide supplemental oxygen as needed. If tension pneumothorax is suspected, treat immediately with needle decompression or chest tube placement. For needle decompression, a large caliber intravenous catheter is inserted in the second intercostal space in the mid-clavicular line, avoiding the inferior aspect of the rib. A chest tube will be required after needle decompression. This is usually placed in the fifth intercostal space just anterior to the mid-axillary line. Prepare to intubate the trachea if the patient has signs of respiratory distress, hypoventilation, extreme hyperventilation, profound hypoxemia, massive chest injury, or signs of abnormal breathing secondary to central nervous system injury, alcohol, or drugs.

**Table 2.3.** Glasgow Coma Scale (GCS). The GCS score is the sum of the best scores in each of three categories

| Category | Action | Score |
|---|---|---|
| Eye-opening response | Spontaneous | 4 |
| | To speech | 3 |
| | To pain | 2 |
| | None | 1 |
| Verbal response | Oriented to name | 5 |
| | Confused | 4 |
| | Inappropriate speech | 3 |
| | Incomprehensible sounds | 2 |
| | None | 1 |
| Motor response | Follows commands | 6 |
| | Localizes to painful stimuli | 5 |
| | Withdraws from painful stimuli | 4 |
| | Abnormal flexion (decorticate posturing) | 3 |
| | Abnormal extension (decerebrate posturing) | 2 |
| | None | 1 |

- Circulation (Chapters 4–6): STOP any external bleeding! In trauma patients, shock indicates loss of blood volume until proven otherwise by ongoing evaluations. Because the brain is very susceptible to a lack of oxygen supply, level of consciousness is one of the best indicators of the adequacy of oxygenation and perfusion. Examine skin color, including mucous membranes, capillary refill, and peripheral and central pulses. Pulse rate, quality, and regularity should be assessed. Patients taking beta-adrenergic blocking agents may not manifest a tachycardic response to hemorrhage. In addition, not all patients in hemorrhagic shock have tachycardia – bradycardia may be observed when profound shock is present. Initiate resuscitation immediately if the patient presents with signs of shock (altered level of consciousness, weak pulses, delayed capillary refill, pale skin color, low blood pressure). In patients with shock or hypothermia, non-invasive blood pressure and pulse-oximetry may not be functional. Therefore, one should be prepared to insert an arterial catheter for direct blood pressure monitoring and blood gas analysis.

- Disability: Is the patient alert on arrival? Can they speak or communicate in any way? Are they appropriate? Do they appear altered by alcohol or drugs? If not previously performed, the GCS score should be obtained (Table 2.3). An abnormal level of consciousness should prompt a re-evaluation of the patient's oxygenation, ventilation, and perfusion. The presence of intoxication (drugs or alcohol) or hypoglycemia may also alter the GCS score and prompt the early use of diagnostic tests such as CT scans of the head and spine. In addition to the GCS score, pupil size and reactivity, as well as extremity movements should be checked. The presence of lateralizing or focal signs suggestive of central nervous system injury should prompt early head CT.

- Exposure: At this point in the initial evaluation, the patient must be completely exposed to examine for any signs of injury. Note that trauma patients are at risk for hypothermia and care must be taken to quickly place warm blankets over patients after exposure and examination, and to maintain a warm environment.

**Resuscitation phase:** Upon completion of the rapid primary survey, and during the secondary survey, the anesthesiologist has a role in supporting ongoing resuscitation of the unstable trauma patient, including:

- Ensuring all monitors are placed and functional, including the establishment of invasive arterial monitoring as indicated.
- Placing adequate IV access, including central access if peripheral access is deemed to be inadequate or if central access is needed for surgical procedures.
- Ensuring blood is drawn for type and cross-match and baseline hematologic tests including pregnancy test (when applicable).
- Establishing a definitive airway (intubation) when indicated.
- Selecting and initiating an appropriate level of ventilatory support to maintain adequate oxygenation and normocapnia.
- Administering warmed isotonic crystalloids as boluses if no radial pulse is present or the patient has an altered level of consciousness consistent with hypoperfusion.
- Preparing to transfuse warmed uncross-matched type O packed red blood cells to patients demonstrating signs of progressive shock and continued blood loss.

**Secondary survey:** A systematic detailed head-to-toe physical exam should follow the primary survey and initial resuscitation phase to uncover injuries missed during the primary evaluation. An "**AMPLE**" history should be obtained at this time – *A*llergies, *M*edications, *P*ast medical history/pregnancy, *L*ast meal, *E*vents related to the injury. It is during this phase that many surgical conditions such as facial fractures, orthopedic injuries, and spinal fractures are discovered and consultations are initiated to facilitate subsequent repair. A helpful mnemonic that is used by emergency medical response teams to facilitate the secondary survey is "**DCAP-BTLS**": **D** – Deformity, **C** – Contusions, **A** – Abrasions/avulsions, **P** – Punctures/penetrations, **B** – Burns/bleeding/bruising, **T** – Tenderness, **L** – Lacerations, **S** – Swelling.

- **Neuro**: A more thorough neurological exam (including a GCS score if not already done) should be performed to include motor and sensory responses in all extremities.
- **Head**: Examination of the head should be performed looking for wounds, lacerations, contusions, and fractures. Identify signs of basilar skull fracture including cerebrospinal fluid, or blood from nose or ears. Eyes should be examined again for pupil symmetry and reactivity to light. The face should be examined for fractures, lacerations, or contusions, and the mouth and oropharynx for bleeding.
- **Neck**: Examination of the neck should be performed while maintaining a neutral alignment; examine the anterior and posterior aspects for wounds, lacerations, contusions, and bony abnormalities. Carefully replace the cervical collar after neck inspection. Determine if the trachea is midline and evaluate for crepitus, which may indicate an airway injury.
- **Chest**: Palpate for deformity and examine for contusions and wounds. Note any asymmetrical chest movements that may be indicative of a flail chest. Breath sounds should be re-evaluated for equality, especially if the trachea has been intubated.
- **Abdomen**: Examine for bruising (i.e., seatbelt sign), lacerations, tenderness to palpation, and distension.
- **Pelvis**: The pelvis should be palpated for discomfort or instability, but not excessively manipulated.

- **Extremities**: Palpate all four extremities for lacerations, wounds, and fractures or deformities. If any fractures are diagnosed, distal pulses must be examined by palpation or Doppler ultrasound.
- **Additional evaluation**: Roll the patient to examine the back for contusions, lacerations, and any bony abnormalities along the spine. The entire length of the spine should be carefully examined for step-offs and palpated for tenderness in any region. A rectal exam should be performed to determine rectal tone and presence of blood. Identify any trauma to the external genitalia and examine for blood at the urethral opening prior to insertion of a bladder catheter.
- **Tests**: At this point in the evaluation, chest and pelvic radiographs should be ordered as well as a FAST exam to determine the presence of intra-abdominal free fluid suggestive of hemorrhage (discussed below). If the patient is hemodynamically stable, consideration for CT imaging may be undertaken. The head, neck, chest, abdomen, and pelvis should be scanned as deemed necessary by the trauma team. CT scanning has replaced cervical spine X-rays at many trauma centers.

**Additional considerations**: Early decision-making regarding the need for operative interventions, particularly in the setting of blunt abdominal and pelvic trauma, relies heavily on non-invasive evaluation of these regions. Three particular modalities may impact on surgical decision-making including the FAST exam, CT imaging, and angiography.

*FAST exam*: In patients with major trauma, the FAST exam is frequently the initial imaging examination since it is readily available, requires minimal preparation time, and may be performed with portable equipment that allows greater flexibility in patient positioning. It is important for the anesthesiologist to be familiar with the FAST exam since this may influence an early decision for going to the OR. During the exam, four views are evaluated to determine the presence of abnormally large intraperitoneal collections of free fluid or the presence of a pericardial effusion. Typical sites of fluid accumulation in the presence of a solid organ injury are Morison's pouch (liver laceration), the pouch of Douglas (intraperitoneal rupture of the urinary bladder), and the splenorenal fossa (splenic and renal injuries). FAST is also used to exclude injuries to the heart and pericardium (see Chapter 10) but is not reliable in the detection of bowel, mesenteric, and bladder injuries. CT is better suited for the evaluation of these possible injury sites. If there is time after the initial FAST survey, ultrasound examination may be extended to rule out pneumothorax or for vascular access or other interventional procedures. When the anesthesiologist is alerted that a positive FAST has been identified, it is important to know what view was positive and how much free fluid was noted. A stable patient may still be a candidate for a rapid CT scan to better differentiate the nature of the injuries as well as to evaluate for significant intracranial pathology prior to surgery.

*CT imaging*: Since the FAST exam has poor sensitivity for the detection of most solid organ injuries, the initial survey is followed by a more thorough examination with multi-detector CT unless the patient is hemodynamically unstable. With improvements in CT accessibility, speed, and image quality over the last decade, many surgeons will send the hemodynamically stable, blunt injury patient directly to CT imaging and forego the FAST exam. In such instances, the time to definitive diagnosis and final management decisions can be reduced significantly although this practice varies greatly. In the hemodynamically unstable patient with a negative FAST exam, and no clear diagnosis, CT scanning may provide additional information. In this setting, the anesthesia provider may need to accompany the patient to the scanner to provide ongoing resuscitation and ventilatory management. If the trachea has not been intubated, definitive airway control may be warranted prior to patient transfer to the imaging suite.

The ability of multi-detector CT angiography (CTA) to identify vascular injury (e.g., carotid dissection, sites of active hemorrhage, aortic dissection, damage to peripheral vessels) has also improved over the last decade and is frequently included as part of the initial CT protocol. In most trauma centers, CTA is the first-line assessment tool for vascular injury. CTA affords a rapid, accurate, non-invasive method of detecting vascular injury and appropriately triaging patients for further evaluation or immediate intervention.

*Angiography*: Although now more frequently used as follow-up to initial CTA, angiography still plays an important role in the early management of the trauma patient. Interventional radiology procedures such as embolization and the placement of endovascular grafts and stents have altered the need for operative interventions in many conditions. Selective arterial embolization that does not cause ischemia or infarction to uninvolved vascular distributions allows surgery to be avoided or provides hemodynamic stability prior to open operation. For example, many splenic injuries with active hemorrhage can be controlled through angiography with embolization without need for an emergent laparotomy (see Chapter 17). Similarly, aortic injuries can frequently be managed non-operatively with endovascular stent placement (see Chapter 16). Because the actively bleeding patient may be unstable during an interventional radiology procedure, involvement of the anesthesia team to provide ongoing resuscitation is invaluable. This requires the availability of portable anesthesia equipment and familiarity with this out-of-the-OR location.

## Prioritization of surgical management

At any point during the initial evaluation and management of the trauma patient, the need for surgical intervention may arise. Table 2.4 provides an algorithm for prioritizing surgical management in the trauma patient with the understanding that individual situations will vary according to available resources and the patient's response to therapy. The trauma patient will often present to the OR with the need for more than one surgical procedure, by more than one surgical service. Frequently, there are a combination of injuries requiring emergency surgery and injuries that can be repaired at a later date in a more elective fashion. The anesthesiologist plays an important role in determining which procedures to perform, in which order, and which procedures should be postponed until the patient is more stable.

Emergent cases must reach the OR as soon as possible. While surgical airway access and resuscitative thoracotomy usually occur in the resuscitation or trauma unit, immediate follow-up in the OR will be necessary should the patient survive. Also considered emergent are any exploratory surgeries (laparotomy or thoracotomy) in a hemodynamically unstable patient, and craniotomy in a patient with a depressed or deteriorating mental status. Limb-threatening orthopedic and vascular injuries should undergo surgical exploration as soon as necessary diagnostic studies have been performed. Urgent cases are not immediately life-threatening, but require surgery as soon as possible to reduce the incidence of subsequent complications. Examples include exploratory laparotomy in stable patients with free abdominal fluid; irrigation, debridement, and initial stabilization of open fractures; and repair of contained rupture of the thoracic aorta not amenable to endovascular repair. Early fixation of closed fractures, especially spine and long-bone fractures, has been shown to benefit trauma patients by reducing the incidence of subsequent pulmonary complications

**Table 2.4.** Surgical priorities in the trauma patient

| Priority | Problem | Potential procedures |
|---|---|---|
| Highest | Airway management | Endotracheal intubation<br>Cricothyroidotomy<br>Mechanical ventilation |
| | Hemo-pneumothorax | Needle decompression<br>Tube thoracostomy |
| | Control of exsanguinating hemorrhage | Exploratory thoracotomy or laparotomy<br>Pelvic external fixation<br>Neck exploration<br>Pericardial window |
| | Intracranial injuries<br>Epidural hematoma<br>Subdural hematoma with mass effect<br>Increased intracranial pressure | Intracranial mass excision<br>Decompressive craniectomy |
| | Threatened limb or eyesight<br>Open globe injury<br>Traumatic near-amputation<br>Peripheral vascular trauma<br>Compartment syndrome | Repair open globe injury<br>Repair/complete traumatic near-amputation<br>Repair vascular trauma<br>Fasciotomy of compartment(s) |
| | Control of ongoing hemorrhage | Exploratory thoracotomy or laparotomy<br>Wound management |
| | High risk of sepsis<br>Perforated bowel or stomach<br>Massive soft tissue contamination | Exploratory laparotomy<br>Wound management |
| | Spine injury | Spinal decompression |
| | Early patient mobilization | Closed long-bone fixation<br>Spinal fixation |
| Lowest | Better cosmetic outcome | Facial fracture repair<br>Soft tissue closure |

(see Chapter 18). Definitive repair within 24 hours is recommended in otherwise stable, non-brain-injured patients. Non-urgent cases are those that can be safely delayed until a scheduled OR time is available. Face, wrist, and ankle fracture fixation are not time-dependent although early surgery will shorten the patient's length of stay. These surgeries are commonly postponed, and may be undertaken days to weeks following injury, when tissue edema has resolved and the patient is otherwise stable.

A key element requiring attention by the anesthesiologist and surgeon is the extent of surgery to be performed in a patient with multiple injuries. The concept of "damage control" has revolutionized surgical thinking in the past decade. With damage control surgery, the focus is on limiting initial therapeutic procedures to those required for hemostasis while delaying reconstructive procedures until adequate resuscitation has been achieved. In a typical example, the surgeon treating an unstable blunt trauma patient might perform an exploratory laparotomy, rapid splenectomy, staple resection of injured bowel (without attempt at re-anastomosis), ligation of bleeding large vessels, and packing of all four abdominal quadrants. The abdomen would be left open under a sterile watertight dressing and the patient taken to the intensive care unit (ICU) for continued resuscitation and stabilization. Angiographic embolization might be used to facilitate liver and retroperitoneal hemostasis during this time. Following resolution of shock; warming; and normalization of laboratory values, the patient would return to the OR in 24–48 hours for debridement of non-viable tissue, reconstruction of the bowel, placement of enteral feeding access, and abdominal closure. The concept of damage control may also be applied to orthopedic injuries where initial external fixation of the pelvis and long bones is adequate for temporary stabilization of fractures without imposing the additional physiologic burdens of intra-medullary nailing or open fixation. While objective indicators of the need for damage control have not been established, this approach should be considered in any patient with persistent hypotension, elevated lactate, or transfusion requirement in excess of one blood volume.

## Teamwork and crisis resource management (CRM) in trauma

The trauma team is ideally suited for the application of teamwork and CRM principles as espoused by a number of experts in the field of team training. The trauma team typically comprises a multi-disciplinary group of individuals from the fields of surgery, anesthesiology, emergency medicine, radiology, nursing and support staff, each of whom provide simultaneous inputs into the assessment and management, with their actions coordinated by a team leader. The goals of the team are to rapidly resuscitate and stabilize the patient, identify and treat life-threatening problems, prioritize and determine the nature and extent of the injuries, and prepare the patient for transfer to the next phase of care, which may be the OR, ICU, or another facility. A well-structured team aims to provide rapid input to the management of the critically injured patient without the need to contact and request the presence of individual team members. The leader of the trauma team must be experienced in the diagnosis and management of trauma patients and the likely pitfalls associated with dealing with severely injured patients. They must also be comfortable directing and responding to other team members, all the while demonstrating good communication and leadership skills. Most commonly, the leader is a surgeon or an emergency medicine physician depending on local availability or ACS trauma center status. As a component of the trauma service, the trauma team has been independently shown to reduce time in the resuscitation or trauma department, reduce missed injuries, and speed the evaluation and treatment process, all of which contribute to mortality reduction.

Beyond the structure of the trauma team, training and auditing are critical to optimizing performance. Extrapolation from the realm of CRM training in anesthesiology suggests that these same principles can be effective in the training and improvement of trauma team responses.

## Key points

- Trauma is a disease that touches all ages and classes of patients, from young and vigorous to elderly and frail.
- The anesthesiologist, as perioperative physician, is in the ideal position to understand and apply new techniques and processes in the resuscitation of the traumatically injured patient throughout the course of their care.

- As a member of the trauma team, the anesthesiologist can bring together an understanding of the physiology of trauma, principles of airway management and resuscitation, and CRM.
- Care of the trauma patient requires the anesthesiologist to be comfortable working outside of the traditional OR to include the emergency department, radiology suite, and ICU.
- The proper application of damage control principles requires input from all members of the trauma team, particularly the anesthesiologist.

# Further reading

1. American College of Surgeons, Committee on Trauma. *Advance Trauma Life Support for Doctors: ATLS® Student Course Manual*. Chicago, IL: American College of Surgeons; 2008.

2. Dutton R, McCunn M, Grissom T. Anesthesia for trauma. In: Miller RD, Eriksson LI, Fleisher LA, Wiener-Kronish JP, Young W, eds. *Miller's Anesthesia*, 7th edition. New York, NY: Elsevier; 2009.

3. Georgiou A, Lockey DJ. The performance and assessment of hospital trauma teams. *Scand J Trauma Resusc Emerg Med* 2010;**18**:66–73.

4. Grissom TE, Dutton R. Anesthesia for trauma and acute care. In: Fleischer LA, ed. *Anesthesia and Uncommon Disease*. Philadelphia, PA: Saunders-Elsevier; 2005.

5. Heller K, Reardon R, Joing S. Ultrasound use in trauma: the FAST exam. *Acad Emerg Med* 2007;**14**:525. Available at: http://onlinelibrary.wiley.com/doi/10.1197/j.aem.2007.01.009/suppinfo. Accessed June 22, 2011.

6. Nicholson AA. Vascular radiology in trauma. *Cardiovasc Intervent Radiol* 2004;**27**:105–20.

7. Shapiro MJ, Morey JC, Small SD, et al. Simulation based teamwork training for emergency department staff: does it improve clinical team performance when added to an existing didactic teamwork curriculum? *Qual Saf Health Care* 2004;**13**:417–21.

8. Uyeda JW, Anderson SW, Sakai O, et al. CT angiography in trauma. *Radiol Clin North Am* 2010;**48**:423–438.

| Chapter |
| --- |
| **3** |

# Airway management

Christian Diez and Albert J. Varon

## Introduction

Airway management of trauma patients may take place in a variety of settings including a designated resuscitation area, emergency room (ER), operating room (OR), intensive care unit (ICU), computed tomography (CT) suite, or prehospital setting. Although the mechanism or severity of injury may be unpredictable, the control of the airway in these patients is a skill in which one must feel comfortable and remain in control, regardless of the situation confronted or physical setting.

The majority of tools and algorithms used for the trauma airway are similar to those used in a non-emergency scenario, but with some modifications. One should always be well equipped, be familiar with available devices, and be able to adapt to rapidly evolving situations. An essential difference between the trauma airway and the non-emergency setting is that awakening the severely injured patient after a failed asleep intubation (or canceling the procedure) is rarely, if ever, an option.

## Airway

The Advanced Trauma Life Support (ATLS) course developed by the Committee on Trauma of the American College of Surgeons helps physicians maximize their resuscitative efforts, and avoid missing life-threatening injuries, by using an organized approach to trauma care. The course includes guidelines for initial airway and ventilatory management and instructs clinicians on how to recognize common pitfalls in the care of trauma patients (see Chapter 2).

Before a patient's arrival, prehospital personnel should convey vital patient information to include mechanism of injury, patient age, level of consciousness or Glasgow Coma Scale (GCS) score (see Table 2.3), vital signs, interventions required, and estimated time of arrival, all of which can aid in airway management preparation and planning. Upon a patient's arrival, immediate assessment of ventilatory status is essential. A simple question such as "What is your name?" can provide a wealth of information. A positive, appropriate verbal response indicates, for example, that the airway is patent, ventilation intact, and circulation is currently adequate for brain perfusion. On the other hand, an incoherent response, or lack thereof, will alert the clinician that one or several issues may be present. Upon patient arrival, if airway or breathing is of concern, one should immediately prepare to obtain a definitive airway – defined as a cuffed tracheal tube below the level of the vocal cords.

*Essentials of Trauma Anesthesia*, ed. A. J. Varon and C. E. Smith. Published by Cambridge University Press.
© Cambridge University Press 2012.

Patients may arrive with oropharyngeal or nasopharyngeal airways in place. An oral airway can be very stimulating; if a patient is seemingly tolerating the airway well, this may provide a clue that tracheal intubation should be immediately performed. Questions regarding why an airway was inserted, or whether the patient received any medications during transport, can help complete the clinical picture.

Several devices in the prehospital setting may help achieve ventilation. The bag-valve-mask (BVM), laryngeal mask airway (LMA), esophageal-tracheal combitube (Combitube), and the laryngeal tube airway (LTA) are examples of airway devices commonly used by prehospital personnel. The airway provider must be familiar with these devices and understand their capabilities, advantages, disadvantages, and how to safely replace them with a definitive airway.

A new tool in the eighth edition of ATLS (although not new for airway specialists) is the tracheal tube introducer, also known as the "gum elastic bougie." The incorporation of the tracheal tube introducer into ATLS is the result of its success in aiding tracheal intubation in other settings, especially with cervical spine precautions. Many institutions have incorporated algorithms that include a bougie if a tracheal tube cannot be inserted on the first attempt.

ATLS guidelines list the following as indications for securing a definitive airway in the trauma setting:

- Apnea
- Inability to maintain a patent airway
- Protection from aspiration
- Potential airway compromise
- GCS score $\leq 8$
- Inability to maintain oxygenation

In addition, tracheal intubation is sometimes performed to prevent a patient from self-harm or to allow proper medical evaluation; the literature has listed these as "discretionary indications" for tracheal intubation.

Tracheal tube placement should include adequate preoxygenation, rapid-sequence induction (RSI), cricoid pressure (CP), and in-line cervical spine immobilization (when indicated) (Figure 3.1). Confirmation of correct tracheal tube placement may occur by

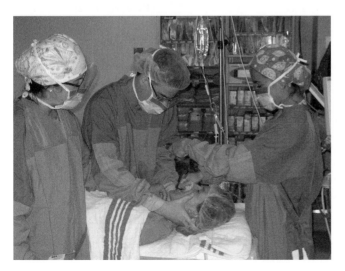

**Figure 3.1.** Rapid-sequence induction, cricoid pressure, and in-line cervical spine immobilization technique for tracheal intubation in a trauma patient with suspected cervical spine injury.

several methods including end-tidal carbon dioxide by capnography (or, if unavailable, by semi-quantitative colorimetry), bilateral breath sounds, absence of gastric sounds, bilateral chest expansion, fogging of the tracheal tube, maintenance of oxygenation by pulse oximetry, direct confirmation by fiberoptic endoscopy, or direct visualization of lung expansion during emergency thoracotomy. When perfusion is present, capnography is the most reliable method for confirmation of tracheal tube placement.

Because the option of awakening a severely injured patient is seldom feasible when there is inability to ventilate or intubate, the ability to obtain a surgical airway should be readily available.

## Equipment and medications

There are several factors that influence the choice of equipment (e.g., laryngoscope blade, tracheal tube) and medications (e.g., induction agent, neuromuscular blocking drug (NMBD)) to secure a patient's airway. Mechanism of injury, vital signs, age, and body size are just a few factors that need to be taken into consideration. A variety of equipment should be readily available to facilitate securing the airway in a timely and safe manner. Such equipment may be placed in an airway tray or cart at locations where tracheal intubations often occur. An advantage of having everything in a single airway tray or mobile cart is that it can be taken to other sites where resources might be scarce or distant. Table 3.1 lists suggested basic equipment for most tracheal intubations in adults.

## RSI: anesthetic agents and NMBDs

Emergency airway medications should include an induction agent and two fast-acting NMBDs such as succinylcholine and rocuronium. These medications should be readily available and easily retrieved.

Every induction agent has advantages and disadvantages. These may relate to characteristics of the medication itself or how it needs to be handled or dispensed. Medications that need to be drawn instead of preloaded require additional time and supplies for preparation. When determining which induction agent is the most appropriate in the trauma setting, drug dosage may be more important than the specific medication used. All of the commonly used induction drugs have the ability to be used in the trauma setting including propofol, etomidate, and ketamine (thiopental is currently not being manufactured in the United States). Most trauma patients will undergo RSI resulting in amnesia and intubating conditions within 30–60 seconds. Propofol may cause profound hypotension in hypovolemic patients and is not recommended in this setting. Etomidate carries the advantage of provoking less hemodynamic changes in comparison to the other induction agents. Some clinicians have challenged the use of etomidate for RSI due to the concern that it may induce adrenal suppression, even after a single dose. Despite this concern, etomidate remains the most frequently used agent for RSI outside of the OR. Ketamine may cause tachycardia and hypertension from endogenous catecholamine release; this side effect may be advantageous in the trauma setting, especially in the setting of cardiac tamponade. However, concerns of myocardial depression in the catecholamine-depleted patient, increased intracranial pressure, and increased intra-ocular pressure may be important considerations when selecting this drug for RSI. In the multiple-trauma patient, who is often in extremis, it is important to

**Table 3.1.** Basic equipment for tracheal intubation in adults

| |
|---|
| Bag-valve-mask system |
| Peep valve |
| Laryngoscope handle |
| Laryngoscope blades (curved #3–4, straight #2–3) |
| Tracheal tube, low-pressure cuff (sizes 6.0–8.5 mm) |
| Tracheal tube stylets |
| Tracheal tube introducer ("gum elastic bougie") |
| Oral airways (various sizes) |
| Nasal airways (various sizes) |
| Supraglottic airway (LMA, laryngeal tube, etc.) |
| Tape |
| $CO_2$ detector |
| Pulse oximeter probe |
| Suction catheters (12–14 Fr.) |
| Magill forceps |
| Tongue blades |
| "C" batteries (spare for laryngoscope handle) |
| Lubrication jelly |
| 10 cc syringe |
| Rigid (Yankauer) suction tip |

recognize that conventional drug doses for induction of anesthesia need to be reduced since all induction drugs have the potential for causing hypotension and cardiovascular collapse in this setting.

Most NMBDs can be used for RSI if a large enough dose is given (see Chapter 7). In clinical practice, succinylcholine (depolarizing NMBD) and rocuronium (non-depolarizing NMBD) are used most often. Succinylcholine has withstood the test of time as the most reliable NMBD for fast onset of ideal intubating conditions. While understanding the many concerns and contraindications for succinylcholine's use is beyond the scope of this chapter, suffice it to say that one should always know the side effects of any drug one administers. Acute burns and acute paralysis are not absolute contraindications to succinylcholine administration, although its use is contraindicated after 24–48 hours of sustaining such injuries due to the risk of hyperkalemia. Furthermore, succinylcholine is relatively contra-indicated when severe hyperkalemia is suspected (e.g., rhabdomyolysis, renal failure). The recommended dose of succinylcholine for RSI has been cited to be at least 0.6 mg/kg for ideal intubating conditions within 60 seconds. Commonly utilized doses include a range of 1.0–1.5 mg/kg. Increasing the dose of succinylcholine above 0.6 mg/kg provides a faster onset (30–45 seconds) and longer duration (5–10 min) of paralysis. If the ability to ventilate the lungs or intubate the trachea is of concern and an NMBD is needed, one may prefer the least possible dose that provides adequate paralysis to avoid a longer and potentially harmful block. However, patients could still be at risk of hypoxemia if there is failure to intubate and/or ventilate, regardless of the dose of succinylcholine administered.

The availability of a non-depolarizing drug for RSI is crucial in the trauma setting since succinylcholine is contraindicated in certain patients. The aforementioned succinyl-choline contraindications and electrical burns are common reasons for using rocuronium instead of succinylcholine for RSI. A rocuronium dose of 0.9 to 1.2 mg/kg should be used for adequate intubating conditions within 60 seconds of administration. After rocur-onium is given for RSI, the option of having the patient return to spontaneous ventilation if the airway cannot be secured is not feasible due to rocuronium's duration of action (45–60 minutes). Therefore, alternative plans for securing the airway and ensuring ventilation (including the use of a surgical airway) must be formulated before proceeding with RSI.

## Oxygenation and cricoid pressure

The process of securing the trauma patient's airway can lead to unexpected challenges. Often patients are uncooperative and their pathology imposes a significant time constraint lending itself to a less than ideal situation.

RSI is the most commonly used method for securing a definitive airway in trauma and emergency settings. The reasons for this preference include the presence of unidentified injuries, hemodynamic instability, unknown or unreliable fasting history, and severe stress and inflammation leading to delayed gastric emptying and risk of aspiration. Preoxygenation before induction should take place whenever possible. This may be difficult in situations where a patient is uncooperative, combative, or has severe facial deformities that impede proper mask seal. When preoxygenation is inadequate or not possible, BVM ventilation (while applying CP) should be used through induction to maintain oxygenation. This is especially important in patients with traumatic brain injury, where maintenance of cerebral perfusion pressure and oxygenation take precedence over the potential risk of aspiration if BVM ventilation results in stomach insufflation. Therefore, it is prudent to provide small positive pressure breaths during RSI to any patient at risk of oxygen desaturation.

The effectiveness of CP in preventing aspiration continues to be debated. Sellick demonstrated that application of pressure to the cricoid ring could obstruct the esophagus as it became pinned between the cricoid cartilage and a vertebral body. Some investigators have suggested that CP may displace the esophagus laterally and not compress it because often the esophagus does not lie directly between the cricoid and the spine. However, magnetic resonance imaging studies have shown that the lumen of the alimentary tract behind the cricoid cartilage (i.e., the postcricoid hypopharynx) is compressed regardless of the position of the cartilage relative to the vertebral body. Other investigators have demon-strated that CP decreases lower esophageal sphincter tone making regurgitation into the esophagus more likely than without CP. In addition, healthcare personnel frequently apply CP incorrectly by applying pressure to the wrong location (e.g., thyroid cartilage) or applying pressure that is too soft or too hard. Distortion of the airway and worsened laryngoscopic view has been well documented with CP. Despite these concerns, CP con-tinues to be the mainstay for RSI in which aspiration is a concern due to its low risk/benefit ratio. CP should be applied throughout induction and attempts at intubation. However, if manipulation or removal of CP is necessary to facilitate intubation or insert an LMA, it should be altered or removed, as being able to secure the airway and provide ventilation is paramount.

## Cervical spine immobilization

Many trauma patients that arrive to the emergency department or trauma center have a cervical collar in place. Prehospital personnel place cervical collars for a variety of reasons including mechanism of injury, signs of neurologic deficit, or prehospital protocol. Hard collars are applied to prevent further damage of a patient's cervical spine during transport. During the assessment of the trauma patient the cervical spine may be cleared clinically. Two common reasons for a cervical collar to remain in place are signs of a cervical injury or inability to clinically "clear the spine." This may be due to a patient being combative, intoxicated, obtunded, or having distracting injuries.

When tracheal intubation is required in a patient with high suspicion for cervical spine injury, a safe approach in a cooperative patient is to proceed with an awake intubation under topical anesthesia. The use of a fiberoptic endoscope facilitates an awake intubation with minimal neck movement and allows the cervical collar to remain in place. This permits assessment of the patient's neurologic status during and immediately after intubation. An awake fiberoptic intubation also allows securing the airway in a potentially difficult intubation without abolishing the patient's ability to breathe spontaneously. Unfortunately, awake intubation can only be performed in a small number of trauma patients. Many times the reason a patient requires tracheal intubation is the same reason an awake intubation is impractical.

When the airway needs to be secured in a patient with suspected cervical injury and awake intubation is not possible, manual in-line immobilization (MILI) should be applied during the RSI process. This requires an additional person to hold the cervical spine in place to prevent the person securing the airway from significantly extending or flexing the cervical spine. Cervical collars do not reliably immobilize the neck during the intubation process and may significantly impede mouth opening. Therefore, the anterior portion of the cervical collar is temporarily removed and MILI applied during RSI.

The use of MILI has recently come into question. Studies have shown that it may lead to an inferior view causing the person intubating to apply greater laryngoscopic pressure, which may be transferred to surrounding tissues including the cervical spine. Secondly, an inferior view may lead to a longer time or failure to secure the airway. Although these are legitimate concerns, MILI is still recommended by ATLS guidelines and commonly applied in patients with suspected cervical injury. At this time there are no outcome data suggesting that direct laryngoscopy with MILI is inferior to any other method, including fiberoptic. Lastly, as was noted for CP, MILI may be reduced if its use impedes tracheal intubation.

## ASA difficult airway algorithm modified for trauma

The American Society of Anesthesiologists' (ASA) difficult airway algorithm offers an excellent guideline for the approach to the difficult airway and can easily be modified for trauma patients (http://www.asahq.org/For-Members/About-ASA/ASA-Committees/Committee-on-Trauma-and-Emergency-Preparedness.aspx). These modifications are necessary because the urgency and circumstances of the trauma setting may require deviations from the original algorithm.

The first modification pertains to awake intubation versus intubation after induction of general anesthesia. In a controlled setting, recognition that a patient may have a difficult airway should prompt the practitioner to consider an awake intubation. Although this is also true in the trauma setting, these patients may be uncooperative or unstable for awake intubation and would therefore be automatically allocated into the intubation after induction category. Induction of general anesthesia in a patient that may have a difficult airway is a challenging approach. However, an awake procedure requires a cooperative and stable patient.

A second modification to the algorithm relates to a patient who is recognized as having a difficult airway and is a candidate for an awake intubation. If non-invasive methods to secure the airway are unsuccessful, invasive airway access may be the only other option because canceling the procedure or other options may not be feasible if such a patient requires a secure airway for operative or non-operative interventions.

The third major modification pertains to the patient in whom general anesthesia has been induced but the initial intubation is unsuccessful. In the trauma setting, awakening the patient is rarely an option and therefore one must continue down the algorithm. The rest of the algorithm coincides with the non-emergency pathway until the end where awakening the patient and other options are again not possible. The most likely solution in such instances would be a surgical airway. Attempts to ventilate should continue during surgical airway placement. Obtaining a surgical airway may sometimes not be rapid and therefore any amount of ventilation can help. For example, if intubation through an LMA is unsuccessful, it may be advantageous to continue ventilation attempts via the LMA while surgical airway access is obtained.

Establishing an institutional trauma airway protocol that takes into consideration available personnel and resources may enhance the safety and effectiveness of airway management in trauma patients. At the Ryder Trauma Center, we have implemented a trauma airway management algorithm that takes into consideration our trainees, faculty, and institutional resources. (Figure 3.2)

## Videolaryngoscopy

A variety of videolaryngoscopes are currently available. Their popularity is due to their ability to improve the laryngoscopic view (when compared to conventional laryngoscopy) and their increased portability as newer technologies become available. Although there are insufficient data on the clinical utility of these devices in trauma patients, some information can be derived from other studies. When compared to direct laryngoscopy, use of the Glidescope (Verathon Inc., Bothell, Washington, USA) was reported to have no significant difference in cervical spine motion when MILI was applied in patients undergoing elective surgery. Conversely, the Airtraq laryngoscope (King Medical Systems, Newark, Delaware, USA) has been reported to produce less cervical motion than the Macintosh laryngoscope (Welch Allyn, Skaneateles Falls, New York, USA) in elective cases.

Several limiting factors exist when reviewing available data on videolaryngoscopes. As previously mentioned, currently there are no outcome data suggesting that direct laryngoscopy with MILI is inferior to any other method. Further, although videolaryngoscopes have been shown to provide better glottic view than other devices, this does not always translate into an easier intubation. Intubation may still be difficult despite a good view

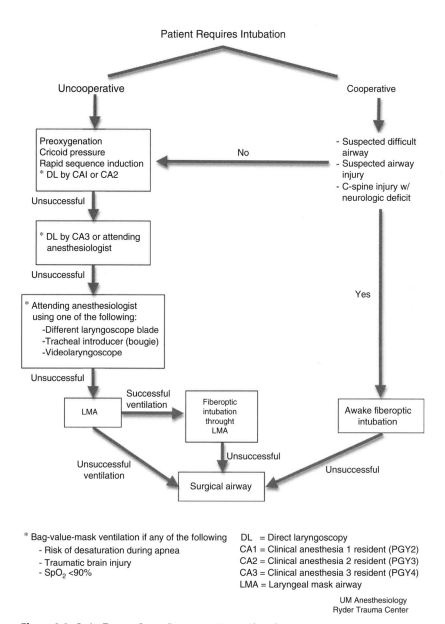

**Figure 3.2.** Ryder Trauma Center Emergency Airway Algorithm.

because the tube or stylette insertion path may not line up with the view obtained by a videolaryngoscope. Another potential difficulty is the oral insertion of fixed-angle videolaryngoscopy devices (e.g., Glidescope) in patients receiving MILI. Finally, the presence of blood, emesis, or airway injury may disrupt the videolaryngoscopic view. Therefore, although the advent of new videolaryngoscopes continues to expand the armamentarium of the airway specialist, these devices have not yet replaced direct laryngoscopy in the trauma setting.

# Tracheal tube introducers

Tracheal tube introducers have grown in popularity and importance in the trauma setting. These devices, which have a coude tip, allow the anesthesiologist to advance the introducer into the trachea despite a limited glottic view, which may be common in the trauma setting due to MILI or CP. As noted above, ATLS current guidelines describe the use of these introducers to facilitate intubation in the difficult airway.

A non-coude tip introducer is the Aintree intubation catheter (Cook Critical Care, Bloomington, Indiana, USA). Although this is not used to gain entry into the trachea during a difficult direct laryngoscopy, it may be used as a bridge to convert a supraglottic airway into a secure airway with a tracheal tube (discussed in more detail later). One of the main characteristics of an Aintree catheter is its hollow center that can accommodate a flexible fiberoptic scope or allow oxygen insufflation. This introducer is shorter than conventional hollow catheters that serve as airway exchange catheters. Due to its shorter length, it allows a fiberoptic scope to protrude through it and offer visibility beyond the catheter.

# Supraglottic devices

The use of supraglottic devices has greatly increased in the last 25 years. Their use varies from rescue devices in a difficult airway scenario to primary airway devices in elective surgical procedures. In 2003, the ASA difficult airway algorithm incorporated the use of the LMA in the "cannot intubate, cannot ventilate" scenario. The use of supraglottic airways has now also been incorporated into ATLS. In the trauma setting, supraglottic airways are most frequently encountered when patients arrive in the emergency department. Airway specialists must recognize these airways, know their function and capabilities, determine if they provide adequate ventilation, and have the skill set to safely exchange them for a definitive airway. This may entail using an airway exchange catheter (AEC) to remove the supraglottic airway followed by tracheal intubation over the AEC, or leaving a supraglottic airway in place temporarily to provide ventilation until a surgical airway can be emergently obtained.

Three commonly encountered supraglottic airways are the LMA, Combitube, and the LTA (King Systems Corporation, Noblesville, Indiana, USA). Although this list does not include all the variations of these airways or all supraglottic airways available, we will discuss these three in more detail.

## Laryngeal mask airway

The LMA is available with several different commercial modifications. These modifications have been made for the LMA to facilitate positive pressure ventilation, serve as an intubating conduit, or allow gastric suctioning while in place. However, the basic design and purpose involves a blindly placed device with a ventilating port that should sit above the glottic opening. The device has been used for many years and in many countries in a broad scope of practice.

As previously stated, in trauma scenarios an airway secured with a cuffed tracheal tube is paramount. Yet, being thoroughly familiar with the LMA is important as patients may arrive in the emergency room with this device and because the LMA can also serve as a rescue airway in the "cannot intubate, cannot ventilate" scenario.

Prehospital personnel should be asked for information to find out if the LMA was placed as the initial airway or as a rescue device after multiple failed attempts. If after failed

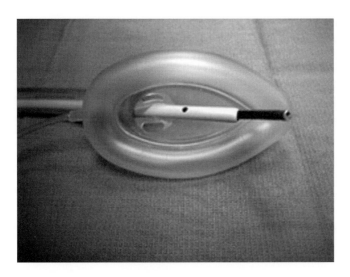

**Figure 3.3.** Fiberoptic endoscope protruding through an Aintree exchange catheter. These are passed through the fenestration of a size 5 laryngeal mask airway to facilitate the exchange of a supraglottic airway to a tracheal tube.

attempts, one should ask about the view obtained with laryngoscopy, and limitations encountered (e.g., large amount of blood or emesis). Finally one should ask if the LMA allowed adequate ventilation. The answers to these questions can lay the groundwork on how the airway should be exchanged.

Several options exist to safely exchange the LMA for a tracheal tube. The first is to simply remove the LMA and then insert a tracheal tube via direct laryngoscopy – the most expeditious method. This option may be pursued if the patient's airway does not appear to be difficult and the LMA was inserted without failed attempts. A second option is to remove the LMA and use a videolaryngoscope for tracheal tube placement. The caveat is that a soiled airway may be difficult to visualize with these devices and their narrow optic field may result in a greater incidence of obstructed views.

A third option is to use the LMA as a conduit for intubation, as first described by its inventor Dr. Archie Brain. Unfortunately, it may be initially unclear what size tracheal tube may fit through a specific LMA. Each LMA variation and size may accommodate different sized tubes through its lumen. In addition, many LMA products have aperture bars at the ventilation opening that greatly limit the size of the tracheal tube able to pass through. One solution to these problems is to pass a small diameter tube under fiberoptic guidance into the trachea, confirm placement, remove the LMA, and then exchange the smaller tube for an appropriately sized tube over an AEC. Fiberoptic guidance is recommended when using an LMA as a conduit for tracheal intubation in the trauma patient. Blind intubation attempts through a standard LMA may increase the risk of damage in patients with airway injury or increase the risk of aspiration due to inadvertent gastric insufflation after failed intubation attempts.

The Aintree AEC adds an attractive option when using the LMA as a conduit for intubation. Unlike other AECs, the Aintree catheter can accommodate a fiberoptic endoscope through its hollow core and shorter length (Figure 3.3). To exchange the LMA for a tracheal tube, the Aintree catheter is advanced under fiberoptic guidance through the aperture bars and glottic opening, the fiberoptic scope and LMA are removed, and an appropriately sized tracheal tube is then advanced over the catheter. Fiberoptic endoscopy can be performed without interrupting ventilation if a dual-axis swivel adapter is inserted between the LMA and the ventilation device. The Aintree AEC can be used for oxygen insufflation after the LMA is removed if unexpected difficulty is encountered inserting the tracheal tube. Exchanging an LMA over an Aintree AEC allows direct visualization, insertion of an appropriate sized tube, and maintenance of oxygenation throughout the process. However, since additional equipment is needed, this technique is reserved for patients who appear to have a difficult airway and time is available to gather the necessary equipment.

Videolaryngoscopy (or rigid fiberoptic laryngoscopy – Wuscope, Bullard) may also facilitate the exchange of a supraglottic airway (or tracheal tube) once an AEC has been inserted by any technique. A videolaryngoscope allows direct visualization of the tracheal tube passage through the glottis over the AEC.

Finally, another option is to leave the LMA in place and obtain a surgical airway. If the patient is receiving adequate ventilation, the surgical airway can be performed semi-urgently but in a more controlled setting. This option often requires discussing with the surgeon the risks and benefits of attempting to exchange the LMA versus those of a surgical airway.

## Esophageal-tracheal Combitube

The Combitube (Tyco-Healthcare-Kendall-Sheridan, Mansfield, MA) has been used as an airway rescue device since its description by Dr. Michael Frass in 1987. The device is inserted blindly into the oropharynx and ventilation occurs via one of its ports. After the Combitube is inserted, the distal and proximal cuffs are inflated with 10–12 cc and 60–80 cc of air respectively, and the ability to ventilate is confirmed. Since the Combitube will be inserted into the esophagus most of the time, the blue port labeled #1 is checked first. If ventilation is confirmed by the presence of breath sounds and end-tidal carbon dioxide ($CO_2$), then the device is used to provide supraglottic ventilation through its side ports. If ventilation cannot be obtained via port #1, then port #2 is checked. If breath sounds and end-tidal $CO_2$ are present through port #2, then the Combitube has been inserted into the trachea and ventilation can be provided through that port.

The use of the Combitube as the supraglottic rescue device of choice has decreased over the years due to its complexity (multiple ports, multiple syringes, multiple pilot balloons), lack of pediatric sizes, and the introduction of other supraglottic devices into clinical practice. Cases of severe oropharyngeal trauma, esophageal rupture, and studies citing easier placement of other supraglottic airways when compared to the Combitube have also caused its decline in popularity. On the other hand, when the Combitube is placed into the esophagus it has the advantage of allowing passage of a catheter through port #2 for gastric suctioning.

When a patient arrives in the emergency room with a Combitube, clinicians must determine its location (esophagus or trachea) and have a plan to exchange the airway. If the Combitube is in the esophagus it cannot be used as a conduit for tracheal tube insertion. To exchange the device in such instances, one can deflate the large proximal (oropharyngeal) cuff, move the tube aside, and attempt to intubate the trachea via direct laryngoscopy, videolaryngoscopy, or fiberoptic endoscopy. Once the proximal cuff is deflated, ventilation through port #1 will no longer be possible. Therefore, personnel and equipment should be ready for intubation before deflating the proximal cuff. Leaving the distal (esophageal) cuff inflated in place keeps gastric contents from entering the oropharynx. However, due to the size of the device, the Combitube often needs to be completely removed for tracheal intubation to be successful. If the Combitube was inserted in the trachea, then an AEC can be used to exchange the device. One method is to place a pediatric AEC via the ventilating port (in this case port #2), remove the Combitube after deflating both cuffs, and insert a tracheal tube over the AEC.

## Laryngeal tube

The LTA is also a supraglottic airway that has undergone several modifications over the past few years. The LTA is inserted blindly into the pharynx and a single pilot balloon is inflated, which fills both the proximal and distal cuffs. In contrast to the Combitube, the LTA must always be inserted into the esophagus to provide supraglottic ventilation. The lungs are ventilated via its sole ventilating port. Newer models (King LTS-D) have a gastric suctioning port that facilitates the placement of a standard sized orogastric tube. One disadvantage is the inability to reliably use the laryngeal tube as a conduit for tracheal tube insertion. Although one study reported the use of the Aintree catheter for this purpose, others have reported failures to use introducers through the LTA for airway exchange. Therefore, to secure the airway, the LTA should be removed after deflating the cuffs and intubation performed via laryngoscopy, videolaryngoscopy, or fiberoptic endoscopy. If tracheal intubation is not possible, one should consider inserting an LMA for immediate ventilation and then using the LMA as a conduit for tracheal tube placement.

## Fiberoptic endoscopy

The fiberoptic bronchoscope (FOB) is an invaluable tool for managing patients with a difficult airway and is the most versatile of the intubating tools currently available. The capabilities of this device include the following:

1.  Aids in establishing an airway in awake and asleep patients.
2.  Can be used to place an airway orally, nasally, or transtracheally
3.  May help confirm position of a tracheal tube.
4.  Facilitates lung isolation (e.g., double lumen tube, bronchial blocker).
5.  Can be used to diagnose or evaluate the extent of an airway injury and place a tracheal tube beyond the level of the injury.

In the trauma setting, the decision to proceed with awake versus asleep fiberoptic intubation is similar to the non-trauma scenario. Awake fiberoptic intubation is safer when difficult ventilation is suspected or if the patient has a full stomach. With patient cooperation and adequate anesthetic topicalization, the trachea of most patients can be intubated in a safe manner. However, because patient cooperation can be a significant challenge in the trauma setting, the awake fiberoptic intubation approach is limited to cooperative patients. Asleep fiberoptic intubations are also infrequently performed in the trauma setting due to the risk of aspiration, except when used as a rescue technique (e.g., through an LMA) or during a "rapid-sequence" fiberoptic intubation (described below).

The main caveat of using an FOB in trauma patients is visualization. A difficult airway in this setting frequently involves bleeding, secretions, or emesis. The suction capability of the FOB may help in such circumstances, however, it is not always sufficient to clear the airway. Even small amounts of fluid can obstruct the view and render the FOB useless. Although the FOB may not be the first tool in mind for securing the airway of a trauma patient, it should be considered an essential tool as a rescue aid and as a diagnostic and therapeutic device.

# Surgical airway

Although the incidence of failed intubation requiring emergency surgical airway is exceedingly low when anesthesiologists participate in the care of trauma patients (0.3%), the ability to rapidly obtain a surgical airway is essential in this setting. Once a decision is made to proceed with RSI, there must be a commitment of the entire team to obtain an airway, as awakening a patient or canceling a case is rarely an option.

Cricothyroidotomy – This is classified into the percutaneous and open methods. The percutaneous method involves the Seldinger technique using a percutaneous cricothyroidotomy kit. The percutaneous method may be more appropriate for airway personnel with less experience at obtaining open surgical airways. The most common method for surgeons to establish an emergency airway is the open technique. This involves using the thyroid cartilage as a landmark, making an incision inferiorly until the cricothyroid membrane is opened and an airway is inserted (e.g., a 6.0 mm tracheal tube). The open technique is the fastest method for obtaining a surgical airway.

Tracheostomy – Although a tracheostomy can be a life-saving procedure, it is not the most rapid method for obtaining a surgical airway. When compared to a cricothyroidotomy, a tracheostomy may have fewer long-term complications. However, the increased time and risk of bleeding outweigh this benefit in the emergency setting.

# Penetrating neck injury

Airway management in patients with penetrating neck injury represents a special challenge not only because these patients may have injuries that may impede tracheal intubation, but also because insertion of a tube into the trachea may worsen the injury.

There is no uniformly agreed upon preferred method of airway management in patients with penetrating neck injuries. The small number of patients included in most series, the prolonged periods over which large series were reviewed, and the diverse nature of these injuries precludes formulating a single method of choice. Most authors agree that blind intubation methods (e.g., blind nasotracheal intubation) should not be used in these patients because further injury or complete airway obstruction may be induced.

At the Ryder Trauma Center, patients with penetrating neck injuries that require airway intervention undergo tracheal intubation by one of the following methods:

- Awake fiberoptic intubation
- "Rapid-sequence" fiberoptic intubation
- RSI
- Awake orotracheal intubation
- Surgical airway (rare)

Factors that determine which of the above methods is selected for a particular patient include urgency of the situation, likelihood of airway injury, patient cooperation, type of injury, and the presence of significant bleeding or airway obstruction.

Awake fiberoptic intubation is the safest method for most patients and should be considered in all cooperative patients with a high suspicion of airway injury. This method allows for evaluation of injuries at or below the glottis and positioning of an endotracheal tube distal to the injury. However, awake fiberoptic intubation is usually not possible in combative patients, or when immediate airway access is required (e.g., in the moribund patient).

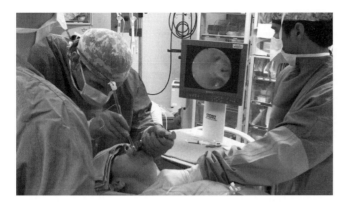

**Figure 3.4.** A "rapid-sequence" fiberoptic intubation can be used for patients with a high suspicion of airway injury when an awake fiberoptic intubation is not possible. RSI is followed by direct larngoscopy and insertion of a bronchoscope through the larynx. A tracheal tube is advanced over the endoscope. This allows clinicians to diagnose airway injury as the intubation is being performed and placement of a tracheal tube distal to the injury.

A "rapid-sequence" fiberoptic intubation technique may be used in combative patients who do not otherwise appear "difficult to intubate." In this technique, RSI is followed by standard laryngoscopy and insertion of a bronchoscope through the larynx to rapidly evaluate for the presence of injury or blood below the vocal cords. The bronchoscope tip is placed distal to the injury and the tracheal tube is then introduced over the endoscope. The cuff of the tracheal tube should be positioned below the injury to prevent air leak and enlargement of the laceration (Figure 3.4).

A standard RSI is used for patients that have normal anatomy, minimal risk for airway injury (e.g., "slash injury" behind sternocleidomastoid), and high risk for bleeding if coughing or straining occurs.

An awake orotracheal intubation is the most expeditious approach when immediate control of the airway is required in a moribund or apneic patient or in cases of massive upper airway bleeding.

If any of the above methods fail, a surgical airway should be immediately established. As noted above, the surgical airway of choice in a true emergency setting is a cricothyroidotomy. However, this procedure may result in complete disruption of the airway in cases of laryngotracheal dissociation. Tracheostomy will often be chosen in such cases. Finally, patients with an overt airway injury communicating with the skin can also undergo intubation through the open wound.

# Key points

- The ASA difficult airway algorithm provides an excellent guideline for the approach to the difficult airway, but needs to be modified for trauma patients.
- If non-invasive methods to secure the airway are unsuccessful in a trauma patient, invasive airway access may be the only other alternative, since awakening the patient or canceling the case is rarely an option.
- RSI is the most commonly used method for securing the airway in trauma patients.
- Small positive pressure breaths are recommended during RSI for any patient at risk of rapid oxygen desaturation.

- Cricoid pressure and MILI continue to be recommended for RSI in the trauma setting. However, these interventions may be reduced if they impede tracheal intubation.
- The incorporation of the tracheal tube introducer ("gum elastic bougie") into ATLS guidelines is the result of its success in aiding to secure a difficult airway in other settings.
- The use of supraglottic airways has increased in the prehospital trauma setting. These airways should be exchanged for a definitive airway as soon as is safely possible.
- Although videolaryngoscopes have expanded the armamentarium of anesthesia providers, the role of these devices in the management of trauma patients has yet to be determined.
- The fiberoptic bronchoscope is the most versatile of the intubating tools currently available for managing patients with a difficult airway.

## Further reading

1. American College of Surgeons, Committee on Trauma. *Advance Trauma Life Support for Doctors: ATLS® Student Course Manual.* Chicago, IL: American College of Surgeons; 2008.

2. Crosby ET. Airway management in adults after cervical spine trauma. *Anesthesiology* 2006;**104**:1293–1318.

3. Desjardins G, Varon AJ. Penetrating neck injuries. The Miami experience. *Resuscitation* 2001;**48**:71–75.

4. Diez C, Varon AJ. Airway management and initial resuscitation of the trauma patient. *Curr Opin Crit Care* 2009;**15**:542–547.

5. El-Orbany M, Connolly LA. Rapid sequence induction and intubation: current controversy. *Anesth Analg* 2010;**110**:1318–1325.

6. Manoach S, Paladino L. Laryngoscopy force, visualization, and intubation failure in acute trauma: should we modify the practice of manual in-line stabilization? *Anesthesiology* 2009;**110**:6–7.

7. Rice MJ, Mancuso AA, Gibbs C, et al. Cricoid pressure results in compression of the postcricoid hypopharynx: the esophageal position is irrelevant. *Anesth Analg* 2009;**109**:1546–1552.

8. Robitaille A, Williams SR, Tremblay MH, et al. Cervical spine motion during tracheal intubation with manual in-line stabilization: direct laryngoscopy versus Glidescope videolaryngoscopy. *Anesth Analg* 2008;**106**:935–941.

9. Stephens CT, Kahntroff S, Dutton RP. The success of emergency endotracheal intubation in trauma patients: a 10-year experience at a major adult trauma referral center. *Anesth Analg* 2009;**109**:866–872.

10. Turkstra TP, Pelz DM, Jones PM. Cervical spine motion: a fluoroscopic comparison of the AirTraq laryngoscope versus the Macintosh laryngoscope. *Anesthesiology* 2009;**111**:97–101.

# Shock, resuscitation, and fluid therapy

Roger Shere-Wolfe and Yvette Fouche

## Shock

Shock has long been recognized as a state of extreme pathophysiologic and metabolic derangement. As early as 1800 John Collins referred to it as a "momentary pause in the act of death," and Samuel Gross later termed it a "rude unhinging of the machinery of life." Many of the greatest luminaries in medicine were intrigued by shock and investigated it. During World War I Walter Bradford Cannon thought that it was caused primarily by "wound toxins," and identified acidosis as a key feature. A generation later Alfred Blaylock focused on hypovolemia as a key element of shock, which he characterized in 1937 as "a peripheral circulatory failure resulting from a discrepancy in the size of the vascular bed and volume of the intravascular fluid."

Our current understanding of shock is that of a microcirculatory disorder in which a variety of etiologies result in failure of adequate oxygen delivery or utilization at the cellular level, and which is perpetuated by cellular and humoral responses. Causes may include:

- Loss of circulating blood volume due to hemorrhage
- Cardiac failure
- Lack of vasomotor tone
- Obstruction to venous return (e.g., cardiac tamponade, tension pneumothorax)
- Impaired cellular utilization of oxygen (e.g., cyanide toxicity)

Shock results in a profound physiologic response that may initially compensate for the underlying deficit, but which may also produce adverse systemic effects. Prolonged shock results in a cumulative "oxygen debt," severe metabolic and physiologic derangement, and ultimately disruption of end-organ integrity and homeostasis. Once the cause of shock is fixed, it is still necessary to correct the associated derangements and restore normal function, which is often referred to as "repaying" the oxygen debt.

Shock may result from a variety of precipitating insults, but in the setting of acute trauma and injury should be presumed to be hemorrhagic until proven otherwise. In a patient with suspected shock, the clinician should rapidly look for potential causes. Life-threatening hemorrhage may occur in one of five places:

- Chest
- Abdomen

*Essentials of Trauma Anesthesia*, ed. A. J. Varon and C. E. Smith. Published by Cambridge University Press.
© Cambridge University Press 2012.

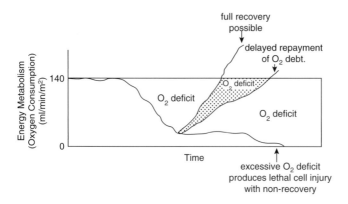

**Figure 4.1.** Cumulative effect of oxygen debt.

- Retroperitoneum (including the pelvis)
- A soft tissue compartment (as with long-bone fractures)
- Externally ("the street")

It is a cardinal sin to overlook a potential source of hemorrhage. Nevertheless, the clinician must also be vigilant in addressing potential non-hemorrhagic causes of shock. In the acutely injured patient these may include readily correctable insults such as tension pneumothorax and cardiac tamponade. Neurogenic shock from central nervous system injury and cardiogenic shock from blunt cardiac injury (see Chapter 16) or underlying cardiac disease must also be considered. More than one source of shock may be present.

It is key to understand that shock is a microcirculatory rather than a macrocirculatory disorder. It is a problem of blood flow (usually) to end organs, not of blood pressure (BP), especially not as measured in a major vessel such as the brachial artery. A patient can have a BP of 80/40 mmHg with perfectly normal perfusion (as do many patients under general anesthesia for elective surgical procedures), but a patient can have a BP of 120/80 mmHg and be in profound shock. Indeed, the majority of shock presents as compensated shock, in which the body is able to maintain the illusion of macrocirculatory stability due to compensatory increases in heart rate and vasoconstriction of "ischemia tolerant" vascular beds. Even compensated shock, if it persists for long enough, can cause end-organ dysfunction – the so-called "occult hypoperfusion syndrome". However, in extreme cases – such as hemorrhage of 30% circulating blood volume or greater – hypovolemia, hypoperfusion and organ derangement overwhelm compensatory mechanisms, resulting in uncompensated shock manifesting as circulatory instability. If not corrected quickly enough, this will progress to irreversible shock, in which the cumulative effects of prolonged hypoperfusion overwhelm the body's ability to respond to resuscitative efforts, even after the precipitating insult has been corrected. Patients in irreversible shock inevitably die. How quickly the patient develops irreversible shock depends on the depth and magnitude of shock and the individual's physiologic reserve, but the concept of the "Golden Hour," formulated over 40 years ago by R. Adams Cowley, is largely based on the observation that time is of the essence, and that the trauma provider is in a race against time to diagnose and treat shock before it becomes irreversible. Figure 4.1 illustrates the "area under the curve" nature of progressive shock.

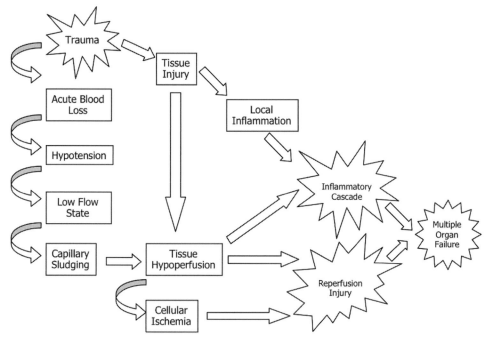

**Figure 4.2.** Pathophysiology of traumatic shock.

## Pathophysiology

The pathophysiology of shock is complex, and beyond the scope of this chapter except for a very brief discussion. Figure 4.2 provides a simplistic schematic of the patho-physiology of hemorrhagic shock. All traumatic injuries combine components of tissue injury and blood loss, both of which may contribute to a variable degree towards shock.

- Uncorrected acute hemorrhage leads to hypotension resulting in a low flow state, capillary sludging, and tissue hypoperfusion.
- This results in cellular ischemia and edema due to impaired energetics and loss of endothelial integrity.
- Capillary swelling and endothelial damage may impair microcirculatory flow long after the correcting insult has been addressed (the "no reflow" phenomenon).
- If shock progresses to the irreversible stage, ischemia and impaired cellular energetics will lead to a generalized loss of cellular membrane integrity and endothelial disruption.

The intricate interactions between ischemia, endothelial cell biology, and the coagulation system are just beginning to be understood, but this most commonly manifests clinically as the "lethal triad" of hypothermia, coagulopathy, and acidosis.

Direct tissue injury may lead to hypoperfusion and ischemia, and will also trigger a local inflammatory response, which is synergistic with that produced by hemorrhage. If the magnitude of these insults is sufficient, a systemic inflammatory response will be generated with widespread release of mediators – such as cytokines, kinins, and components of the coagulation system – and activation of the immune system. Reperfusion may also lead to release of free radicals and inflammatory mediators with systemic effects. The cumulative effect of this cascade will be the development of organ failure. This may occur acutely – as in irreversible shock, with the patient succumbing within hours – or over a prolonged period of time, as with occult hypoperfusion syndrome.

The anesthesiologist caring for the severely injured patient must have a basic understanding of this pathophysiology:

- Inadequate resuscitation leads to prolonged shock and either death from irreversible shock or subsequent multiple organ failure.
- Resuscitation to macrocirculatory stability does not necessarily mean that microcirculatory flow has been re-established, and the patient is still prone to end-organ ischemia and organ failure.

However, resuscitation is itself a process fraught with peril, in which reperfusion may exacerbate the response to injury. In addition, over-resuscitation can both lead to increased hemorrhage in the patient in whom source control has not been achieved, and in exacerbation of the physiologic response to injury. The anesthesiologist must be aware of the potentially adverse effects of therapy – including fluids, blood products, and pharmacologic agents – and balance these carefully against the risks of under-resuscitation.

## Diagnosis and recognition

Recognition of the shock state is essential for timely intervention and therapy. Unfortunately, the degree of shock cannot be determined by BP alone as shock is often compensated or "occult," and signs and symptoms may be subtle until patients exhaust their physiologic reserves and progress to uncompensated shock. In young patients especially, blood loss up to 40% of the normal circulating volume can occur before the limits of compensation are reached and hypotension or vascular collapse occurs.

The astute clinician should always be vigilant in searching for potential signs and sources of shock. Clinical signs may include:

- Tachycardia
- Tachypnea
- Impaired mentation (ranging from agitation and combativeness to confusion and lethargy)
- Cyanosis
- Pallor
- Diaphoresis
- Decreased capillary refill
- Decreased BP
- Narrow pulse pressure
- Difficulty obtaining a pulse oximetry signal
- Decreased urine output
- Hypothermia

Since many of these signs are non-specific and can be influenced by confounding factors, clinical judgment is paramount. Different types of shock often manifest different clinical pictures – the patient with spinal shock is generally warm, vasodilated, and bradycardic,

**Table 4.1.** ATLS classification of hemorrhagic shock. ATLS guidelines classify hemorrhagic shock based on the estimated percentage circulating blood volume lost and the corresponding signs and symptoms. Class I and II generally present as "compensated" or "occult" shock, with relatively normal hemodynamics, despite significant hypoperfusion. Uncompensated shock generally indicates a profound level of underlying physiologic perturbation and derangement

|  | Class I | Class II | Class III | Class IV |
|---|---|---|---|---|
| **Blood loss** | < 15% | 15–30% | 30–40% | >40% |
| **Heart rate (bpm)** | < 100 | >100 | >120 | >140 |
| **Blood pressure** | Normal | Normal | Decreased | Decreased |
| **Pulse pressure** | Normal | Decreased | Decreased | Decreased |
| **Respiratory rate** | 14–20 | 20–30 | 30–40 | >35 |
| **Urine output (mL/hr)** | >30 | 20–30 | 5–15 | Negligible |
| **Mental status** | Normal | Anxious | Confused | Lethargic |

Abbreviation. ATLS: Advanced Trauma Life Support.

whereas the patient with hemorrhage is generally cool, vasoconstricted, and tachycardic. Septic shock generally produces a warm, vasodilated but tachycardic picture. Mixed patterns can be particularly challenging. Nevertheless, recognizing shock before the patient has lost the ability to compensate generally provides a greater window for therapy and subjects the patient to less physiologic derangement.

Hemorrhage is the most common cause of shock in the traumatic setting, the second most common cause of mortality from injury, and the most common treatable cause. As previously mentioned, shock in the setting of trauma should be presumed to be hemorrhagic until proven otherwise. The Advanced Trauma Life Support (ATLS) training course classifies hemorrhagic shock into four categories based on the degree of hemorrhage, as listed in Table 4.1. Patients in class I and II hemorrhagic shock (less than 25% loss of circulating blood volume) generally present with normal BP and only mild tachycardia. Patients with 30% or greater loss of circulating blood volume rapidly lose their ability to compensate. It is important to realize that the patient who presents in uncompensated shock has already been subject to a severe "dose" of shock sufficient to overwhelm their physiologic ability to compensate, requiring prompt and aggressive intervention. The patient should be assumed to have a significant source of hemorrhage, which must be quickly identified. In some cases, the source will be obvious. Ultrasound examination and plain film radiographs may rapidly indicate other sources. Immediate life-saving interventions such as airway management, thoracostomy tube insertion, application of a pelvic binder, and establishment of venous access can be performed in the trauma bay while evaluation is in progress (see Chapter 2). If a clear site of massive hemorrhage is detected (e.g., by a positive ultrasound exam or massive chest tube output), then immediate operative intervention for source control is indicated. In other cases, and if the patient is more stable, angiographic intervention may be preferable. In either case, once shock is recognized and the cause identified, source control becomes paramount and must be coordinated with resuscitative efforts. Delaying intervention to perform additional studies may place the patient at greater risk for developing irreversible shock, and over-aggressive resuscitation before source control has been established may precipitate greater hemorrhage.

Laboratory values may assist in the diagnosis of shock and in assessing the degree and progression of shock, but they are generally not immediately available, and are not a substitute for clinical judgment. Lactate levels, base deficit, pH, serum osmolarity, and coagulation parameters should all be taken into consideration. The evolution of point-of-care devices may allow for the bedside determination of many of these parameters and guide diagnosis and therapy. The bleeding patient bleeds whole blood, so the admission hematocrit generally is fairly normal even in patients with massive hemorrhage; it is only after these patients become normovolemic by fluid administration that a decrease in hematocrit becomes manifest.

## Fluid therapy

Fluids have long been a mainstay for the treatment of shock. Even non-hemorrhagic sources of shock generally respond, at least transiently, to fluid administration. However, fluid administration should not be a substitute for treating the underlying cause. Anaphylactic, neurogenic, and septic shock result from vasodilation producing a discrepancy between the vascular bed and the circulating blood volume, and are treated with a combination of fluids and vasopressors in addition to source management. Obstructive shock – as in cardiac tamponade or tension pneumothorax – acutely decreases venous return and the resulting hemodynamic instability is magnified in patients with a low preload. In such instances, fluid therapy is utilized while correcting the underlying cause. Even patients in cardiogenic shock will respond to fluids up to a point, as defined by their Starling curve. In the case of hemorrhagic shock, it is obvious that acute loss of circulating blood volume resulting in hypoperfusion must somehow be replaced, in addition to correcting the underlying insult.

The history of fluid resuscitation – including the use of crystalloids, colloids, and blood components – parallels that of shock. During the Vietnam War, Shires and colleagues developed models of resuscitation using balanced crystalloid solutions and defined the basic compartments into which fluids distributed. This work led to the standard "3:1" ratio for crystalloid replacement of blood loss, and was based on animal models using controlled hemorrhage. This work exerted a profound influence, and large volume crystalloid resuscitation quickly became standard care. Only in the past decade has the pendulum swung away from this approach.

How much and what kind of fluid is used to resuscitate clearly depends on the injury, the timing of fluid administration, and the patient. ATLS guidelines currently recommend isotonic crystalloids as the first line of therapy, suggesting a 1–2 L crystalloid bolus with monitoring of the patient's hemodynamic response to assess whether there is significant ongoing blood loss (Table 4.2). Fluid administration is clearly beneficial to the patient who has lost blood but is not actively bleeding. This patient may have suffered hypotension acutely, but due to the compensatory vasoconstriction may be normotensive at the time of treatment. A fluid challenge will produce an immediate increase in blood pressure. As intravascular volume improves, the vascular system relaxes and tissue perfusion is improved. Patients with ongoing bleeding will manifest transient or no discernible improvement, indicating a need for hemostasis. However, while crystalloid bolus may be appropriate for patients in class I and II shock, it is probably deleterious to rely only on this strategy in patients with significant ongoing hemorrhage or in profound (class III or IV) hemorrhagic shock. Patients with this degree of shock should be treated with fluids that have either $O_2$ carrying capacity or the ability to support hemostasis (see Chapter 6).

**Table 4.2.** Responses to initial fluid resuscitation. ATLS guidelines utilize patients' response to initial crystalloid bolus (2000 mL lactated Ringer's in adults, 20 mL/kg in children, over 10 to 15 min) to classify their estimated blood loss and likelihood of ongoing hemorrhage and need for intervention

|  | Rapid response | Transient response | No response |
| --- | --- | --- | --- |
| **Vital signs** | Return to normal | Transient improvement; recurrence of hypotension and tachycardia | Remain abnormal |
| **Estimated blood loss** | Minimal (10%–20%) | Moderate and ongoing (20%–40%) | Severe (> 40%) |
| **Need for more crystalloid** | Low | High | High |
| **Need for blood** | Low | Moderate–high | Immediate |
| **Blood preparation** | Type and cross-match | Type-specific | Emergency blood release |
| **Need for operative intervention** | Possibly | Likely | Highly likely |
| **Surgical consultation** | Yes | Yes | Yes |

Abbreviation. ATLS: Advanced Trauma Life Support.

# Timing and rate of fluid administration

Prior to the advent of surgical hemostasis, over-aggressive fluid administration can be deleterious, as outlined in Figure 4.3. BP will rise acutely, which will lead to increased bleeding from open vessels and will break loose fragile clots. Fluids will also dilute necessary clotting factors thereby reducing or preventing intrinsic clot formation. The overall effect will be a rise in BP followed by a second drop as bleeding accelerates. If more fluids are administered without addressing the cause/source, a vicious cycle is created that leads to exsanguination and vascular collapse. This is the "transient responder" described in the ATLS curriculum and represents a surgical emergency. Effective treatment in the patient actively bleeding consists of definitive control of hemorrhage facilitated by tolerance of mild to moderate hypotension until hemostasis is achieved, as discussed in more detail below.

Both animal and human models of the timing of fluid administration with respect to intrinsic hemostasis suggest that hemostasis is a flow- and time-dependent phenomenon related to the rate of hemorrhage:

- "Fast bleeders" tend to form clots and "self-resuscitate" more quickly than "slow bleeders." Therefore, the rate of fluid administration during resuscitation may affect the stability of immature clots.
- Slow bleeders will take longer to become hypotensive and a rapid bolus will inhibit a further drop in BP, therefore delaying the process of clot formation.

Fast bleeders will become hypotensive sooner and initiate the clotting process sooner. This has been demonstrated in several small animal studies. However, in clinical practice trauma patients do not invariably re-bleed when the BP returns to normal. This may be due to clot stabilization over time or to surgical or angiographic hemostasis.

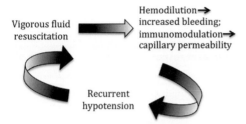

**Figure 4.3.** "Fluid creep." Over-aggressive administration of fluids leads to hemodilution and clot disruption, with transient improvement of hemodynamics but increased bleeding. Immunomodulatory effects of resuscitation fluids may also exacerbate the inflammatory response of injury, leading to increased capillary permeability, with extravasation of fluid. The result is recurrent hypotension, leading to more fluid administration, and a vicious cycle.

Animal models have shown that the risk of death in uncontrolled hemorrhage appears to be related to the severity of hemorrhage. In severe hemorrhage, fluid resuscitation reduces the risk of death, but in less severe hemorrhage, the risk of death is increased. Aggressive fluid resuscitation increases hydrostatic pressure and leads to destabilization of premature clots, increased blood loss, dilution of clotting factors, and decreased oxygen-carrying capacity of blood. This suggests that the risk–benefit ratio of fluid resuscitation is finely balanced. Animal studies show a benefit to small volume, hypotensive resuscitation in reducing the risk of death. Human studies have been equivocal and failed to show a difference in outcomes in small volume hypotensive resuscitation versus normotensive resuscitation. This suggests that animal models do not reflect the complexity of multiple injuries or comorbidities in humans. Revised ATLS guidelines, reflecting more recent thinking, emphasize control of bleeding first with more judicious early fluid resuscitation.

## Fluid alternatives for small volume resuscitation

Because of the above data suggesting that large volume fluid resuscitation in active hemorrhage may be deleterious, an evolving alternative approach to large volume fluid with isotonic crystalloids is small volume resuscitation using a hypertonic solution. Hypertonic solutions such as 3% saline act as magnets drawing fluid from tissues into the bloodstream, and thereby increase circulating volume. Small volume resuscitation is recommended by the Committee on Fluid Resuscitation for Combat Casualties. Although small volume resuscitation is currently approved for use in several European countries, it is currently not a part of the ATLS guidelines. Crystalloid undergoes an exponential departure from the vascular space with a half-life of only 17 minutes. The distribution of intravascular to interstitial fluid is anywhere between 1:3 and 1:10. This necessitates infusing larger volumes of crystalloid than the perceived blood loss in order to achieve homeostasis. As previously mentioned, in hemorrhagic shock, this could jeopardize early tenuous clot formation. Other potential complications include pulmonary edema (fluid being re-distributed to the low capacitance vessels of the pulmonary vasculature), increased total body water, hypoalbuminemia, coagulopathy, abdominal compartment syndrome, cardiac dysfunction, gastrointestinal ileus, and potential disruption of bowel anastomoses. In contrast, when hypertonic fluids are administered they undergo a longer exponential decay from the vascular space, yielding a distribution of intravascular to interstitium of less than 1:1.5. Small volume resuscitation is not a definitive therapy and must be followed by conventional therapy once the source of bleeding has been controlled and the patient has achieved initial hemostasis. Hypertonic solutions have been shown to improve microvascular flow, control intracranial pressure, and stabilize arterial pressure and cardiac output, with no deleterious effects on immune function or coagulation. Meta-analyses of clinical studies, however, show no significant difference in survival outcomes for resuscitation with hypertonic solutions. Further, there was no survival benefit with hypertonic saline for the initial resuscitation of adult patients with hemorrhagic shock or traumatic brain injury (*Resuscitation Outcomes Consortium Study*).

Several colloid solutions are commercially available in the United States, which include albumin, hydroxyethyl starch, and dextran. Colloids have been shown to improve microvascular perfusion and may have anti-inflammatory properties, although the latter has not been confirmed in large studies. Furthermore, colloids are expensive, may bind serum ionized calcium, decrease circulating immunoglobulins, and can lead to coagulopathy in doses greater than 30 mg/kg. Meta-analyses of clinical studies show no improvement in outcome when trauma patients are resuscitated with colloids as compared to crystalloids.

## Resuscitation from hemorrhage

The goals of resuscitation are complex, and may vary based on status of surgical hemostasis and nature of the injury. Goals include:

- Maintaining adequate perfusion pressure to the brain and other vital organs
- Avoiding irreversible shock
- Preventing clot disruption and worsening hemorrhage
- Restoring circulating volume
- Restoring the microcirculation
- Modulation of the immune and inflammatory response
- Restoring end-organ integrity and homeostasis

Figure 4.4 illustrates a simplified algorithm for managing the patient in hemorrhagic shock. Recognition of the shock state and identification of the potential causes is paramount. Correction of mechanical causes such as tension pneumothorax and cardiac tamponade may be performed in the resuscitation bay in parallel with the ABCs and secondary survey (see Chapter 2). Once a patient has been identified as being in shock and a potential etiology identified, treatment and resuscitation become priorities. Even in patients with apparent hemodynamic stability it may be advisable to secure the airway early on, before uncompensated shock sets in, and to establish large-bore central or peripheral access and possibly invasive BP monitoring (see Chapter 5). In cases of compensated shock where bleeding does not appear to be severe, judicious crystalloid resuscitation may be appropriate. In patients with uncompensated shock and likely massive hemorrhage, hemostatic resuscitation with blood and clotting products should be initiated as soon as possible.

## Early resuscitation

In instances of profound hemorrhagic shock, early resuscitative efforts must be coordinated with surgical efforts to achieve source control. This may be achieved rapidly (e.g., application of a pelvic binder in the resuscitation bay, ligation of splenic artery in the operating room) or may be extremely difficult to accomplish in the case of diffuse or anatomically

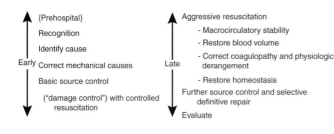

**Figure 4.4.** Early versus late resuscitation: basic approach.

challenging injuries. Prior to the establishment of adequate surgical hemostasis, the anesthesiologist must navigate the narrow territory between inadequate resuscitation leading to irreversible shock and over-aggressive fluid resuscitation leading to clot disruption, hemodilution, and worsening hemorrhage. The anesthesiologist must not strive for "optimal" resuscitative goals, since achieving these may conflict with the goal of minimizing ongoing hemorrhage, but rather for minimally acceptable signs that the patient is not going into irreversible shock. In patients without obvious cardiopulmonary disease and without evidence of traumatic brain injury, mild hypotensive resuscitation to a systolic pressure of 80–90 (or to a palpable radial pulse) may be beneficial. A heart rate less than 120 generally suggests that the patient is moving away from uncompensated (class III/IV) shock. Achieving a pH somewhere around 7.20 (in the 7.10–7.25 range) is probably indicative of a minimally acceptable level of microvascular perfusion, and the presence of urine output and a working pulse oximeter may also suggest that basic tissue perfusion is being achieved. Measurements of red cell and clotting factor levels are extremely dynamic during this period, but a hematocrit $> 25\%$ should be attainable.

Fluids should be limited to small boluses to the extent necessary to maintain adequate perfusion without worsening hemorrhage. In cases where the patient is extremely unstable, surgical packing may allow the anesthesiologist to "catch up" to a point that allows further exploration. The patient in hemorrhagic shock compensates by vasoconstriction, and is severely volume depleted. Although the anesthesiologist ultimately aims at converting that patient to a vasodilated, volume repleted ("anesthetized") state, this process is fraught with peril while the patient continues to bleed and must be carefully matched with surgical hemostasis. Anesthetic agents should be cautiously added in as much as tolerated, but with the understanding that over-aggressive administration may precipitate cardiovascular collapse. Narcotics such as fentanyl blunt the sympathetic response to injury with minimal direct vasodilation or cardiovascular depression, and may be preferable to inhalational anesthetics. The hemodynamic response to anesthetic agents may also be used to assess the patient's underlying volume status and surgical progress towards source control. As hemorrhage is controlled and the patient is volume resuscitated, larger doses of anesthetic agents should be tolerated without major hemodynamic perturbation.

Fluids should be the mainstay of maintaining perfusion. Vasopressors generally do not improve microcirculatory perfusion, may merely mask the depth of underlying shock, and should be reserved as a last resort in patients who do not respond to fluids. Failure of the patient to stabilize under such circumstances may be due to irreversible shock, but is also suggestive of ongoing hemorrhage from other sources or shock from another mechanism. This should prompt an aggressive search for the underlying cause. Failure to identify and treat such a cause subjects the patient to a greater dose of shock and an increased risk of progressing to irreversible shock or subsequent organ dysfunction.

## Late resuscitation

Once surgical hemostasis has been achieved, resuscitation should aim at the complete restoration of macro- and micro-circulatory stability and of end-organ homeostasis. This is generally achieved with additional fluid resuscitation to restore circulating blood volume in combination with anesthetic agents to vasodilate and open up circulatory beds and promote microvascular perfusion. Macrocirculatory goals include a stable systolic BP > 100 mmHg and a heart rate less than 100 bpm. Urine output should be normal. A normal pH as well as normalization of lactate and base deficit levels is suggestive of restored microvascular perfusion. Aggressive correction of any residual hypothermia and coagulopathy should also be priorities during this phase of resuscitation.

How much fluid loading is beneficial is still a matter of debate. Previously, observations that survivors tended to exhibit normal or elevated ("supranormal") cardiac output led to the practice of volume loading and the use of inotropes to achieve pre-specified goals for oxygen delivery and cardiac function. This approach has been criticized for leading to an unacceptably high rate of intra-abdominal hypertension and pulmonary dysfunction. Fluids – including blood products and hemostatic agents – may also have immunomodulatory effects that may be synergistic with the effects of shock and reperfusion, and which may impact on the subsequent development of organ dysfunction and sepsis.

## Damage control resuscitation

It is generally possible to predict early which patients are likely to have severe hemorrhage requiring massive transfusion and develop life-threatening coagulopathy. A number of scoring systems to predict the need for massive transfusion have been described, and most depend on readily available data on or shortly after admission.

Patients in class III and IV hemorrhagic shock are most likely coagulopathic on presentation to the trauma center, even if their admission coagulation studies are normal. Recent studies suggest that traumatic coagulopathy is not merely a dilutional phenomenon, but an early manifestation of physiologic derangement in severe hemorrhagic shock (see Chapter 6). Prompted by these studies, some trauma centers have moved away from the use of crystalloid and colloid solutions to the use of "hemostatic" resuscitation. Because the patient with severe hemorrhage loses cells and clotting factors at such a rapid rate, waiting for laboratory results to guide resuscitation invariably results in under-resuscitation and significant coagulopathy. The "damage control resuscitation" paradigm outlined in Table 6.1 severely limits crystalloid administration and uses empiric ratios of blood products to support hemostasis early on. Laboratory values are repeated every 30–60 minutes to monitor progress and guide resuscitation.

## Key points

- Shock from hemorrhage is the leading cause of potentially preventable injury mortality.
- Hypoperfusion leads to homeostatic derangement and a cumulative "oxygen debt" that becomes irreversible if not treated in a timely fashion; patients presenting with profound hemodynamic instability already have received a significant "dose" of shock.
- Resuscitative efforts – including fluids for volume resuscitation – must be closely coordinated with surgical efforts to achieve source control, and should

promote hemostasis, circulatory stability, homeostasis, and the restoration of end-organ integrity.

- The approach to resuscitation and therapeutic endpoints is evolving, as we better understand the complex pathophysiology of shock and its interaction with resuscitative practices.

## Further reading

1.  American College of Surgeons, Committee on Trauma. *Advance Trauma Life Support for Doctors: ATLS® Student Course Manual.* Chicago, IL: American College of Surgeons; 2008.

2.  Alam HB, Rhee P. New developments in fluid resuscitation. *Surg Clin N Amer* 2007;**87**:55–72.

3.  Bikovski RN, Rivers EP, Horst HM. Targeted resuscitation strategies after injury. *Curr Opin Crit Care* 2004;**10**:529–538.

4.  Cotton BA, Guy JS, Morris JA, Abumrad NN. The cellular, metabolic, and systemic consequences of aggressive fluid resuscitation strategies. *Shock* 2006;**26**:115–121.

5.  Dawes R, Thomas GO. Battlefield resuscitation. *Curr Opin Crit Care* 2009;**15**:527–535.

6.  Dutton RP. Current concepts in hemorrhagic shock. *Anesth Clin* 2007;**25**:23–34.

7.  Moore FA, Mckinley B, Moore EE. The next generation of shock resuscitation. *Lancet* 2004;**363**:1988–1996.

8.  Pruitt BA. Fluid resuscitation of combat casualties. Conference proceedings: June 2001 and October 2001. *J Trauma* 2003; **54**:S1–S2.

9.  Cotton BA, Reddy N, Hatch QM, *et al.* Damage control resuscitation is associated with a reduction in resuscitation volumes and improvement in survival in 390 damage control laparotomy patients. *Ann Surg* 2011;**254**:598–605.

# Chapter

# 5

# Vascular cannulation

Shawn Banks and Albert J. Varon

## Introduction

Appropriate vascular access is fundamental in the management of trauma patients to provide volume replacement, administer medications, monitor hemodynamic parameters, and collect samples for laboratory testing. This chapter will review the most commonly encountered vascular access techniques used in trauma patients. Indications, risks, benefits, and potential complications will be summarized for each.

## General considerations

### Factors influencing flow

- Increasing the radius of an intravenous (IV) catheter exponentially increases flow
- Increasing the length of an IV catheter increases resistance and decreases flow

Based on the Hagen–Poiseuille equation there are numerous factors that influence the pressure differential ($\Delta P$) across a tube. These include the flow rate (Q), length of tube (L), radius of tube (r), and viscosity of the fluid ($\mu$).

$$\Delta P = 8\,\mu\,LQ/\pi\,r^4$$

A simple rearrangement of the formula solving for flow rate (Q) illustrates the drastic influences that length and radius have on the maximum achievable volumetric flow through a particular vascular access catheter.

$$Q = \Delta P(\pi\,r^4)/8\,\mu\,L$$

Changes in catheter radius are directly proportional to changes in flow by the fourth power. For example, flow would theoretically be increased by a factor of 16 by doubling the radius of a catheter. Changes in length are inversely proportional to changes in flow.

## Ultrasound guided procedures

- Ultrasound decreases the time and number of needle punctures required to successfully cannulate a vessel.
- Healthcare agencies have advocated for increased use of ultrasound to improve patient safety.

*Essentials of Trauma Anesthesia*, ed. A. J. Varon and C. E. Smith. Published by Cambridge University Press.
© Cambridge University Press 2012.

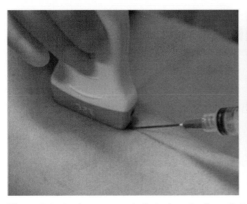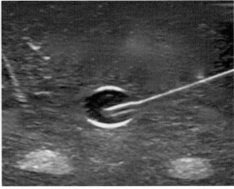

**Figure 5.1.** In-plane approach. Entire length of needle is visible when held parallel to long axis of probe.

Techniques for using ultrasound imaging for vascular cannulation have been described since the 1970s and in recent years have gained popularity among healthcare providers, particularly for obtaining central venous access. Ultrasound can be used to scout the patient's anatomy and mark an appropriate needle insertion site, or for real-time guidance of needle placement. In one prospective study comparing real-time and scout-only to landmark techniques, the success of cannulation on first needle pass was twice as frequent using the scout technique, and even higher in the real-time guided group. Time to successful cannulation was also reduced in both ultrasound groups. Ultrasound imaging may be of particular benefit in the trauma patient when coexisting injuries prohibit routine patient positioning for landmark techniques. Location of deep veins may also be easier with the assistance of imaging when patients have very low intravascular volumes and effectively smaller vein diameters. The use of ultrasound guidance for vascular cannulation has been identified by the Agency for Healthcare Research and Quality as a practice that should be employed to improve patient care and should be considered for trauma patients when practical. In the recent Practice Guidelines for central venous access, the consultants and American Society of Anesthesiologists (ASA) members agree that ultrasound imaging should be used for internal jugular vein cannulation.

When used for needle guidance, techniques are often described as "in-plane" or "out-of-plane," which indicates the needle's position relative to the ultrasound beam.

In-plane guidance refers to maintaining the needle position parallel to the long axis of the ultrasound probe, and entirely within the ultrasound beam. This allows the user to view the entire length of the needle and tip as it is advanced into the desired structure (Figure 5.1).

Out-of-plane guidance indicates that the needle is advanced perpendicular to the long axis of the ultrasound probe. The user will not be able to view the entire needle as it is advanced, as only a small cross-section of the needle will be visible at any time (Figure 5.2).

## Venous access

Access to the venous system can be achieved either peripherally or centrally. Peripheral access refers to the insertion of venous catheters of any length that terminate outside of the thorax; central access catheters terminate within the thorax.

### Peripheral venous access

- Peripheral IV lines are usually easier and faster to obtain in trauma patients.
- Peripheral IV lines may allow for higher flow rates than certain central lines.

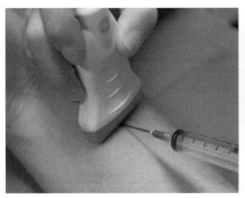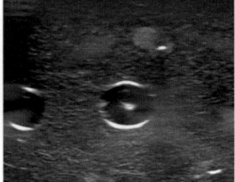

**Figure 5.2.** Out-of-plane approach. Cross-section of needle shaft visualized within vessel lumen, position of needle tip not continuously in view.

**Table 5.1.** Approximate crystalloid flow rates of various catheters based on major manufacturer specifications

| Size | 18 ga | 16ga | 14 ga | 8.5 Fr | 16 ga |
|---|---|---|---|---|---|
| | Peripheral venous catheter | Peripheral venous catheter | Peripheral venous catheter | Pulmonary artery catheter introducer | Lumen of central line |
| Length (cm) | 3 | 3 | 3 | 10 | 15 |
| Flow to gravity (mL/min) | 100 | 200 | 350 | 700 | 60 |
| Flow at 300 mmHg pressure (mL/min) | 200 | 500–600 | 1000 | 1800–1900 | 300 |

Catheterization of peripheral veins is by far the most common means of achieving venous access among all patients. The insertion of peripheral IV catheters can be performed quickly, with little preparation, and has a relatively low risk of serious complications. It is also possible to achieve very high flow rates when administering IV fluids through peripheral venous catheters, usually higher than those achievable through central catheters of the same diameter (Table 5.1). This is mainly due to the influence of length on the rate of flow, as described in the preceding section.

Though virtually any peripheral vein can be cannulated with an appropriately sized catheter, most peripheral IVs are placed in the upper extremities. The antecubital veins are often selected in emergency situations due to their large size and prominence. Antecubital IVs may be more affected by positioning of the arms than other locations and recognition of extravasation of IV fluids may be delayed due to the compliance of the surrounding compartment.

- Short IV catheters in the external jugular may increase the risk of catheter dislodgement and extravasation.

External jugular veins can be successfully cannulated with short, peripheral IV catheters. This practice may be useful for short-term management when other peripheral veins cannon be accessed, but there is an increased likelihood of unintentional catheter migration out of the vessel lumen due to patient movement. One should consider using longer catheters in the external jugular vein if the IV catheter is to be used outside of the OR or without close monitoring. It is possible to thread a longer catheter into the central compartment, as the external jugular eventually terminates into the subclavian vein.

## Central venous access

- Maximum barrier precautions and sterile technique should be used at all times.
- Emergency lines placed without ideal sterile conditions should be replaced *as a priority*, as soon as patient condition allows.
- Blood color and flow pulsations are not reliable indicators of arterial versus venous needle placement in hypotensive trauma patients.

In the trauma patient, IV fluid resuscitation is the most common indication for central venous catheter placement. Other indications include secure delivery of concentrated or vasoactive medications and to facilitate the introduction of other instruments or monitors into the heart or pulmonary circulation. Standard care requires that central venous lines be placed using maximum barrier precautions and sterile preparation. This includes skin preparation with antiseptic (2% chlorhexidine-based preparation), full patient draping, operator hand sanitization, and sterile gown, gloves, cap, and mask. Only in the most extreme situations should these standards be violated. Any central line placed without strict adherence to complete sterile technique should be removed as soon as an alternate line can be secured.

General complications associated with line placement in any central vein include bleeding with hematoma formation, accidental arterial puncture or catheterization, catheter-related bloodstream infections, arteriovenous fistula formation, pneumothorax, and extravasation.

The most widely utilized techniques for placing central venous catheters are based on modifications of the Seldinger method. This requires needle-cannulation of the desired vessel, placement of a guide wire through that needle, dilation of the subcutaneous tissue and vein, and threading the IV catheter over that guide wire into the vessel lumen. Initial cannulation of the desired vein is performed using either anatomic landmarks or ultrasound imaging as a guide to needle placement.

It is advisable to use additional tests to confirm venous placement of the needle before the tissue is dilated and the catheter threaded. Confirmatory tests include transduction of a venous waveform, venous manometry, blood gas analysis, ultrasound visualization of the guide wire in the vein, and echocardiographic visualization of the guide wire in the superior vena cava. Manometry, which is the simplest of these techniques, consists of aspiration of blood into a 20-inch IV extension tubing and visualization of a descending column of blood while the IV tubing is held vertically. Though no single test precludes the possibility of a misplaced needle, using one or more verification techniques may reduce the risk of accidental arterial insertion.

## Site of venous catheterization

- Resuscitation lines should be placed above the diaphragm, particularly if abdominal vascular injuries are suspected.

Each catheter insertion site has certain advantages and disadvantages, and all of these must be carefully considered in the context of the patient's injuries. The ideal position of a catheter placed for volume resuscitation will allow for uninterrupted delivery of IV fluids to the heart. For example, if a patient has sustained abdominal gunshot wounds, then it may be advisable to avoid femoral venous access. This reduces the possibility of loss of resuscitation fluids through any intervening vascular injuries. One should also be mindful of the continuum of the trauma patient's care and consider optimal line placement for extended intensive care unit use and associated infectious risks.

### Subclavian vein

- Maintains better patency in severe hypovolemia.
- Remains accessible when patient is in cervical collar.
- May reduce risk of catheter-related bloodstream infections.

The subclavian vein is a preferred site due to easily identifiable landmarks, relatively stable anatomic position based on patient position, and lower likelihood of collapse in low-volume states. The procedure does not necessarily require manipulation of the spine, which is undesirable in patients with high suspicion of spine injuries. The subclavian site is also associated with a lower incidence of catheter-related bloodstream infections. There is a potentially higher risk of pneumothorax associated with subclavian vein cannulation; other complications include hemothorax and thoracic duct injury. In the event of accidental subclavian artery puncture, direct pressure cannot be applied to the vascular structures due to the overlying clavicle.

### Patient positioning

The subclavian vein may be approached from above or below the clavicle, but the infraclavicular approach is most common (Figure 5.3). With the patient supine and the ipsilateral arm adducted, the operator must first identify the patient's clavicle from medial to lateral and divide its length into thirds. The needle is inserted one centimeter below the clavicle at the junction of the outer third and middle two thirds. The needle tip is aimed toward the sternal notch and slowly inserted at an angle that passes just below the clavicle. Some operators prefer to first contact the inferior edge of the clavicle, then slowly "walk off" the bone to prevent too steep an angle of insertion, as the pleura lies just deep to the subclavian vein. The needle is advanced with constant aspiration until venous blood freely returns. A guide wire is then threaded through the needle and the catheter is inserted by the Seldinger method. The line may become kinked or occluded if the entry point is too close to the clavicle and forms a sharp angle as it dives beneath the bone.

Ultrasound for subclavian placement is challenging due to the overlying clavicle. Its best application is for the supraclavicular approach to the subclavian vein. In this approach, the subclavian vein is visualized at the lateral border of the lateral head of the sternocleidomastoid muscle (SCM) near its insertion to the clavicle. The needle is directed toward the junction of subclavian vein and internal jugular veins using a longitudinal, in-plane approach.

### Internal jugular vein

The internal jugular vein is often selected for central line placement due to its large diameter and relatively superficial location. The area is also compressible in the event of accidental arterial puncture and the incidence of pneumothorax is thought to be lower than with the

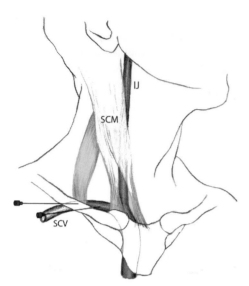

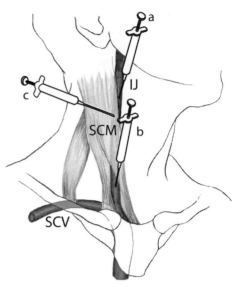

**Figure 5.3.** Alternative needle positions for subclavian vein cannulation. IJ = internal jugular vein; SCM = sternocleidomastoid; SCV = subclavian vein. Image by D. Lorenzo.

**Figure 5.4.** Alternative approaches to internal jugular vein cannulation. (a) Anterior approach. (b) Middle approach. (c) Posterior approach. IJ = internal jugular vein; SCM = sternocleidomastoid; SCV = subclavian vein. Image by D. Lorenzo.

subclavian approach. Jugular venous distension is considerably diminished in hypovolemic patients, which may make line placement more difficult when using blind techniques. Skin hygiene and dressings may be more difficult to maintain for these catheters after placement.

The patient is ideally positioned supine, feet elevated above the head, with the head turned away from the intended side of placement. Turning the head may not be advisable in trauma patients with suspected cervical spine injuries. The positions for needle insertion are in relation to the SCM. The internal jugular vein may be approached anterior to the SCM, between the sternal and clavicular heads of the SCM, or posterior to the SCM (Figure 5.4). As the internal jugular and carotid artery descend the neck toward the thorax, the vein usually moves from a position directly anterior to the carotid to a more lateral position; lower insertion points would theoretically decrease the risk of arterial puncture. For blind puncture in the middle and anterior approaches, the needle is inserted at a 30–45 degree angle aiming toward the patient's ipsilateral nipple, taking care to avoid the carotid pulsation. Constant aspiration is applied until there is free flow of venous blood, a guide wire is threaded, and a catheter placed using the Seldinger method.

Ultrasound guidance is particularly useful for placing internal jugular lines when the cervical spine cannot be manipulated. The ultrasound probe is placed on the neck perpendicular to the path of the vessels to provide a cross-sectional view. Patent veins are readily compressible compared to arteries, and arterial walls appear much thicker than those of veins. The Valsalva maneuver may enhance venous distension. In general, when the image of the target vessel is centered on the ultrasound monitor, the probe will be centered directly over that vessel. The needle is inserted out-of-plane at a 45-degree angle at the midline of the probe. Compression of the overlying tissues will be evident as the needle is advanced, but the needle tip will not routinely be visualized. With constant aspiration, the needle is advanced until venous blood is obtained. After the guide wire is threaded, ultrasound can then be used to confirm endovascular location of the wire.

### Femoral vein

- Femoral venous access is not ideal for patients with abdominal injuries; blood return to the heart may be impaired by intervening vascular injuries.
- Femoral lines may be associated with higher rates of venous thrombosis in long-term use.

The femoral vein may be selected due to its accessibility, compressible location, and reliable anatomic orientation. It is not a central line by definition. Concerns for infection and venous thrombosis have generally discouraged its long-term use in critically ill patients, but it may be appropriate for short-term resuscitation goals. This site also carries the risk of retroperitoneal hematoma formation and abdominal compartment syndrome with extravasation.

The vein is approached 2 cm below the inguinal ligament, just medial to the femoral pulse. The femoral location also lends itself to guidance by ultrasound in either out-of-plane or in-plane approaches.

## Types of central venous catheters
### Small-bore multi-lumen catheters

A variety of small-bore multi-lumen catheters with external diameters in the range of 7 to 8.5 French are available. These devices usually contain 3 to 4 lumens for infusion with internal diameters of 16- to 18-gauge, and the catheters most typically range from 15 to 20 cm in length. Though the internal diameters are equivalent to those of commonly used peripheral IV catheters, the length of these central catheters will significantly decrease flow rate.

These smaller catheters should be considered when a patient requires limited volume resuscitation, or the primary indication for placement is continuous infusion of vasoactive or irritant solutions.

### Large-bore single-lumen catheters ("introducers")

8–9 French single-lumen introducer catheters are primarily designed as conduits for additional instrumentation (e.g., insertion of pulmonary artery catheter or transvenous pacemaker wire), but they are also widely used for large volume fluid resuscitation. High flow rates can be achieved due to their relatively short length (approx. 10 cm) and large central diameter. As a single-lumen catheter, there are no additional side ports for administration of additional medications or infusions. Some manufacturers offer companion multi-lumen catheters that can be inserted through the introducer, but this may significantly reduce the effective internal diameter of the introducer and impede flow during high volume resuscitation.

### Large-bore multi-lumen catheters

Large-bore multi-lumen catheters with external diameters in the region of 12 French are available. These usually include 2 to 3 lumens with internal diameters varying in size from 12- to 14-gauge and overall catheter lengths of approximately 15 cm. Flow is limited to a lesser degree than smaller diameter catheters of equal length because of the exponential reduction in resistance as the radius increases. The presence of additional ports makes it easier to administer additional continuous infusions in the presence of rapid volume resuscitation.

## Intraosseous (IO) access

- Intraosseous lines may provide a delivery route for life-saving medications to patients in whom other types of vascular access cannot be established.
- Slow flow rates through IO lines limit their utility during rapid volume resuscitation.

The delivery of solutions into the circulation via the bone marrow was first described in the 1920s. It has evolved as a second-line, emergency option for vascular access in patients in whom reliable peripheral or central venous access cannot be obtained, particularly in the prehospital setting and in pediatrics.

The venous sinusoids of the medulla of long bones all drain into a central canal which returns blood directly to the venous system via emissary veins. This space remains accessible in hypotensive patients, as it is encapsulated in bone and is non-collapsable. Investigators have studied IO delivery of multiple medications including vasopressors, inotropes, bicarbonate, muscle relaxants, induction agents, and hydroxyethyl starch. In general, the onset times of medications delivered via the IO route are similar to IV.

The maximum achievable IO flow rates are significantly less than IV and limit the utility of the IO line for large volume resuscitation. Based on the average needle diameter in commercially available kits, flow of crystalloid solutions has been reported in the range of 2–3 mL/min at gravity. A number of needle systems and automatic powered needle injectors are commercially available, with needle sizes ranging from 15- to 18-gauge and length adjusted to the estimated weight of the patient.

Though originally described in the sternum, the proximal tibia is now the site of choice for IO cannulation. The classic site of insertion is the medial aspect of the tibia, approximately 2 cm distal to the tibial tuberosity. The needle is directed at a 60–90 degree angle, aimed away from the knee joint and any growth plate (Figure 20.2).

Complications from IO lines include malposition of the needle and extravasation of fluids, fat embolism, compartment syndrome, bone fractures and subsequent abnormal bone growth, infection, and osteomyelitis (rare).

## Arterial access

- Arterial catheters have rates of infection similar to those of central venous catheters.
- Arterial catheters should be placed with sterile conditions, even in emergencies.

Catheterization of the arterial system is indicated when continuous blood pressure monitoring or frequent arterial blood sampling is needed. Trauma patients frequently have large changes in intravascular volume due to bleeding and fluid resuscitation, so it may be useful to choose direct, invasive blood pressure measurement both for reliability and faster recognition of changes in blood pressure. The presence of an arterial catheter in a trauma patient also allows monitoring of arterial pressure variations during mechanical ventilation. The magnitude of these changes is dependent on the fluid status of the patient

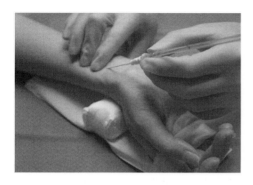

**Figure 5.5.** Radial artery cannulation. Sterile drapes removed for demonstration purposes.

and can predict a patient's response to fluid bolus (see Chapter 9). Electrolyte and gas exchange abnormalities should also be anticipated based on the degree of injury and volume resuscitation; many practitioners use frequent arterial blood analysis to guide therapy accordingly.

Arterial catheterization has historically been considered to have lower rates of catheter-related infections than venous lines, but recent evidence suggests rates of infection are similar regardless of venous or arterial location. The site of arterial catheterization should always be aseptically prepared and draped. The operator should observe sterile technique, including sterile gloves, drape, face mask, eye protection, and cap.

## Sites for arterial catheterization
### Radial artery
The radial artery is a preferred site for catheterization because of its ease of accessibility, superficial location, and the presence of collateral blood flow to distal structures. Complications arising from radial artery catheterization are infrequent. Adequate ulnar artery blood flow may not be present in a minority of patients, so it may be prudent to determine hand perfusion before placing the arterial line. This may prove difficult, if not impossible, in the unconscious or hypotensive patient and should not prevent the practitioner from placing the line, if indicated. The modified Allen test is the most commonly employed technique for assessing collateral flow. The patient is instructed to elevate the hand above the level of the heart and form a fist to remove blood from the extremity. Both the radial and ulnar arteries are then occluded by pressure from the examiner's fingertips and the hand is lowered and relaxed. The examiner then releases the ulnar artery only and watches for reperfusion of the hand and return of capillary blush, which should return in 6 seconds or less.

After site preparation, the radial artery pulse is palpated 3–4 cm proximal to the union of the wrist and hand (Figure 5.5). It may be useful to secure the hand with the wrist extended to stabilize the wrist and better expose the artery, but the hand must be released immediately after the procedure. The artery is approached with a catheter-over-needle device or cannulation needle at a 45 degree angle to the skin. When arterial blood returns through the needle, the angle of insertion can be lowered to 15 degrees and a guide wire inserted. The appropriately sized catheter, most commonly a 20-gauge 4.5 cm, is then passed over the wire using a modified Seldinger technique, the wire removed, and the catheter connected to a transducer system.

### Axillary artery

The axillary artery offers the benefit of fewer artifacts from arm position, a superficial location, and proximity to the central arterial tree. Long-term care and asepsis of the insertion site may be more challenging when compared to other sites. The catheter is inserted using a modified Seldinger technique as described above, but the location will require a longer catheter system of approximately 10–12 cm.

### Femoral artery

The femoral artery can be accessed using the modified Seldinger technique and a long arterial catheter. Placement is relatively easy due to the large arterial diameter and pulses are usually still palpable when the patient is hypotensive. The complications associated with this site include formation of a retroperitoneal hematoma or arteriovenous fistula. Care and asepsis for the insertion site may be challenging in the long term.

### Dorsalis pedis artery

The dorsalis pedis artery is palpated just lateral to the extensor hallicus longus tendon on the dorsum of the foot. The distal location of this site tends to create overestimation of the systolic blood pressure.

### Brachial artery

Use of the brachial artery is often discouraged due to the perception of increased thrombotic complications, though the incidence of these may be no greater than in other cannulation sites. The sequelae of brachial artery thrombosis may be severe due to lack of collateral circulation below this artery.

## Key points

- Increasing the radius of an IV catheter exponentially increases flow and decreases resistance. Conversely, increasing the length of an IV catheter linearly increases resistance and decreases flow.
- Peripheral IV access (large bore) can provide faster flow than some central venous catheters and can be obtained more quickly.
- Sterile procedure for vascular access should not be compromised in trauma patients; catheters placed without ideal conditions should be replaced at the earliest opportunity.
- Central access from above the diaphragm is preferred if abdominal injury is suspected.
- The subclavian vein is preferred over other sites in hypovolemic patients.
- Ultrasound decreases the time and number of needle punctures required to successfully cannulate a vessel, and should be used when practical to improve patient safety.

## Further reading

1. Banks S, Varon AJ. Vascular cannulation. In: O'Donnell JM, Nacul FE, eds. *Surgical Intensive Care Medicine*, 2nd edition. New York, NY: Springer; 2010.

2. Ezaru CS, Mangione MP, Oravitz TM, et al. Eliminating arterial injury during central venous catheterization using manometry. *Anesth Analg* 2009;**109**:130–134.

3. Franklin C. The technique of radial artery cannulation. Tips for maximizing results while minimizing the risk of complications. *J Crit Illn* 1995;**10**:424–432.

4. Lucet J, Bouadma L, Zahar J, et al. Infectious risk associated with arterial catheters compared with central venous catheters. *Crit Care Med* 2010;**38**:1030–1035.

5. *Making Health Care Safer: A Critical Analysis of Patient Safety Practices.* Rockville, MD: Agency for Healthcare Research and Quality; 2001.

6. Milling TJ, Rose J, Briggs WM, et al. Randomized, controlled clinical trial of point-of-care limited ultrasonography assistance of central venous cannulation: The Third Sonography Outcomes Assessment Program (SOAP-3) Trial. *Crit Care Med* 2005;**33**:1764–1769.

7. Trottier SJ, Veremakis C, O'Brien J, Auer AI. Femoral deep vein thrombosis associated with central venous catheterization: results from a prospective, randomized trial. *Crit Care Med* 1995;**23**:52–59.

8. Practice guidelines for central venous access: A report by the American Society of Anesthesiologists task force on central venous access. *Anesthesiology* 2012; **116**:539–573.

**Chapter**

**6**

# Blood component therapy and trauma coagulopathy

Richard Dutton

## Introduction – the pathophysiology of hemorrhagic shock

Hemorrhage is the second leading cause of death after injury, but may be the most preventable. Some patients die within minutes, the result of catastrophic exsanguination from central vessels, and offer little opportunity for resuscitation. In many others, however, death from hemorrhage comes only after the gradual exhaustion of compensatory mechanisms in the face of ongoing blood loss and progressive tissue ischemia. Even when bleeding is controlled, the depth and duration of hypoperfusion – the "dose" of shock – may be large enough that it leads to death days or weeks later from the accumulation of organ system failure and repeated sepsis. Successful resuscitation of the bleeding patient requires understanding of the pathophysiology of shock, knowledge of those therapies most likely to encourage hemostasis, and the willingness to act with speed and precision in the face of the unknown.

Sudden loss of circulating blood volume triggers a predictable cascade of compensatory mechanisms intended to preserve perfusion of the most sensitive tissue beds.

- Release of catecholamines in response to pain and hemorrhage causes vasoconstriction of ischemia-tolerant organs such as the skin, bone, muscles, and intestines.
- Blood flow to the brain is preserved, and blood flow to the heart transiently increased.
- This enables increased heart rate and inotropic state as a means of preserving cardiac output in the face of decreased blood volume.
- It is not until the loss of more than 20% of circulating blood volume (i.e., more than 1 L in a 70 kg adult) that blood pressure begins to fall.
- Once the threshold of compensation is crossed, the consequences of tissue ischemia accumulate quickly. In the hospital setting, these patients are observed to suffer from the "lethal triad" of acidosis, coagulopathy, and hypothermia.
- In the absence of definitive hemostatic treatment, death from hemorrhage is the result of endothelial failure, manifested as progressive unresponsiveness to fluids or pressors, edema, and eventual circulatory collapse.

While the gross signs and symptoms of hemorrhagic shock have been well understood for centuries, it is only recently that the intricate interaction between ischemia, endothelial function, and coagulation has been recognized. In particular, several studies have now observed that shock and tissue injury cause coagulopathy even in the absence of dilution

*Essentials of Trauma Anesthesia*, ed. A. J. Varon and C. E. Smith. Published by Cambridge University Press.
© Cambridge University Press 2012.

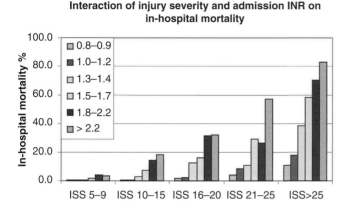

**Figure 6.1.** Interaction of injury severity, coagulation status at admission, and mortality. Note the interaction between injury severity score (ISS) and the presence of coagulopathy (increased international normalized ratio (INR)), as well as the more ominous association between this early coagulopathy and mortality. N = 32,000 trauma center admissions.

with resuscitative fluids. Figure 6.1 illustrates this concept, based on the initial laboratory samples of more than 30,000 trauma admissions to a single urban trauma center. Few of these patients had received more than 500 mL of fluid prior to admission, so dilution was not the cause of this early coagulopathy. The subsequent eloquent work of Brohi and colleagues has identified an early increase in Protein C expression as one cause of the "Acute Coagulopathy of Traumatic Shock," but it is likely that the observed clinical effect is the result of hundreds of biochemical changes in the endothelium and plasma. That an ischemic cell should release fibrinolytic compounds makes intuitive sense, since the overwhelming cause of ischemia for most cells is proximal thrombosis or embolic obstruction. Greater understanding of the complex role that the endothelial cell plays in supporting the liquid phase of coagulation also makes it clear that ischemia leading to dysfunction in the endothelium must also have profound consequences for coagulation.

Improved understanding of the cellular physiology triggered by hemorrhagic shock and ischemia has led to a rethinking of the traditional approach to early trauma care, with increased emphasis on rapid anatomic control of bleeding and early support of the coagulation system. This approach, known variously as "hemostatic resuscitation" or "damage control resuscitation," has evolved through the crucible of recent military conflicts to become the modern standard of care in civilian trauma centers in much of the developed world.

## Goals of early resuscitation

Early resuscitation – defined as the period from injury until definitive anatomic control of the source of bleeding – is characterized by the need to support the circulation in the face of diagnostic uncertainty as to the exact cause and expected duration of hemorrhage. Table 6.1 provides recommendations for early resuscitation focused on preservation and support of the coagulation system.

Anatomic control of the sites of bleeding is the first priority. This begins in the field, with first aid for hemorrhage. Direct pressure on the bleeding wound is the first approach, but is not effective for internal hemorrhage or for badly mangled extremities (e.g., from a motorcycle collision or improvised explosive device blast). Tourniquets, once nearly

**Table 6.1.** Elements of hemostatic or "damage control" resuscitation

- First aid focused on immediate control of hemorrhage by dressings and pressure
  - Consider the use of a tourniquet
  - Consider the use of topical hemostatic dressings
- Expedite anatomic control of bleeding (e.g., surgery or angiographic embolization), if not already in the operating room
- Titrate fluid to restore consciousness, radial pulse, and a systolic blood pressure of 80–90 mmHg until definitive surgical control of bleeding can be achieved
- Fluid treatment is aimed to a systolic blood pressure of at least 100 mmHg in patients with hemorrhagic shock and head or spinal cord trauma
- Early use of plasma and platelets is critical to maintaining clotting capability in the actively bleeding patient
- Monitor ionized calcium and lactate level
- Maintain normothermia
- Once hemostasis is achieved, assess all laboratory and hemodynamic variables and complete resuscitation as needed

abandoned in prehospital care, have seen renewed utility in controlling bleeding from badly and multiply injured extremities. Indeed, the most current field medical training of both the British and American military teaches "CABC," to emphasize control of Catastrophic hemorrhage even before Airway management, Breathing, and Circulation.

The military has also pioneered the use of topical hemostatic agents and dressings to provide rapid control of external bleeding. These products, now in a second generation of development since the start of the War on Terror, are designed to be rapidly placed on a bleeding site, conform to the injury, allow direct pressure, facilitate clotting locally but not systemically, and be removable without further injury when the patient reaches definitive care. Hemostatic dressings typically include a collagen matrix of some sort, impregnated with fibrinogen, thrombin, other clotting proteins, or exothermic drying agents such as zeolite. A complete discussion of topical hemostatics is not possible in this short chapter, but it is likely that these products will see increasing use in civilian prehospital trauma practice in the near future.

Once the patient reaches the hospital, the same prioritization of anatomic control of hemorrhage should apply. Early diagnostic tests focus on the search for sites of internal bleeding (chest X-ray, ultrasound, computed tomography) and then expediting the patient's access to the operating room or to angiographic embolization. Indeed, one of the most important components of hemostatic resuscitation is the conscious decision NOT to perform many otherwise normal diagnostic or therapeutic maneuvers, preferring rapid transport to the operating room for definitive or damage control surgery.

Once they have arrived in surgery, the patient in unstable hemorrhagic shock should be managed with "damage control" principles. Surgery should focus on control of hemorrhage and preservation of life and limb, without digressing for any procedure that can be safely deferred. Injured sections of bowel can be rapidly stapled to limit contamination; temporary shunting may be appropriate for some vascular injuries; external fixation is used to stabilize fractures; and the abdomen (and even chest) can be packed open under a sterile dressing rather than being definitively closed. Anastomosis of the bowels, complex vascular repairs, definitive orthopedics, and even closure of the abdomen can be deferred. The object is to transfer a living and hemostatic patient back to intensive care as soon as possible, where resuscitation can be completed based on laboratory data and advanced hemodynamic monitoring.

During this period the anesthesiologist must manage a highly dynamic patient in empiric fashion, based on a best guess at what course the surgery and resuscitation are going to take. The process is much like driving a car down the highway backwards at night, guessing which way to turn the wheel in order to stay on the road. Sending laboratory studies is like turning on the headlights – it provides a clear view of where the patient has been, but does not shed as much light on what is still to come.

## Fluid and blood products

The need to maintain the patient in a slight hypotensive state until hemorrhage is controlled should not be accomplished by fluid restriction, but rather by an active process of anesthetic administration balanced by carefully titrated fluid administration.

- The goal is to move the patient's physiology from the intense vasoconstriction of hemorrhagic shock to the more vasodilated state associated with major elective surgeries.
- If this can be accomplished without raising the blood pressure so high that re-bleeding occurs, then tissue perfusion can be improved and ischemic cellular injury limited.

One of the enduring controversies of resuscitation science is the best fluid to use in the actively bleeding patient. Hemostatic resuscitation emphasizes the early and aggressive use of blood products – in a ratio of 1:1:1 for red blood cells (RBCs), fresh frozen plasma (FFP), and platelets – over any other fluids, including empiric administration based on an understanding of the patient's physiology and trajectory rather than on laboratory data alone. The goals of this empiric approach are to maintain oxygen delivery, reducing tissue ischemia, and preserve hemostatic function.

Fresh whole blood is the ideal resuscitative fluid for patients in uncontrolled hemorrhagic shock. It contains a more than adequate quantity of RBCs to transport oxygen, as well as 2,3-diphosphoglycerate (2,3 DPG) to facilitate loading and unloading. It contains a physiologic quantity of clotting factors and platelets, unaffected by storage losses, and the combination with RBCs at a high hematocrit will encourage margination of platelets and factors within blood vessels, to further facilitate clotting. Anecdotal evidence from the US military in Iraq and Afghanistan and from the transfusion services of the Israeli Defense Forces indicates that, when available for resuscitation, fresh whole blood produces the best results. Unfortunately, this product is not available in civilian trauma centers in the US. Fractionation of donated blood allows for close matching of a limited national supply to an ever-increasing demand, as well as storage of plasma and RBCs for extended periods. Further, routine nucleic acid testing of donated blood for viral pathogens takes up to 72 hours per unit; beyond the time frame that whole blood (especially the platelets) can be kept functionally viable. Table 6.2 illustrates the difference between whole blood and the components that it eventually becomes. It can be seen from this analysis that even a 1:1:1 ratio of blood bank products, with no exogenous crystalloid added, leads to an infused mixture that is poorly concentrated and on the lower end of physiologically acceptable.

**Table 6.2.** Fresh whole blood versus fractionated blood products. Donated whole blood is diluted with an anticoagulant solution and then centrifuged and fractionated, resulting in the loss of potency when that unit is "reconstituted"

|  | When donated | Individual unit after fractionalization | When given as 1:1:1 |
|---|---|---|---|
| **Total volume** | 500 mL | 450 mL RBC, 200 mL plasma, 50 mL platelets | 700 mL |
| **RBC hematocrit** | 45% | 55% | 28% |
| **Clotting factor activity** | 100% | 90% | 65% |
| **Platelet count** | 300,000/hpf | Millions/hpf | 65,000/hpf |

RBC = red blood cells; hpf = high powered field.

The following fluids, blood products, and derivatives are commonly available in US civilian practice:

- *Isotonic crystalloids* are the first line of therapy for most injured patients, especially in the prehospital environment. While these fluids are routinely beneficial to most trauma patients, their excessive administration is counterproductive in those with uncontrolled hemorrhage. Excessive crystalloid administration will increase blood pressure – and thus blood loss – while contributing to both hypothermia and hemodilution.

- Asanguineous *colloids*, such as albumin, gelatin, or starch solutions, exert a greater oncotic presence than crystalloids and will therefore achieve similar increases in blood pressure with smaller administered volumes. As with isotonic crystalloids, however, administration to the patient with ongoing hemorrhage may be counterproductive.

- *RBCs* should be the first choice of fluid for the seriously injured patient. RBCs carry oxygen, thus reducing ischemia at the tissue level, while preservation of a higher hematocrit facilitates coagulation. Blood typing and cross-matching of donor units produces a typical logistic lag between sending a sample and administering the product of at least one hour in elective cases. In trauma patients, however, the use of uncross-matched type O (universal donor) RBCs is routine and effective, and the military and most major civilian centers have created protocols for rapid delivery of these units to the bedside. One large observational study demonstrated no adverse effects attributable to the early administration of more than 600 units of type O RBCs in a one-year period, even when Rh+ units were administered to Rh- patients.

- *Plasma* fractionated from donated blood contains all necessary clotting and antithrombotic factors, in approximately physiologic concentrations. Plasma units are frozen for long-term storage and must be thawed and ABO-typed before elective administration. Larger hospitals, with greater average demand for plasma transfusion, will pre-thaw some units each day, thus shortening the delivery time in emergency situations. As with RBCs, it is possible to store thawed universal donor (type AB) plasma in the trauma unit, thus making it immediately available for resuscitation in unstable patients. Unlike type O RBCs, however, type AB plasma is a rare commodity, and few blood banks are able to make it freely available. In most civilian trauma programs, therefore, there is a logistic delay in plasma administration of about 30 minutes if the blood bank has pre-thawed units on hand, and 60 minutes if both typing and thawing are required.

- *Platelets* for rapid administration are typically available in concentrated packs pooled from four to six donors, or taken from a single donor by apheresis. A unit of platelets includes a small amount of plasma, and by itself is a relatively concentrated product. Platelets are the blood component with the shortest storage life outside the body, and are thus typically in the shortest supply in the blood bank and nationally. Platelets are also the most sensitive component of blood due to the vicissitudes of storage. Moreover, the benefits of a platelet transfusion can be lost if the product is administered through a filter or complex tubing system that binds most of the active cells. Temperatures ranging from room temperature (20°C) to 42°C are generally not considered to have an activating effect on platelets.

- *Cryoprecipitate* is a pooled product manufactured from the plasma component of donated blood. Cryoprecipitate consists of a higher concentration of certain factors – especially fibrinogen – than a plasma unit. In most situations cryoprecipitate offers no great advantages over plasma, although the role of fibrinogen in early resuscitation has received renewed interest of late, as this seems to be one of the factors that decline most rapidly in severely injured patients. The downside of plasma transfusion to a patient who is already coagulopathic from injury and ischemia is that it is too dilute to help the patient recover normal function. Administration of cryoprecipitate, platelets, and specific clotting factor concentrates can help to overcome this issue and "jump-start" the failing coagulation system.

- *Prothrombin complex concentrates* (PCCs) are also derivative products of plasma, manufactured to contain precise concentrations of important clotting factors. The older products available in the US include these factors in their activated form, and they have been associated with increased risk of thrombotic complications. Newer products have been developed and used in Europe in recent years, but the safety of these PCCs is still controversial and it is not clear when they will be widely available in the US.

- *Specific factor concentrates* are available for many components of coagulation, including Factors VII, VIII, and I (fibrinogen). They are seldom used in trauma patients in the US, because of both expense and a prevailing belief that rapidly bleeding patients require the mixed administration of all factors, rather than just a selection. This opinion may change in the near future, however, based on the greater availability of point-of-care coagulation testing in the emergency department or operating room that can reveal specific factor deficiencies in bleeding patients.

- *Tranexamic acid*, a lysine analogue, inhibits fibrinolysis by blocking the lysine binding sites on plasminogen. There has been increased interest in the use of this hemostatic agent for treatment of coagulopathy in the trauma setting. A large prospective randomized placebo-controlled trial (CRASH-2) demonstrated significant reductions in all-cause mortality and in deaths due to bleeding in trauma patients that received tranexamic acid (1 g loading followed by 1 g over 8 hours). However, the benefit was only seen when tranexamic acid was administered within 3 hours of injury and increased mortality occurred when the drug was given after this period.

# Empiric transfusion ratios

The single greatest controversy in resuscitation research in recent years has been debate over the optimal ratio of RBCs to plasma during early resuscitation. Most trauma specialists agree that empiric therapy is necessitated in seriously injured and shocked patients, because waiting for precise laboratory or diagnostic monitor information may impose a life-threatening delay in care. However, most physicians now also recognize that "blood transplant" is a therapy that should not be undertaken lightly. Numerous observational studies have documented the strong association between the quantity of blood transfused and adverse outcomes, including organ system failure and mortality. While these data are contaminated to a degree by the "Sicker Patients Do Worse" phenomenon (i.e., patients with worse injuries and a higher risk for bad outcome are also more likely to get transfused), there have now been enough carefully controlled studies published that it is hard to argue with the idea that heterologous transfusion is inherently dangerous. This may be the result of subtle allergic reactions or by-products of the storage and reinfusion process (such as cellular debris), but is more likely related to the immune consequences of introducing foreign material and the alteration in inflammatory state that results.

The only patients that should get blood products, therefore, are those who will die or suffer serious morbidity if they do not. Various schemes exist to identify these patients, including combinations of vital signs, injury severity, and admission laboratory values, but for anesthesiologists the most significant variable in the decision to transfuse should be dynamic trends in the patient's blood pressure. Hypotension in an unanesthetized patient likely indicates loss of at least 20% of normal blood volume (e.g., 1000 mL in a 70 kg adult). This patient should respond to bolus administration of fluid with increased blood pressure in the short term, but it is the change that comes next that will be most telling. Patients who have become hemostatic will remain stable following a fluid load; those who become hypotensive again can be considered to be actively bleeding. The introduction of the effects of sedative and sympatholytic medications complicates interpretation of vital sign trends somewhat, but in a way that should still be interpretable by an experienced anesthesiologist. The interaction of vascular capacity (vascular tone) and blood volume is shown in simplified form in Figure 6.2. The goal in the hemorrhaging trauma patient is to move from vasoconstricted (shock) to vasodilated (anesthetized) while avoiding hypertension, so as to minimize re-bleeding.

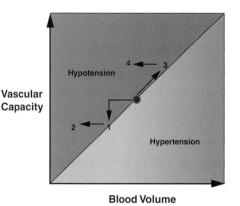

**Figure 6.2.** The physiologic relationship between vascular capacity (vascular tone) and the quantity of blood that fills it. In the normal state (the center dot), volume and capacity are matched. Hemorrhage reduces blood volume, and compensatory vasoconstriction preserves blood pressure (point 1). Bleeding in excess of compensation leads to hypotension (point 2). Anesthesia increases vascular capacity through vasodilation, compensated by fluid administration (point 3). Bleeding while under anesthesia leads to hypotension (point 4).

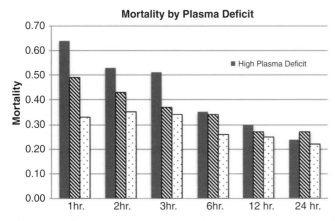

**Figure 6.3.** The association between early plasma use and mortality in rapidly bleeding patients, based on the "plasma deficit," calculated as red blood cell units minus plasma units.

Having thus identified the patient at risk for exsanguinating hemorrhage, what blood products should be administered? Type O RBCs have been used for this purpose for decades, and are known to be safe and beneficial. However, the use of RBCs alone, while adequate to support oxygen delivery, risks exacerbating the dilution of clotting components and potentiating coagulopathy. Hence the recent recommendations for co-administration of plasma. When considering this issue some time ago at the R Adams Cowley Shock Trauma Center we discovered that over the course of a year we had transfused almost equal amounts of plasma and RBCs, and that any patient receiving a massive transfusion – defined as 10 or more units of RBCs – almost inevitably received equal amounts of plasma and platelets. It occurred to us that coagulation might be better preserved by administering the products in a continuous 1:1:1 ratio, rather than giving several units of RBCs, then reacting to laboratory values and pouring in plasma later. This observation, combined with the thought exercise embodied in Table 6.2, prompted our change to 1:1:1 more than a decade ago. This approach has been facilitated in recent years by the blood bank's ability to provide pre-thawed type AB plasma units in the trauma resuscitation unit, for immediate administration with type O RBCs in badly injured and unstable patients.

Research into the benefits of this approach has included more than 20 recent observational series of transfusion patterns and ratios in trauma patients. The raw data show improved survival associated with earlier and higher volume administration of plasma, but the majority of these studies do not control for the so-called "survivor bias." Patients in most centers who are bleeding very rapidly are more likely to receive RBCs than plasma before dying, purely on logistic grounds. If there is no control for the time of death in the observation, then surviving long enough to receive plasma becomes a surrogate for slower bleeding and improved long-term outcome. This literature was summarized in a recent review by Stansbury et al. (reference 7 in Further reading). Studies that have attempted to control for survival bias show that early plasma use is beneficial, but only in the first two hours after injury (see Figure 6.3 and reference 4 in Further reading).

Finally, a recent prospective observational study indicates that a 1:1 FFP:RBC ratio does not provide any additional benefit over ratios of 1:2 to 3:4, and that the hemostatic benefits of plasma therapy are limited to patients with coagulopathy. Currently, the American Association of Blood Banks and the European task force recommend early intervention with FFP but without a preset FFP:RBC ratio.

## Late resuscitation

Once hemorrhage has been definitively controlled, time pressure is greatly relieved and subsequent resuscitation can be guided by laboratory values, invasive hemodynamic monitoring, and individual patient response. The goal in the hemodynamically stable patient is to optimize physiology for long-term survival. This requires providing adequate fluid to restore normal or supranormal tissue perfusion, and may be indicated by maximized cardiac output, return of normal mental status and renal function, and clearance of serum lactate.

Entry into the late resuscitation phase typically implies that coagulopathy has been corrected or averted. Once the patient is hemostatic by clinical observation and continued hemodynamic stability, it is generally not necessary to administer any more plasma or platelets. Elevated prothrombin time and low platelet count will recover spontaneously if the patient is not further stressed, whereas administration of more products in this situation may provoke or exacerbate an immunologic predisposition to organ system failure. The modern trauma anesthesiologist must therefore practice in a conflicting fashion: aggressive with blood products in the unstable patient and stingy with them thereafter.

## Future developments

The science of resuscitation from hemorrhagic shock has changed dramatically in the past two decades, and may change again in the near future. Point-of-care coagulation testing and non-invasive hemodynamic monitors may combine to provide accurate real-time data on the bleeding patient's condition, thus allowing precise administration of blood products, calcium, asanguineous fluids, and factor concentrates in only the amounts that are needed. In the meantime, however, the anesthesiologist must think one step ahead of the patient's clinical course, and aggressively and empirically treat those patients who are unstable and actively bleeding.

## Key points

- Coagulopathy after trauma results from severe tissue injury and shock.
- Coagulopathy is exacerbated by resuscitation with unwarmed fluid and blood products.
- Outcomes are improved by resuscitation focused on early control of hemorrhage and support of coagulation.
- Early use of blood products, at ratios of at least one unit of plasma to two units of RBCs, is associated with improved outcome.
- Early use of the antifibrinolytic agent tranexamic acid has been associated with improved outcomes.
- Use of specific clotting factor concentrates early in resuscitation may benefit some patients, but remains controversial.

# Further reading

1. Bolliger D, Gorlinger K, Tanaka KA. Pathophysiology and treatment of coagulopathy in massive hemorrhage and hemodilution. *Anesthesiology* 2010;**113**:1016–1018.

2. CRASH-2 trial collaborators. Effects of tranexamic acid on death, vascular occlusive events, and blood transfusion in trauma patients with significant haemorrhage (CRASH-2): a randomised, placebo-controlled trial. *Lancet* 2010;**376**:23–32.

3. Davenport R, Manson J, De'ath H, et al. Functional definition and characterization of acute traumatic coagulopathy. *Crit Care Med* 2011;**39**:2652–2658.

4. de Biasi AR, Stansbury LG, Dutton RP, et al. Blood product use in trauma resuscitation: plasma deficit versus plasma ratio as predictors of mortality in trauma. *Transfusion* 2011;**51**:1925–1932.

5. Hess JR, Lindell AL, Stansbury LG, Dutton RP, Scalea TM. The prevalence of abnormal results of conventional coagulation tests on admission to a trauma center. *Transfusion* 2009;**49**:34–39.

6. Spinella PC, Holcomb JB. Resuscitation and transfusion principles for traumatic hemorrhagic shock. *Blood Rev* 2009;**23**:231–240.

7. Stansbury LG, Dutton RP, Stein DM, et al. Controversy in trauma resuscitation: do ratios of plasma to red blood cells matter? *Transfus Med Rev* 2009;**23**:255–265.

Chapter

7

# General anesthesia for trauma

Michael D. Bassett and Charles E. Smith

Trauma affects all ages, from newborns to the elderly. It is the leading cause of death in the United States between the ages of 1 and 45 years and the third leading cause of death overall (see Chapter 1, Figure 1.1). Anesthesiologists are involved with trauma patients beginning with airway management and shock resuscitation, continuing with intraoperative care during surgery, and extending on to critical care and pain management postoperatively. Trauma patients present unique challenges to anesthesiologists as their acute injury as well as their chronic comorbid conditions must be both recognized and managed. This chapter will focus on the perioperative care of the trauma patient receiving general anesthesia.

## Preoperative preparation

In the case of a life-threatening injury requiring emergency or urgent surgery with general anesthesia, the time for gathering information about a patient is limited.

- Prior to induction, the medical history should be reviewed including allergies, home medications, past surgeries, and previous anesthetic experiences.
- Important details concerning mechanism of injury and interventions required are usually available from prehospital and emergency department personnel.
- If the patient is unable to provide a medical history and informed consent (unstable or uncooperative, intoxicated, sedated, head injury and altered mental status, trachea already intubated), family members should be contacted and interviewed, if possible.
- Relevant labs should be drawn (complete blood count, basic metabolic panel, type and cross, coagulation profile) and a Foley catheter placed.
- Rapid volume replacement may be necessary for resuscitation.

It is important to establish peripheral intravenous (IV) access, preferably with two large-bore catheters or a central line. Central venous access (e.g., introducer) facilitates administration of large volumes of fluid and offers a safe route to administer emergency medications, inotropes and vasopressors. In addition, central venous pressure monitoring can be employed to aid in directing resuscitation. There are three sites to obtain central access: subclavian vein, internal jugular vein, and femoral vein (see also Chapter 5). The subclavian vein remains patent in shock due to its walls being reinforced with a thick tunica fibrosa that adheres to adjacent ligaments, fascia, and periosteum. In addition, this vein can be cannulated in patients wearing a cervical collar. It has the lowest infection rate of the three sites. Cannulation of the femoral vein avoids the potential for pneumothorax, hemothorax,

*Essentials of Trauma Anesthesia*, ed. A. J. Varon and C. E. Smith. Published by Cambridge University Press.
© Cambridge University Press 2012.

or arrhythmias, and it can be accessed during cardiopulmonary resuscitation. Furthermore, this vein is accessible without any manipulation of the neck. The femoral vein is unsuitable if there are extensive abdominal or lower extremity injuries. The internal jugular vein may not be accessible in a patient with a cervical collar, and rotating or extending the neck for access is not advisable when cervical spine injury is suspected. When possible, an arterial line prior to inducing anesthesia is helpful.

When the trauma patient is stable and there is time for patient preparation, a comprehensive history and physical should be completed and all imaging and laboratory data reviewed. The patient should be medically optimized prior to surgery.

## Operating room setup

In order to effectively manage a trauma patient, the anesthesia provider must first properly set up the operating room (OR). It is helpful to have an OR designated as the "trauma room" with readily available equipment. This is routine at Level 1 trauma centers. Once the OR is designated, it should be warmed to minimize heat loss and improve temperature homeostasis. Several units of type O negative blood need to be immediately available in the OR blood refrigerator in the event that a hemorrhaging patient arrives emergently and their blood type has not yet been established.

A standard setup for an adult trauma includes multiple items.

- There should be a properly functioning anesthesia machine, oxygen supply source, and suction with Yankauer tip.
- The machine should be properly calibrated and checked out.
- There should be a backup E-cylinder oxygen tank in the room that is full and a backup Ambu bag.
- Standard American Society of Anesthesiology (ASA) monitors should be available and properly working.
- There should be various types of prepared airway equipment.
- All IV lines should be flushed with crystalloid and the air evacuated.
- Pressure bags for rapid volume expansion and nasogastric/orogastric tubes for stomach decompression should be available.
- Preassembled kits for intravenous catheters, arterial lines, and central venous lines should be in the room.
- In addition, sterile, calibrated transducers with flushed lines should be in place to connect to the arterial and central venous lines for invasive monitoring.
- Equipment for blood transfusion, including a fluid warmer and blood filter with blood tubing attached to a pump, should be available. Two fluid warmers are sometimes necessary.
- A rapid transfusion device with fluid warming should be ready and primed in cases where substantial blood loss is expected.
- Convective forced air warming blankets and warming pads should be in the room and connected to a power source.

All medications in the room should be labeled with drug, concentration, and date. Induction drugs that should be available include etomidate and ketamine, (or propofol and thiopental if hemodynamically stable). Amnestic drugs include midazolam and scopolamine. If the patient is hypotensive and unstable, scopolamine (0.4 mg IV) is used for amnesia.

Succinylcholine and rocuronium (or vecuronium) should be available for neuromuscular blockade. Fentanyl or morphine should be available for intraoperative and postoperative pain control. Resuscitation drugs include calcium chloride, sodium bicarbonate, phenylephrine, and norepinephrine. Emergency medications include epinephrine, atropine, lidocaine, and vasopressin. In addition, antibiotics should be available for administration prior to incision. Access to recombinant factor VIIa and tranexamic acid should also be available for massively bleeding patients.

The mnemonic "MSMAIDS" is well known and has been used to assist in preparing an OR for all types of surgery (Table 7.1). This mnemonic is easily adapted to assist in preparing the room for a trauma patient:

- M – Machine
- S – Suction
- M – Monitors
- A – Airway
- I – IVs
- D – Drugs
- S – Special

## Monitoring

Standard ASA monitoring includes that qualified anesthesia personnel be present in the room throughout the conduct of all types of anesthesia (see also Chapter 9). In addition, a patient's oxygenation, ventilation, circulation, and temperature are continually evaluated. Oxygenation is evaluated through the use of an oxygen analyzer with a low concentration alarm in every ventilator, a pulse oximeter with variable pitch pulse tone and low threshold alarm, and illumination and exposure of the patient to assess color. Ventilation is measured by chest excursion, auscultation of breath sounds, observation of the reservoir breathing bag, and when an endotracheal tube or laryngeal mask airway is used, continual end-tidal carbon dioxide ($CO_2$) analysis by capnography, capnometry, or mass spectroscopy. In addition, there should be an audible alarm to alert the presence of elevated and decreased end-tidal $CO_2$, as well as detect mechanical disconnection from the breathing circuit. Circulation is measured by continuous electrocardiogram (ECG), and blood pressure and heart rate determination at least every five minutes. Temperature is measured continuously. These are the minimum for monitoring patients. In emergency situations, as is often the case in trauma patients, life support measures take precedence over standard monitoring. However, once the patient is stabilized, appropriate monitoring should be instituted. Trauma patients are often unstable and will require additional monitoring for their care (Table 7.2).

## General anesthesia

Anesthetic and adjunct drugs need to be tailored to five major clinical conditions in trauma patients:

- Airway management
- Hypovolemia
- Head injury
- Cardiac injury
- Burns

**Table 7.1.** Trauma operating room setup for anesthesia providers

| Mnemomic: MSMAIDS | Item | Comments |
|---|---|---|
| Machine | Anesthesia machine | Confirm that the anesthesia machine has been checked out, properly calibrated, and has a breathing circuit attached. In addition to machine oxygen supply, there should be a portable E-cylinder oxygen tank as well as an Ambu bag. |
| Suction | Suction | There should be a properly working suction source with Yankauer tip attached, independent of the surgical/nursing unit. |
| Monitors | Oxygen analyzer EKG Heart rate Respiratory rate Pulse oximeter Blood pressure End-tidal $CO_2$ Temperature | Monitors should be calibrated and working properly. These represent standard monitoring for every case. Trauma patients may require additional monitoring (see Table 7.2). |
| Airway | Airway supplies | There should be multiple different sizes available of masks, oral/nasal airways, cuffed endotracheal tubes, stylets, laryngeal mask airways, and a laryngoscope with multiple blade options. There should also be an endotracheal tube tie in each room. In addition, there should be equipment readily available for difficult intubation such as gum elastic bougie, Glidescope, fiberoptic bronchoscope, transtracheal jet ventilation, cricothyrotomy kit, and tracheostomy kit. |
| IV | IV supplies | There should be large-bore peripheral IV catheters (14- & 16-gauge angiocaths), tourniquets, IV tubing flushed and attached to fluid warmer, arterial line kits, central line kits, Swan Ganz catheter kits, and pressurized transducers flushed and connected to monitor. In addition, there should be an abundant supply of crystalloid fluid in the room, and several units of type O negative blood in a refrigerator nearby. |
| Drugs | Medications | There should be induction agents, volatile anesthetics, opioids, neuromuscular blocking drugs, vasopressors, antibiotics, and emergency medications for each trauma. Certain patients and/or traumas may require specific medications to manage their underlying pathophysiology. Examples include insulin for diabetic patients or mannitol to treat elevated intracranial pressure in head injury patients. |
| Special | Transfusion supplies | There should be blood tubing and filters flushed through with 0.9% saline and attached to a fluid warmer. In addition, a rapid transfusion device, as well as pressure bags, should be ready. |

**Table 7.1.** (*cont.*)

| Mnemomic: MSMAIDS | Item | Comments |
|---|---|---|
| | Temperature | The operating room should be warmed and forced air convective warming blankets available for use. In addition, all linens placed on the patient should be warmed and if possible a gel pad warming mattress placed on the OR table. All IV and blood tubing should be attached to a fluid warmer. |
| | Other | The room should also be stocked with Foley catheters, gastric tubes, temperature thermistors, a peripheral nerve stimulator, and possibly a BIS monitor. An ultrasound machine is useful in the room to assist with arterial and/or central venous access. |

**Table 7.2.** Additional monitors for trauma clinical situations

| Monitors | Clinical situations |
|---|---|
| Central venous pressure | Hypovolemia, shock (all types), pericardial tamponade, myocardial contusion, cardiac valvular injuries, air embolism, pulmonary contusion |
| Pulmonary artery catheter | Myocardial contusion, coronary artery injuries, cardiac valvular injuries, traumatic or preexisting heart failure, pulmonary hypertension, pericardial tamponade, ARDS, differentiation of low pressure and high pressure pulmonary edema, severe COPD, hypovolemic and cardiogenic shock, traumatic placental abruption |
| Mixed venous oximetry | Low perfusion, low cardiac output states |
| Transesophageal echocardiogram | Life-threatening hypotension, myocardial contusion, coronary artery injuries, cardiac valvular injuries, atrial or ventricular septal injuries, aortic dissection, embolism (air, fat, blood), thoracic aorta rupture, hypovolemic and cardiogenic shock (see Chapter 10) |
| Thromboelastogram/ thromboelastometry | Massive transfusion, preexisting coagulation abnormalities |
| Intracranial pressure | Traumatic brain injuries, decreased GCS score |
| Evoked potentials (sensory, motor) | Various surgical procedures where spine, brain, or peripheral nerve function is placed at risk |

Abbreviations: ARDS = acute respiratory distress syndrome; COPD = chronic obstructive pulmonary disease; GCS = Glasgow Coma Scale.

Goals of general anesthesia for trauma consist of maintaining physiologic stability, and providing analgesia, amnesia, unconsciousness, and surgical relaxation (Table 7.3). Care must be taken to avoid aspiration and cervical spine injury.

**Table 7.3.** Goals of general anesthesia for trauma

1. Re-establish and maintain normal hemodynamics
   a. For hypotension, fluids first, then vasopressors
   b. Frequent evaluation of acid-base status, hematocrit, urinary output
   c. Titration of additional anesthetics if satisfactory blood pressure

2. Maximize surgical exposure and minimize bowel edema
   a. Limit fluids according to needs
   b. Limit blood loss by allowing anesthetic catch-up
   c. Optimize neuromuscular blockade
   d. Nasogastric or orogastric tube to decompress bowel
   e. Avoid nitrous oxide

3. Limit hypothermia
   a. Monitor core temperature
   b. Warm all IV fluids and blood
   c. Keep patient covered
   d. Warm the operating room ($> 24°C$)
   e. Apply convective warming blanket over patient
   f. Apply gel pad warming mattress to operating room table

4. Help limit blood loss and coagulopathy
   a. Encourage surgeon to stop and pack if blood loss excessive (damage control)
   b. Frequently monitor hematocrit, ionized calcium, coagulation studies
   c. Provide calcium for large citrated product administration
   d. Administer plasma, platelets, cryoprecipitate, fibrinogen, factor concentrates including recombinant factor VIIa, and tranexamic acid as clinically indicated

5. Limit complications to other systems
   a. Monitor intracranial pressure, maintain cerebral perfusion pressure $> 70$ mmHg
   b. Monitor peak airway pressures and tidal volumes. Be vigilant for pneumothorax
   c. Measure urine output
   d. Monitor peripheral pulses

Modified from Wilson WC. Anesthesia considerations for abdominal trauma. In: Smith CE, ed. *Trauma Anesthesia*. New York, NY: Cambridge University Press; 2008.

# Airway management and anesthetic agents (see also Chapter 3)
## Aspiration prophylaxis

General anesthesia with tracheal intubation is indicated for patients who are unstable, uncooperative, or have multiple injuries.

- A trauma patient is always considered to have a full stomach and be at risk for aspiration. Reasons include ingestion of food or liquids less than eight hours prior to the injury, swallowed blood from nasal or oral injuries, delayed gastric emptying associated with stress of trauma, and administration of oral contrast for abdominal or chest computed tomography (CT) scanning.
- If the patient's airway exam is favorable, rapid sequence induction (RSI) and intubation is preferred following maximal preoxygenation (Table 7.4). Manual in-line cervical stabilization is done, as clinically indicated.

**Table 7.4.** Timing of rapid sequence induction and intubation

| Time (min) | Action |
| --- | --- |
| −3 min to 0 | Preoxygenation (critical step) |
| −3 min (optional) | Precurarization (0.03 mg/kg rocuronium or equivalent) |
| −1 min (optional) | Small dose opioid |
| 0 min | Induction agent |
| At loss of consciousness | Cricoid pressure^<br>Neuromuscular blocking agent:<br>– succinylcholine, 1 mg/kg, if no precurarization, or<br>– succinylcholine, 2 mg/kg, if precurarization, or<br>– rocuronium, 1 mg/kg<br>No manual ventilation* |
| + 0.75 to 1.5 min (when blockade complete) | Laryngoscopy and intubation |
| After tracheal intubation | Release of cricoid pressure, confirm end-tidal carbon dioxide |

^ Cricoid pressure may distort the airway and increase tracheal intubation difficulty.

* Manual ventilation of the lungs using low inflation pressures (< 20 cm $H_2O$) is done if the patient is inadequately preoxygenated or is at risk of becoming hypoxic or hypercarbic (modified RSI).

Modified from Donati F. Pharmacology of neuromuscular blocking agents and their reversal in trauma patients. In: Smith CE. *Trauma Anesthesia*. New York, NY: Cambridge University Press; 2008.

- When performing RSI, etomidate and ketamine are advantageous over propofol and thiopental due to less cardiovascular and respiratory depression
- Succinylcholine (1–2 mg/kg IV) is the neuromuscular relaxant of choice due to its rapid onset (less than 1 minute) and short duration (5–10 minutes)
- Succinylcholine does have some undesirable side effects (increased intragastric pressure, intraocular pressure, and intracranial pressure [ICP], as well as exaggerated potassium release in patients with certain neuromuscular disorders and burns) and is contraindicated in some patients (Table 7.5)
- If succinylcholine is contraindicated, rocuronium, 1 mg/kg IV, has a rapid onset (1–1.5 minutes) without those undesirable effects
- Rocuronium's longer duration of action can be disadvantageous if intubation and ventilation prove impossible. In these cases alternative methods of securing the airway must be available, including cricothyrotomy or tracheostomy. It is helpful to have a surgeon on standby prepared for this situation
- The value of cricoid pressure has been questioned in recent years due to its ability to:
  - compress the glottis
  - distort the airway
  - displace the esophagus
  - worsen the laryngeal view during intubation

A gastric tube should be placed after tracheal intubation to decompress the stomach. If there is one in place prior to induction of anesthesia, it is reasonable to suction the stomach

**Table 7.5.** Succinylcholine and adverse effects in trauma

| Effect | Diminished by precurarization | Made worse by | Comments |
|---|---|---|---|
| **Common side effects** | | | |
| Fasciculations | Yes | | Especially in muscular individuals |
| Myalgias | Yes | | Especially in muscular and ambulatory individuals |
| Hyperkalemia | No | Burns, spinal cord trauma, crush injuries | Previously hyperkalemic patients might be at risk. Increased risk with acidosis |
| Bradycardia, asystole | No | More common in children, or after 2nd dose succinylcholine | Prevented by atropine |
| Catecholamine release | Yes | | |
| Increased intra-ocular pressure | No | Light anesthesia, inadequate paralysis | |
| Increased intra-cranial pressure | Uncertain | Light anesthesia, inadequate paralysis | Unlikely to be clinically significant in head trauma patients |
| **Rare side effects** | | | |
| Malignant hyperthermia | No | | |
| Masseter spasm | No | | |
| Prolonged blockade | No | | In patients with decreased or atypical plasma cholinesterase activity |
| Rhabdomyolysis | No | Muscle dystrophy, corticosteroid therapy | Risk of hyperkalemic cardiac arrest |
| Anaphylaxis | No | | |

Modified from Donati F. Pharmacology of neuromuscular blocking agents and their reversal in trauma patients. In: Smith CE. *Trauma Anesthesia.* New York, NY: Cambridge University Press; 2008.

and leave the tube in prior to induction. In a traditional RSI, no attempts to ventilate should be made until the endotracheal tube is secured in the trachea. However, if preoxygenation is insufficient (uncooperative patient, respiratory distress) or laryngoscopy proves difficult and oxygen desaturation occurs, mask ventilation should be done. Ventilation and oxygenation always take precedence over the risk of regurgitation and aspiration.

If the patient's airway exam is not favorable and the patient is awake, alert, and cooperative, an awake intubation can be done. Uncooperative, combative patients with anticipated difficult airways may need IV sedation before manipulating the airway. If there is concern of airway injury, spontaneous ventilation is maintained provided the patient is cooperative, stable, and is not in respiratory distress. A surgical airway or rapid sequence fiberoptic intubation may be necessary.

## Cervical spine precautions

Blunt trauma patients are assumed to have cervical spine injury until proven otherwise. Distracting injuries, intoxication, and altered mental status can make clearing the cervical spine difficult prior to proceeding to the OR for surgical management. These patients will arrive in the OR with a cervical collar and on a backboard. This directly impacts central line placement, patient positioning, and intubation. The anesthesiologist must be aware of the stability of the cervical spine for every trauma patient. Almost any manipulation of the airway has the potential to exacerbate a spinal cord injury. If time permits, imaging studies of the patient's cervical spine should be reviewed. In patients with neurological symptoms or a known spinal cord injury, awake fiberoptic intubation is a prudent choice in a cooperative patient. A neurolological exam should be completed following intubation, prior to induction of anesthesia. In other patients, RSI with inline cervical stabilization is preferred.

## Airway compromise

If after performing an airway exam there is doubt about the ability to intubate the trachea following induction of anesthesia, consideration should be given towards securing the airway with topical anesthesia and mild sedation; induction agents and neuromuscular relaxants should be avoided before the airway is secured. If time permits, lateral neck radiographs, CT scanning, and endoscopy can be used to better define airway anatomy. Intubation technique (conventional laryngoscopy, Glidescope, flexible fiberoptic) is determined by skills, judgment, experience, and available equipment.

## Hypovolemia and anesthetic agents (Tables 7.6, 7.7)

Anesthetic agents affect the cardiovascular system in various ways:

- Direct cardiovascular depressant effects.
- Inhib compensatory hemodynamic reflexes such as central catecholamine output and baroreceptor reflexes that maintain blood pressure in hypovolemia.
- Baroreceptor depression is typically greater for the inhalational agents compared to the intravenous agents.
- Accurate estimation of the degree of hypovolemia and a reduction in the dose of anesthetic medications is important in these patients.
- The presence of hypotension reflects uncompensated hypovolemia and anesthetic agents almost invariably produce further deterioration of blood pressure.
- In the presence of ongoing hemorrhage, the airway may need to be secured with minimal anesthesia and succinylcholine, even though this approach may result in recall.

A small dose of scopolamine (0.4 mg IV) prior to induction may help to decrease this complication. Midazolam can be used as well for amnesia. Furthermore, if time permits, a bispectral index (BIS) monitor can be quickly placed and intubation can proceed when the value decreases below 60. In hypotensive patients, etomidate or ketamine are the preferred

**Table 7.6.** Physiologic effects of non-volatile anesthetic agents

| | Propofol | Etomidate | Ketamine | Thiopental | Midazolam |
|---|---|---|---|---|---|
| Induction dose (IV) | 1–2.5 mg/kg | 0.2–0.5 mg/kg | 1–2 mg/kg | 3–5 mg/kg | 0.1–0.3 mg/kg |
| Mechanism of action | Interacts with GABA receptor and prolongs duration of the opening of chloride channels | Increases the affinity of GABA receptor complex for GABA; disinhibitory effects on extrapyramidal motor activity control | Dissociates the thalamus from the limbic cortex; NMDA receptor antagonist; interacts with opioid receptors, monoaminergic receptors, muscarinic receptors, and voltage sensitive calcium channels | Decreased rate of dissociation of GABA from its receptor; directly activates chloride channels; selectively decreases transmission through sympathetic nervous system ganglia | Enhancement of the chloride channel functioning on GABA receptors on postsynaptic nerve endings in the cerebral cortex |
| Mean arterial pressure | Decreased | Unchanged to mild decrease | Increased | Decreased | Decreased |
| Heart rate | Unchanged | Unchanged to mild increase | Increased | Increased | Unchanged to mild increase |
| Ventilatory depression | Yes | Mild | No | Yes | Yes |
| Cerebral oxygen consumption | Decreased | Decreased | Increased | Decreased | Decreased |
| Intracranial pressure | Decreased | Decreased | Increased | Decreased | Decreased |
| Cerebral blood flow | Decreased | Decreased | Increased | Decreased | Decreased |
| Other effects | Severe hypotension common if shock, rapid awakening, antiemetic, antipruritic | Nausea and vomiting common, adrenocortical suppression | Bronchodilator, analgesic effects, emergence delirium, increased secretions, direct myocardial depressant effects unmasked by exhaustion of catecholamine stores | Severe hypotension common if shock | Anxiolytic, specific antagonist (Flumazenil) |

Abbreviations: GABA = Gamma-aminobutyric acid; NMDA = N-Methyl-D-aspartate.

**Table 7.7.** Physiologic effects of volatile anesthetics

|  | Nitrous oxide | Isoflurane | Sevoflurane | Desflurane |
|---|---|---|---|---|
| MAC (%) | 105 | 1.2 | 2 | 6 |
| Mean arterial pressure | Unchanged to mild increase | Decreased | Decreased | Decreased |
| Heart rate | Unchanged to mild increase | Increased | Unchanged | Increased |
| Cardiac output | Unchanged to mild increase | Unchanged | Decreased | Unchanged to mild decrease |
| Myocardial contractility | Depressed | Depressed | Depressed | Depressed |
| Ventilation | Unchanged to mild decrease | Decreased | Decreased | Decreased |
| Cerebral oxygen consumption | Increased | Decreased | Decreased | Decreased |
| Intracranial Pressure | Increased | Increased | Increased | Increased |
| Cerebral blood flow | Increased | Increased | Increased | Increased |
| Comments | Avoid in early pregnancy due to possible teratogenic effects to fetus; avoid in patients with pneumothorax, intestinal obstruction, intracranial air, air embolism, tympanic membrane grafting due to its ability to diffuse into air-containing cavities | Bronchodilator; more pronounced fall in minute ventilation than other volatile anesthetics; coronary vasodilator and concern for coronary steal syndrome | Non-pungent which makes it a good choice for inhalational inductions; bronchodilator; emergence delirium in pediatrics; increases heart rate at 1.5 MAC | Poor choice for inhalational induction due to pungency and airway irritability; wake-up times faster than isoflurane; emergence delirum in pediatrics |

Abbreviations: MAC = minimum alveolar concentration.

induction agents rather than propofol or thiopental. Propofol decreases arterial blood pressure by causing a decrease in systemic vascular resistance (SVR), cardiac contractility, and preload. The reduction in SVR is due to inhibition of sympathetic nervous system mediated vasoconstrictor activity. The negative inotropic activity of propofol may be caused by inhibition of intracellular calcium intake. In addition, propofol impairs the baroflex response to hypotension. Blood pressure changes are often exaggerated in hypovolemic patients, elderly patients, and patients with compromised left ventricular function. In normal patients, the stimulation produced by direct laryngoscopy and intubation will typically offset the decreases in blood pressure, however this is not always the case with the hypovolemic patient. The hypotension seen with propofol is more pronounced than that seen with thiopental. Thiopental causes a decrease in blood pressure through depression of the medullary vasomotor center and subsequent vasodilation of peripheral capacitance vessels. This causes a peripheral pooling of blood and decreased preload. In normovolemic patients, the decrease in preload is compensated by a rise in heart rate and increased contractility of the heart through compensatory baroreflexes. In the hypovolemic patient, the baroreflexes are inadequate, thus cardiac output and blood pressure may fall significantly due to direct myocardial depression and uncompensated peripheral venous pooling of blood. Etomidate offers greater cardiovascular stability compared to these drugs. A mild decrease in blood pressure reflects a decrease in SVR. Heart rate, cardiac output, and cardiac contractility usually remain unchanged. Ketamine typically increases blood pressure, heart rate, and cardiac output, making it favorable for hypovolemic patients. These effects are due to stimulation of the sympathetic nervous system and inhibition of the reuptake of norepinephrine. However, it is also a direct myocardial depressant, likely due to inhibition of calcium transients. In normal patients, the effect of the catecholamine release masks the cardiac depression and the result is hypertension and tachycardia. In patients who have exhausted their catecholamine stores (rare), the myocardial depressant effects may predominate.

Maintenance of anesthesia in the hypovolemic trauma patient is likewise complicated. Depending on the degree of hemorrhage, minimum alveolar concentration (MAC) may be decreased by as much as 25%. In normal patients, the myocardial depressant effect of nitrous oxide ($N_2O$) is somewhat counterbalanced by its sympathetic stimulation and elevated heart rate, cardiac output, and blood pressure. In the hemorrhaging trauma patient, sympathetic stimulation is already increased and use of $N_2O$ may lead to hypotension as its myocardial depressant effects predominate. Because $N_2O$ leads to elevated catecholamine levels, it may be associated with a higher incidence of epinephrine-induced arrhythmias. In addition, use of $N_2O$ will decrease the fraction of inspired oxygen and may exacerbate hypoxemia in patients with pulmonary and cardiac compromise. Typically $N_2O$ is not used in trauma patients due to concern for undiagnosed pneumothorax and risk of expansion of air-containing cavities. Isoflurane, sevoflurane, and desflurane all decrease arterial blood pressure through reductions in SVR and depression of myocardial contractility. Isoflurane and desflurane both cause an increased heart rate to compensate for the fall in blood pressure and normally maintain cardiac output. Sevoflurane does not show an increase in heart rate until greater than 1.5 MAC is achieved, so cardiac output is not as well maintained with this drug. In the hypovolemic patient who is already tachycardic, use of these volatile anesthetic drugs may impair cardiac output and organ blood flow, leading to cardiovascular collapse. They should be used in low concentrations or, in the most unstable of trauma patients, not at all.

# Head injury and general anesthesia

Anesthetic agents used in the management of traumatic brain injuries should produce the least increase in ICP, the least decrease in mean arterial blood pressure, and the greatest reduction in cerebral metabolic rate of oxygen ($CMRO_2$). Hypotension produced by anesthetic agents can contribute to the development of cerebral ischemia and thus must be used in reduced dosages or avoided (see also Chapter 13). Thiopental, propofol, midazolam, and etomidate produce dose-dependent reductions in cerebral spinal fluid formation, cerebrovascular constriction causing decreased cerebral blood flow, and decreased $CMRO_2$. Ketamine on the other hand increases $CMRO_2$ and causes increased cerebrovascular constriction, thus increasing ICP and making it an inappropriate choice for trauma patients with head injuries. The drop in ICP seen with thiopental is typically greater than the decline in arterial blood pressure, therefore cerebral perfusion pressure is maintained (cerebral perfusion pressure is the difference between mean arterial pressure and ICP or jugular venous pressure if this value is greater than the ICP). The decrease in cerebral blood flow with thiopental is not detrimental to the patient as cerebral oxygen consumption is decreased to a greater amount. Thiopental may help protect the brain from transient episodes of focal ischemia, but it will not help with global ischemia. Propofol results in more profound hypotension than thiopental on induction and thus may lead to detrimental decreases in cerebral perfusion pressure in patients with elevated ICP. If this drug is used, steps must be taken to support mean arterial pressure. Midazolam reduces cerebral blood flow, cerebral oxygen consumption, and ICP but not to the extent that thiopental does. Etomidate is similar to thiopental in terms of decrease in cerebral blood flow, cerebral oxygen consumption, and ICP. It has minimal cardiovascular changes, so cerebral perfusion pressure is well maintained. Regardless of what induction agent is used, one must be careful to ensure that cerebral perfusion pressure is not compromised by the cardiovascular depressant effects of the induction agents. This problem can be tempered by appropriate doses of opioids (fentanyl 2–3 mcg/kg IV) to decrease the amount of induction agent required. Opioid administration may also help prevent myoclonus (which will raise ICP) sometimes seen following etomidate administration. However, myoclonus is better prevented by appropriately timed administration of neuromuscular relaxants.

Laryngoscopy and tracheal intubation can increase ICP; thus, it is important to establish an adequate depth of anesthesia prior to intubation. Succinylcholine causes a transient increase in ICP, which has not been shown to be detrimental to cerebral blood flow or cerebral perfusion pressure in patients with traumatic head injury. None of the non-depolarizing agents increase ICP. All of the inhalational anesthetics can increase ICP by cerebral vasodilation, thus increasing cerebral blood flow and volume. However, cerebral autoregulation, responsiveness to arterial $CO_2$, and $CMRO_2$ are reduced. Inhalational anesthetics decrease $CMRO_2$ while increasing cerebral blood flow. This is in contrast to thiopental, which decreases both $CMRO_2$ and cerebral blood flow. Amongst the volatile anesthetics, isoflurane has the least vasodilatory effect on cerebral blood flow, while sevoflurane has been shown to best preserve cerebral autoregulation. $N_2O$ may increase ICP through cerebral vasodilation when administered concurrently with the inhalational anesthetics if the arterial $CO_2$ is normal or elevated. This effect may be eliminated if the patient is hyperventilated or receives barbiturates. The effect of $N_2O$ on $CMRO_2$ is variable, with both increases and decreases observed. Although $N_2O$ is probably safe in patients with minimal ICP elevation, it is generally avoided by the authors in trauma patients.

## Cardiac injury and anesthetic agents

Patients that present with traumatic blunt and penetrating cardiac injuries have complicated physiological states that must be managed carefully while undergoing general anesthesia (see also Chapter 16). Blunt cardiac injuries are a spectrum of injuries diagnosed by non-specific arrhythmias or regional wall motion abnormalities on echocardiography (see

Chapter 10). Cardiac dysfunction may result. Valves may be disrupted. Injury of the coronary arteries may occur, and the interventricular or interatrial septum may rupture. In those that suffer from a blunt cardiac injury, it is advisable to maintain cardiac contractility and lower pulmonary vascular resistance. Medications such as milrinone may need to be administered to accomplish this goal. In addition, maintenance of anesthesia through intravenous anesthetics and opioids may be necessary to avoid the myocardial depression seen with inhalational anesthetics. If possible, it is advisable to restore intravascular volume prior to administering anesthetic medications, and maintain SVR.

In patients that present with traumatic pericardial tamponade, the goal is to maintain cardiac contractility, preload, and cardiac output. These patients typically present with hypotension and tachycardia. They have a fixed stroke volume due to the pericardial effusion. Any decrease in heart rate must be promptly corrected in order to maintain cardiac output. If general anesthesia is required for evacuation of the effusion, the patient should be prepped and draped prior to administration of induction agents in order to facilitate rapid relief of tamponade. Hemodynamic collapse may occur with institution of positive pressure ventilation. Ketamine is the induction agent of choice due to its catecholamine release. In the authors' experience, hypotension is rare following administration of ketamine in patients with cardiac tamponade. Indeed, the hypotension most frequently occurs with institution of positive pressure ventilation. Therefore, positive end expiratory pressure and high airway pressures should be avoided until the tamponade is relieved. Other induction agents like propofol and thiopental can depress cardiac contractility and cause vasodilation and are best avoided in patients with tamponade physiology.

The most common great vessel injury following blunt chest trauma is aortic dissection, typically at the ligamentum arteriosum. If associated with aortic insufficiency or dissection into the coronary arteries, it is a surgical emergency. Otherwise, endovascular repair under controlled conditions is preferred (see Chapter 16). It is important to maintain tight blood pressure and heart rate control to decrease the chance of further dissection. Induction of anesthesia should proceed in a cautious manner. Beta-blockers are effective in preventing heart rate increases and increased dP/dT during laryngoscopy and intubation. Doses of induction drugs may need to be decreased to prevent severe hypotension. Conversely, hypertension from direct laryngoscopy, transesophageal echocardiography probe insertion, or sternotomy can be attenuated with opioids and nitroglycerin. These patients may require deep hypothermic cardiac arrest in order to fix their injury.

## Anesthetic agents and burns

Patients that present with burns have a hypermetabolic state and often require multiple operations (see also Chapter 19). These patients must be immediately evaluated for any airway involvement. Airway obstruction can result from direct injury, smoke inhalation injury, as well as edema. Burns of the head and neck, singed nasal hairs, or soot seen in the mouth or throat are very concerning and should prompt immediate evaluation for intubation. A normal airway can deteriorate very rapidly to a cannot oxygenate, cannot ventilate situation. Furthermore, burn patients may have very high levels of carbon monoxide, which can lead to hypoxemia. The pulse oximeter, however, may still read 100% as it cannot detect a difference between oxyhemoglobin and carboxyhemoglobin. A co-oximeter should be used to measure the carboxyhemoglobin level. These patients should be treated with 100% oxygen until clinically significant carbon monoxide intoxication is ruled out. Depending on burn size, they often require massive fluid resuscitation, temperature management, fluid control, management of electrolytes and coagulopathy, and medication adjustments. The doses of induction agents should be decreased while resuscitating the patient to prevent hemodynamic depression. On the other hand, burn patients often require very high doses of opioids to manage their pain. Their response to neuromuscular blockers is unaltered in the first 24 hours following the burn, but changes drastically after that period secondary to upregulation of acetylcholine receptors. Succinylcholine should be avoided 24–48 hours after burns due to the risk of producing exaggerated potassium release and life-threatening hyperkalemia. Resistance develops to the non-depolarizer muscle relaxants following the first week, and increased doses of these medications are required.

## Maintaining normothermia

Hypothermia in trauma patients is a common finding and is typically multi-factorial in nature. Causes include cold environment, alcohol intoxication, shock, burns, surgical procedures with large exposed surface areas, and abnormalities in thermoregulation. It can also be caused or exacerbated by infusion of cold fluids or blood. Induction of general anesthesia results in peripheral vasodilation that causes heat to distribute to the periphery. This results in a decrease in the core temperature of 1.0–1.5°C in the first hour and a slower decrease after that time. Hypothermia is responsible for many negative effects including cardiac depression, myocardial ischemia, arrhythmias, peripheral vasoconstriction, decreased tissue oxygen delivery, blunted response to catecholamines, metabolic acidosis, increased blood viscosity, decreased function of coagulation factors, impaired platelet function, decreased hepatic metabolism of drugs, impaired wound healing, and impaired resistance to infections (Table 7.8). During shock, measurement of core temperature is preferred as blood is diverted away from the periphery to the core organs. Measurement of core temperature can be accomplished through thermistors in the distal esophagus, naso-pharynx, pulmonary artery, and tympanic membrane. Measurement of temperature sub-lingually, rectally, in the axilla, and of the bladder is considered intermediate and less accurate in trauma patients.

Various methods have been used to prevent hypothermia or re-warm an already hypothermic trauma patient (Table 7.9). One of the most overlooked, underutilized, and simple methods is to increase the temperature of the OR above 24°C prior to induction for all trauma patients. A reusable gel warming pad system can be placed on the OR table (very useful for supine surgeries). The gel pad temperature is set at 39–42°C. Heat is transferred to the patient's dorsal surface via the circulating water within the encapsulated gel pad. Convective warming blankets are routinely applied over non-surgical sites. Administration of warm IV fluids and blood using thermally effective high-capacity warming systems is an effective method of heat conservation and is routinely done. In the authors' practice, every IV site should be connected to a fluid warmer to minimize the risk of iatrogenic hypothermia from infusion of unwarmed crystalloids, colloids, and blood products.

## General anesthesia and damage control surgery

It is often difficult to differentiate whether injury severity, hemorrhagic shock, resuscitation with fluid and blood products, coagulopathy, and hypothermia are caused by the trauma or are the result of treatment. Hypothermia below 34°C, coagulopathy, and acidosis (pH < 7.10) is known as the lethal triad and marks the limits of patient tolerance to definitive

**Table 7.8.** Consequences and complications from hypothermia

| System affected | Examples |
|---|---|
| Impaired cardiorespiratory function | • Cardiac depression<br>• Myocardial ischemia<br>• Arrhythmias<br>• Peripheral vasoconstriction<br>• Decreased tissue oxygen delivery<br>• Increased oxygen consumption during rewarming<br>• Blunted response to catecholamines<br>• Increased blood viscosity<br>• Acidosis<br>• Leftward shift of hemoglobin-oxygen dissociation curve |
| Impaired coagulation | • Decreased function of coagulation factors<br>• Impaired platelet function |
| Impaired hepato-renal function and decreased drug clearance | • Decreased hepatic blood flow<br>• Decreased clearance of lactic acid<br>• Decreased hepatic metabolism of drugs<br>• Decreased renal blood flow<br>• Cold-induced diuresis |
| Impaired resistance to infections (pneumonia, sepsis, wound infections); impaired wound healing | • Decreased subcutaneous tissue perfusion mediated by vasoconstriction<br>• Anti-inflammatory effects and immunosuppression<br>• Decreased collagen deposition |

Modified from Soreide E, Smith CE. Hypothermia in trauma. In: Smith CE. *Trauma Anesthesia*. New York, NY: Cambridge University Press; 2008.

**Table 7.9.** Methods of re-warming

| Category | Methods | Comments | Re-warming rate ($^\circ$C/h) |
|---|---|---|---|
| Passive external | Blankets | Remove patient from cold environment, dry off wet skin. Warm the room ($> 24°C$) | 0.5–2.5 |
| | Humidifier inspired air | Reduces evaporative heat loss | Variable |
| Active external | Forced air (convective warming) | Risk of temperature after-drop and re-warming hypotension. May be difficult to apply because of requirement for surgical exposure. Thermoregulatory vasoconstriction limits transfer of heat | 0.5–2.5 |
| | Circulating warm water blankets, gel pads, conductive fabric warming, radiant warmer | Risk of burns, temperature after-drop, and re-warming hypotension | Variable |

**Table 7.9.** (cont.)

| Category | Methods | Comments | Re-warming rate (°C/h) |
|---|---|---|---|
| Active internal | Warm (42°C) humidified air | Insulates respiratory tract and prevents respiratory gas-related heat loss. Low heat transport capacity | 0.5–1.2 |
| | Warm (42°C) intravenous fluids | Especially useful in the resuscitation of hypothermic trauma victims. Rapid infusion maximizes heat delivery. Effective at preventing heat loss from IV fluids: in adult, 2 L crystalloid at 20°C corresponds to 0.6°C decrease in core temperature; 2 L cold blood corresponds to 0.9°C decrease in core temperature | Variable |
| | Body cavity lavage with warm fluid (gastric bladder, colon, pleural, peritoneal) | Limited data, risk of mucosal injury, risk if aspiration with gastric lavage | Variable |
| Extracorporeal | Hemodialysis and hemofiltration | Widely available, rapid initiation, requires adequate blood pressure | 2–3 |
| | Continuous arteriovenous re-warming | Rapid initiation, trained perfusionist not required, less available, requires adequate blood pressure | 3–4 |
| | Cardiopulmonary bypass | Provides full circulatory support, allows oxygenation, less available, requires trained perfusionist and heparinization, delays in initiation | 7–10 |

Modified from Aslam AF, Aslam AK, Vasavada BC, Khan IA. Hypothermia: evaluation, electrocardiographic manifestations, and management. *Am J Med* 2006;**119**:297–301.

surgical repair (Figure 7.1). One of the major goals of resuscitation of a hemorrhaging trauma patient is to avoid the development of the lethal triad, as each insult exacerbates the other and can lead to life-threatening bleeding. However, if it occurs, the anesthesia provider needs to alert the surgical team to this situation and the patient should undergo an abbreviated surgery, known as damage control surgery. This applies for laparotomy, thoracotomy, and orthopedic procedures. The goal with damage control surgery is to stop the bleeding and prevent any ongoing contamination. The wound is packed and the patient is transported to the intensive care unit (ICU). In the ICU, the patient will be re-warmed, resuscitated, and have any ongoing coagulopathy corrected. Once the patient is more stable, definitive surgical repair can be completed, typically a day or two later.

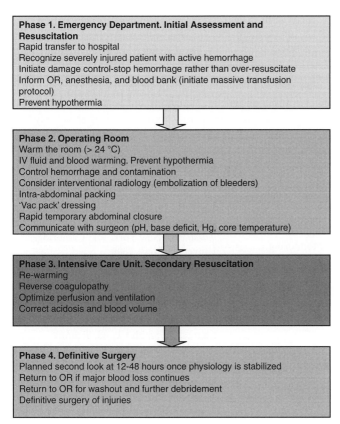

**Figure 7.1.** The four phases of damage control in trauma. OR = operating room; IV = intravenous; Hg = hemoglobin. Modified from Parr MJA, Buehner U. Damage control in severe trauma. In Smith CE. *Trauma Anesthesia*. New York, N.Y. Cambridge University Press, 2008.

# Key points

- Standard monitoring and secure venous access is critical for providing general anesthesia for trauma patients. Invasive monitoring is frequently required
- When time permits, history and physical should be completed, all imaging and laboratory data reviewed, and the trauma patient should be medically optimized prior to surgery
- Trauma patients are generally considered to have full stomachs and are at increased risk of aspiration during general anesthesia
- Trauma patients are likely to have exaggerated response to anesthetic agents in the setting of moderate to severe blood loss. Extreme caution should be used in the setting of shock
- For patients with traumatic brain injury, anesthetic agents should be selected to produce the least increase in intracranial pressure, the least decrease in mean arterial blood pressure, and the greatest reduction in cerebral metabolic rate
- Patients with tamponade physiology should be prepped and draped prior to administration of induction agents in order to facilitate rapid relief of tamponade.

Hemodynamic collapse may occur with institution of positive pressure ventilation. Ketamine is the induction agent of choice due to its catecholamine release

- Succinylcholine should be avoided 24–48 hours after burns due to receptor upregulation and risk of hyperkalemia
- Burn patients often require high doses of opioids for adequate pain control
- Hypothermia often complicates trauma patient management and is associated with increased morbidity and mortality. Preventive measures need to be instituted early, including warming the operating room ($> 24°C$), heating IV fluids to normothermia, and convective and/or gel pad warming.
- Damage control surgery is necessary to prevent the lethal triad of hypothermia, coagulopathy, and acidosis

# Further reading

1. American Society of Anesthesiologists. Standards for Basic Anesthetic Monitoring. *Effective date* July 1, 2011.

2. Barash PG, Cullen BF, Stoelting RK, Cahalan M, Stock MC, eds. *Clinical Anesthesia*, 6th edition. Philadelphia, PA: Lippincott Williams & Wilkins; 2009.

3. Donati F. Pharmacology of neuromuscular blocking agents and their reversal in trauma patients. In: Smith CE, ed. *Trauma Anesthesia*. New York, NY: Cambridge University Press; 2008.

4. Kaplan J. *Essentials of Cardiac Anesthesia*. Philadelphia, PA: Saunders Elsevier; 2008.

5. Miller R, ed. *Miller's Anesthesia*, 6th edition. Philadelphia, PA: Elsevier Churchill Livingstone; 2005.

6. Morgan GE, Mikhail MS, Murray MJ. *Clinical Anesthesiology*, 4th edition. New York, NY: McGraw Hill; 2006.

7. Parr MJA, Buehner U. Damage control in severe trauma. In: Smith CE, ed. *Trauma Anesthesia*. New York, NY: Cambridge University Press; 2008.

8. Smith CE, ed. *Trauma Anesthesia*. New York, NY: Cambridge University Press; 2008.

9. Soreide E, Smith CE. Hypothermia in trauma. In: Smith CE, ed. *Trauma Anesthesia*. New York, NY: Cambridge University Press; 2008.

10. Stoelting RK, Miller RD. *Basics of Anesthesia*, 4th edition. Philadelphia: Elsevier Churchill Livingstone; 2000.

11. Wilson WC. Anesthesia considerations for abdominal trauma. In: Smith CE, ed. *Trauma Anesthesia*. New York, NY: Cambridge University Press; 2008.

12. Wilson WC, ed. *Trauma: Emergency Resuscitation, Perioperative Anesthesia, Surgical Management*. Volume 1. New York, NY: Informa Healthcare; 2007.

Chapter

# 8

# Regional anesthesia for trauma

Sripad Rao, Megan Gatlin, and Ralf E. Gebhard

## General considerations

Peripheral nerve blocks are frequently utilized for elective surgical procedures in ambulatory or inpatient settings. While the benefits of nerve block anesthesia are well described in the anesthesia and orthopedic literature, fewer investigations describe the performance of peripheral nerve blockade in the trauma population. However, based upon the experience of the United States Armed Forces, and on recent reports of the successful use of nerve blocks in major earthquake victims, it appears that regional anesthesia techniques can not only be successfully utilized in trauma, but may be the preferred anesthetic choice in austere environments.

## Regional anesthesia: concerns in the trauma patient
### Obtaining informed consent

Due to the nature of the physician-trauma patient encounter, obtaining informed consent may be challenging. Since peripheral nerve blocks offer substantial benefits for the patient and may even result in better surgical outcomes (e.g., continuous sympathetic blockade to prevent vasospasm after digital reattachment), alternative paths to obtaining consent may be indicated. If patients are not able to provide consent, one of the following options may prove feasible:

- Obtain consent from proxy or family member.
- Consider a two-physician consent in emergency cases, should benefits of regional blockade be expected to be substantial.
- Postpone peripheral nerve block procedure until consent can be obtained.

### Hemodynamic instability

Depending on the injury pattern and other factors, trauma patients may demonstrate substantial hemodynamic instability. In such scenarios, the addition of a regional anesthetic technique can further contribute to hypotension, especially if the technique is associated with extensive lower body sympathectomy. Regional blockade can also unmask relative hypovolemia by blunting the patient's normal sympathomimetic stress response. The following strategy appears appropriate in cases of existing hemodynamic instability or suspected hypovolemia:

- Avoid neuraxial blockade.
- Select a peripheral nerve block technique with low or no risk of significant sympathectomy or accidental epidural local anesthetic spread (e.g., femoral nerve block or fascia iliaca block would be more desirable than lumbar plexus block).
- If circumstances allow, normalize patient's volume status.

## Coagulation status

There are well-recognized guidelines by the American Society of Regional Anesthesia and Pain Medicine (ASRA) regarding the performance of neuraxial regional anesthetic techniques in patients receiving prophylactic or therapeutic anticoagulation. However, relatively little is known regarding the use of regional anesthetic techniques in patients in whom the coagulation status has been altered by trauma and significant blood loss requiring aggressive fluid replacement. In such scenarios the following precautions should be considered:

- Obtain coagulation studies in cases associated with major blood loss and fluid replacement therapy, including platelet count, prothrombin time, international normalized ratio, and partial thromboplastin time.
- Carefully weigh benefits of regional anesthesia versus risks of hematoma formation.
- Consider using ultrasound to decrease the risk of accidental puncture of blood vessels adjacent to nerve structures.
- Consider choosing "shallow" nerve block approaches over "deeper" techniques to allow for the ability to compress the site in case of accidental blood vessel puncture.
- Consider application of ASRA guidelines for any nerve block catheter in close proximity to the spine (e.g., lumbar plexus or paravertebral nerve block catheter) in order to avoid untoward outcomes, such as epidural hematoma formation.

## Traumatic nerve injury

Occasionally, a trauma patient will present with traumatic nerve injuries. This may complicate the decision to perform a regional anesthetic technique, since the question may later arise whether nerve damage preexisted or was caused, or exacerbated, by the regional anesthetic. However, such concerns would preclude trauma patients with injury-related nerve damage from the benefits of regional anesthesia, especially peripheral nerve blockade techniques. A strategic approach to balance these concerns includes the following:

- Examine patient for preexisting nerve damage prior to performing a regional anesthesia technique.
- Review surgical notes for evidence of nerve injury.
- Document any abnormal findings and discuss with surgical colleagues in case of discrepancy between your assessment and their findings.
- Do not perform regional technique if patient has signs of neuraxial or complex plexus injury.
- If possible, perform regional anesthetic in clear distance from site of suspected nerve damage.

## Risk of infection

Infection and sepsis are feared complications in any severely injured patient. The anesthesiologist should take careful precautions in order to minimize the risk of infection, as follows:

- Use aseptic technique for any single shot technique and full barrier precautions for any continuous catheter placement.
- Do not introduce nerve block needles or place continuous catheters in areas where the skin is not intact.
- Management of a continuous catheter technique requires daily rounds and inspection of catheter site. Replace any dressing that is wet or not intact. The patient may experience pain at the catheter insertion site as an early sign of local infection prior to the development of redness and swelling.

## Compartment syndrome

Of great concern to orthopedic surgeons is the development of a compartment syndrome (e.g., after intramedullary nailing of long-bone fractures). For early detection and timely intervention, surgeons rely on the patient as a monitor to alert healthcare personnel by reporting significant ischemic pain in the involved extremity. Consequently, surgeons have expressed significant concerns over whether peripheral nerve blocks, especially nerve block catheters, may mask a compartment syndrome. Similar concerns were raised when other advances in perioperative pain management, such as patient controlled analgesia (PCA), were introduced into clinical practice. However, ischemic pain is usually not well controlled by peripheral nerve blockade. Indeed, discrepancies between an apparently functioning nerve block and new-onset patient complaints of pain have frequently alerted the medical staff of a developing underlying problem. Suggestions to address the concerns of performing peripheral nerve blocks in patients at risk for compartment syndrome are as follows:

- Together with our surgical colleagues, identify patients at risk.
- Educate colleagues regarding ischemic pain.
- Consider additional methods of monitoring such as measurement of compartment pressures.
- Consider short-acting local anesthetics for the initial block, place a nerve block catheter and infuse with normal saline (this will create a "free interval" to allow for assessment). After surgical clearance (e.g., 24 hours postoperative), bolus catheter with local anesthetic and start local anesthetic infusion.
- If the peripheral nerve is blocked with long-acting local anesthetics or a nerve block catheter is placed in patients at risk, notify the surgeon immediately if there is new onset of pain or apparent discrepancy between the expected level of pain control and the achieved level of pain control.

## Ultrasound in regional anesthesia

With the advent of new technology, the use of ultrasound-guided regional anesthesia has enabled the operator to identify the target and adjacent structures when performing peripheral nerve blocks. In addition, the needle can be visualized on its path towards the nerve; the spread of local anesthetic solution can similarly be observed. Consequently, ultrasound guidance for performance of peripheral nerve blocks has become more widely used either as the sole technique or in combination with nerve stimulation.

Even though there is evidence of faster onset to sensory and motor blockade with the use of the ultrasound-guided technique, there is little evidence to show improved readiness for surgery, increased block success rate, or decreased incidence of complications. The use of low-volume anesthetic techniques for supraclavicular or interscalene blocks may be beneficial with regard to block-related side effects such as hemidiaphragm paralysis.

## Physics of ultrasound

Frequency ranges used in medical ultrasound are 2.5 to 15 MHz. Ultrasound frequency range can be adjusted on transducers from higher frequencies with shorter wavelength for better resolution, to lower frequencies with longer wavelength for better penetration. The piezoelectric crystals in the probe vibrate to electric charge and emit sound waves that penetrate the tissues and echo back. Reflected waves are then reconverted to electricity, the signal is processed, and an image is displayed.

There is progressive weakening of the signal strength as it passes through tissue by reflection, scatter, refraction, and absorption. Adjusting the screen depth to place the target structures at the center of the screen helps optimize the image.

The ultrasound beam has a width of less than 1.0 mm and can be oriented in relationship to the target to provide a short axis or transverse view, and a long axis or sagittal view. Bone and air cannot be visualized since the probe is calibrated to receive sound speeds at approximately 1500 m/sec. Air and lung transmit sound at approximately 350 m/sec, and bone around 3500 m/sec.

The structures can appear as:

- Blacks: fluid-filled (blood vessels, cysts, ascites)
- Grays: solid organs, soft tissue
- White: denser tissue like muscle
- Black sectors: acoustic shadows from bone
- Fog: noise artifacts from bowel and reverberations

Most ultrasound machines are equipped with color flow and pulse wave Doppler to help distinguish between veins and arteries and determine flow velocities. The colors seen with the flow Doppler are determined by the flow direction. Flow directed away from the probe will result in blue color display; flow towards the probe in red color display (**Blue Away Red Towards = BART**).

It is important to check the depth, frequency, and gain on the ultrasound machine and the orientation of the probe before starting the procedure.

## Needle approaches to nerves

Depending on the alignment of the ultrasound probe in relationship to the target structure, and the alignment of the needle in relationship to the ultrasound probe, there are four possible approaches:

- Short axis – in plane
- Short axis – out of plane
- Longitudinal axis – in plane
- Longitudinal axis – out of plane

### Short axis – in plane

The probe is directed to obtain a transverse view of the target structure. The needle is then introduced parallel to the ultrasound beam. It is important that the needle is inserted below

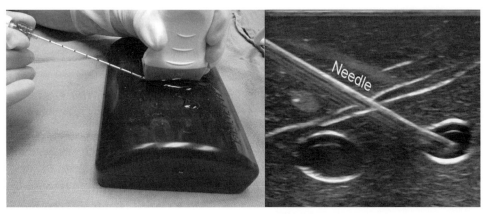

**Figure 8.1.** Short axis: in plane.

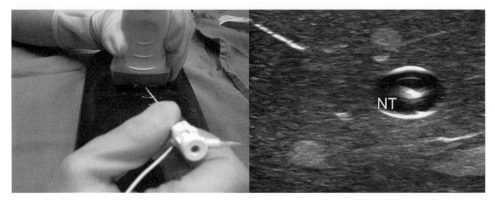

**Figure 8.2.** Short axis: out of plane. NT = needle tip.

the center of the probe since the ultrasound beam generated by the probe is less than 1.0 mm wide. The needle will only be visualized when within the ultrasound beam. This is the most commonly used approach utilized for peripheral nerve blocks since it allows for visualization of the entire needle including the needle tip when the needle approaches the target structure (Figure 8.1).

## Short axis – out of plane

The probe is directed to obtain a transverse view of the target structure. The needle is then introduced at a strict perpendicular angle to the probe at the middle of the probe. Technically, it may be difficult to visualize the needle tip with this approach. It is crucial to aim the probe toward the tip of the needle as it is being inserted. Since the operator will only be able to visualize the needle as a single dot, images of the needle shaft may be mistaken for the needle tip. However, this approach allows for needle direction parallel to the axis of the target structure and may be preferred when nerve block catheters are placed (Figure 8.2).

## Long axis – in plane

The probe is directed to obtain a sagittal view of the target structure. The needle is then inserted parallel to the ultrasound beam. It is important that the needle is inserted below

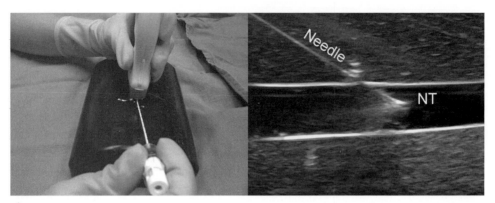

**Figure 8.3.** Long axis: in plane. NT = needle tip.

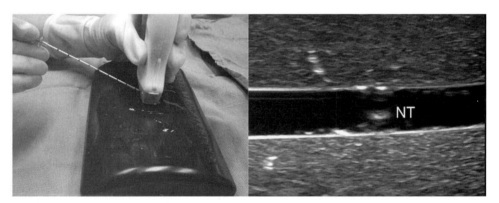

**Figure 8.4.** Long axis: out of plane.

the center of the probe since the ultrasound beam generated by the probe is only approximately 1.0 mm wide. The needle will only be visualized when within the ultrasound beam (Figure 8.3).

## Long axis – out of plane

The probe is directed to obtain a sagittal view of the target structure. The needle is then introduced at a strict perpendicular angle to the probe at the mid level of the probe. Technically, it may be difficult to visualize the needle tip with this approach. It is important to aim the probe towards the tip of the needle as it is being inserted. Since the operator will only be able to visualize the needle as a single dot, images of the needle shaft may be mistaken for the needle tip (Figure 8.4).

## Upper extremity blocks

Extensive understanding of the upper extremity dermatomes (Figure 8.5) and brachial plexus anatomy (Figure 8.6) is essential prior to choosing any upper extremity nerve block technique.

The brachial plexus arises from the ventral rami of the roots from C5 to T1 in the majority of the population and sometimes receives contributions from C4 and T2, resulting

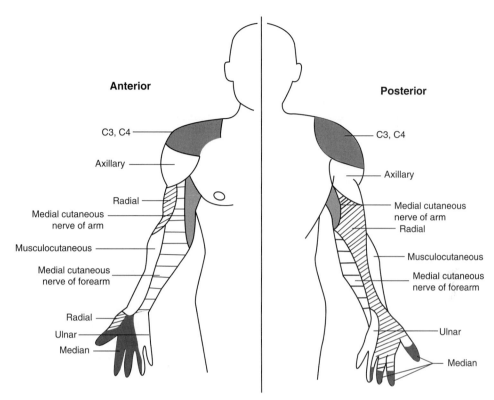

**Figure 8.5.** Upper limb dermatomes.

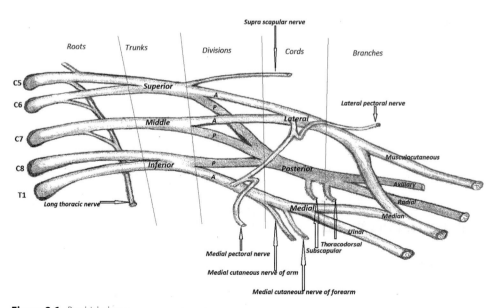

**Figure 8.6.** Brachial plexus.

in a prefixed and a postfixed plexus, respectively. The roots lie posterior to the vertebral artery, an important structure to keep in mind while performing an interscalene block.

The nerve roots emerge between the anterior and middle scalene muscles to form trunks. The suprascapular nerve that supplies the rhomboid muscle, and the sensory innervation to the posterosuperior aspect of the shoulder, arises from C5. The long thoracic nerve that supplies the serratus anterior muscle arises from the C5, 6, and 7 nerve roots. The upper C5 and 6 roots and the lower C8 and T1 roots pair to form the superior and inferior trunks respectively, while the C7 root continues to form the middle trunk. The trunks are formed in the lower posterior triangle, between the sternocleidomastoid and the trapezius muscles, just above the middle third of the clavicle. The trunks continue caudally to the first rib and divide into anterior and posterior divisions. The anterior divisions of the superior and middle trunks join to form the lateral cord and the anterior division of the inferior trunk continues as medial cord while the posterior divisions join to form the posterior cord. These pass under the clavicle and are labeled according to their relationship to the axillary artery. The cords divide at the border of the pectoralis minor muscle into five nerves that pass around the head of the humerus.

The musculocutaneous nerve, from the lateral cord, enters the coracobrachialis muscle and supplies the biceps and brachialis muscle. It then becomes the lateral cutaneous nerve of the forearm, located lateral to the biceps tendon at the elbow. The lateral and medial branches from the lateral and medial cords form the median nerve, which lies superior to the axillary artery in the arm and medial to the brachial artery at the level of the elbow. The posterior cord continues as the radial nerve, which wraps around the humerus and passes posteriorly to the artery. The radial nerve lies between the brachioradialis muscle and the brachialis muscle at the level of the elbow. The medial cord continues as the ulnar nerve between the artery and the vein and lies posterior to the medial epicondyle at the elbow.

Prior to performing a regional anesthetic technique, standard monitors are placed and supplemental oxygen is administered to the patient. A "timeout" is performed. The patient is then appropriately sedated and the site of nerve block and the ultrasound probe are prepped and draped in a sterile manner.

When using a tourniquet, an intercostobrachial nerve (T2) block should be performed by injecting a long-acting local anesthetic subcutaneously starting at the deltopectoral groove all the way to the inferior portion of the arm. The intercostobrachial nerve supplies the inner portion of the upper half of the arm.

## Interscalene block

- Indications: procedures on the shoulder, the lateral part of the clavicle, and the upper arm.
- Anatomy: the roots and trunks of the brachial plexus pass through the interscalene groove at the level of the cricoid cartilage. The groove lies deep and lateral to the clavicular head of sternocleidomastoid muscle between the scalene muscles.
- Landmarks: lateral border of the sternocleidomastoid muscle, accentuated by a head lift with the patient's head turned to the opposite side. Cricoid cartilage, external jugular vein accentuated with a Valsalva maneuver, and scalene muscles accentuated by asking the patient to take a deep breath.
- Technique: with the patient in supine position and the head slightly turned towards the contralateral side, the brachial plexus is identified with the ultrasound probe in the

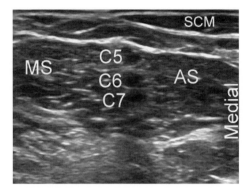

**Figure 8.7.** Interscalene block. SCM = sternocleidomastoid muscle; AS = anterior scalene muscle; MS = middle scalene muscle.

following fashion. A transverse (short axis) view can be obtained with a depth of 3 cm and a frequency of 12–15 MHz. The probe is placed parallel to the clavicle at the level of the cricoid cartilage. Scanning from medial to lateral will identify the carotid artery, the internal jugular vein, the sternocleidomastoid muscle, the anterior scalene muscle, the nerve roots (hypoechoic), and the middle scalene muscle (Figure 8.7). The vertebral artery, which is normally visualized below C6, also appears hypoechoic. Color flow may be used to distinguish the artery from the nerve roots. If the nerve root visualization appears difficult, a scan of the supraclavicular region can be utilized to identify the divisions of the brachial plexus lateral to the subclavian artery (cluster of grapes). The divisions of the brachial plexus can be followed in a cephalad direction until the nerve roots are identified. The phrenic nerve may sometimes be localized between the sternocleidomastoid muscle and the anterior scalene muscle. Individual nerve root identity can be confirmed with nerve stimulation. The usual volume of local anesthetic is between 20 to 30 mL.

- Specific side effects and complications: hoarseness from recurrent laryngeal nerve paralysis, unilateral diaphragmatic paralysis, Horner's syndrome, intravascular injection into vertebral artery, unintentional epidural or subarachnoid block, pneumothorax.

## Supraclavicular block

With the advent of ultrasound, this block has regained popularity because of the proximity of the plexus to the skin and the relatively small volumes of local anesthetic required to block the entire arm. All divisions of the brachial plexus are in close proximity, resulting in a fast onset and dense arm blockade.

- Indications: surgical procedures of the upper arm, elbow, and forearm.
- Anatomy: the divisions of the brachial plexus and the subclavian artery lie superior to the first rib and are located posterior and lateral to the artery. The subclavian vein lies medial to the artery and is separated by the anterior scalene muscle. The pleura is located inferior and posterior to the plexus and can be as close as 1 to 2 cm. Approach is in a lateral to medial direction towards the middle scalene muscle in the posterior triangle of the neck just above the middle third of the clavicle.
- Technique: a transverse (short axis) view can be obtained with an initial depth setting of 4 cm and a frequency of 12–15 MHz with the patient supine and the head turned to the

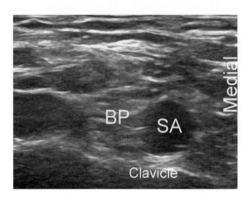

**Figure 8.8.** Supraclavicular block. BP = brachial plexus; SA = subclavian artery.

contralateral side. The probe is placed on the supraclavicular fossa. After identifying the subclavian artery, the divisions of the brachial plexus can be seen just lateral to the artery (Figure 8.8). If the artery is not visible, tilting the probe inferiorly should be attempted. The divisions of the brachial plexus appear as a cluster of grapes. Though not well visualized, fine septae are located between the individual divisions. Multiple injections around the plexus assure a higher block success rate. An in-plane technique is normally preferred, since it is critical to have real-time visualization of the needle tip to avoid accidental pleura puncture. If needle visualization is difficult, the probe can be tilted perpendicular to the patient. The usual volume of local anesthetic is 20 to 30 mL.

- Specific side effects and complications:

  - Pneumothorax. Due to the close proximity of the divisions of the brachial plexus to the pleura, pneumothorax is a serious potential complication of the supraclavicular block. While ultrasound can identify the pleura and allow advancement of the needle towards the brachial plexus while avoiding pleural puncture, visualization of the entire needle is not guaranteed throughout the procedure. Consequently, pneumothoraces have occurred even under ultrasound guidance. Controlled trials comparing different nerve block modalities regarding this complication are not available.

  - Intravascular injection. The suprascapular and transverse cervical arteries appear hypoechoic (i.e., similar to nerve bundles) and are visible around the plexus. Therefore, it is important to use color flow to identify these structures to avoid accidental intravascular injection.

## Axillary block

- Indications: procedures on the elbow, forearm, and hand. This block can also be used for sympathectomy of the upper extremity. This is an excellent block for patients with suspected cervical spine injury, as positioning does not require the neck to be moved. In addition, this block does not carry the risk of accidental phrenic nerve block or pneumothorax.

- Anatomy: the terminal branches of the brachial plexus are blocked at this level. The musculocutaneous nerve branches above the lateral cord and can easily be missed with a single injection around the axillary artery. The musculocutaneous nerve is visualized

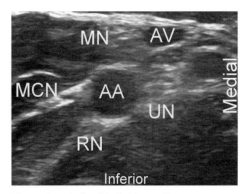

**Figure 8.9.** Axillary block. AA = axillary artery; AV = axillary vein; MCN = musculocutaneous nerve; MN = median nerve; RN = radial nerve; UN = ulnar nerve.

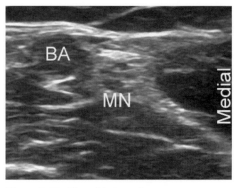

**Figure 8.10.** Elbow block: median nerve. BA = brachial artery; MN = median nerve.

in the belly of the coracobrachialis muscle or at a more distal level within the biceps muscle. The median, ulnar, and radial nerves surround the axillary artery at 10, 2, and 6 o'clock positions, respectively. Multiple anatomical variations in terms of nerve location in relation to the axillary artery have been described.

- Technique: with the patient in supine position and the arm abducted to 90 degrees, the probe is placed perpendicular to the arm as high as possible in the axilla. A short axis (transverse) view can be obtained with the frequency at 12–15 MHz and a depth of 3 cm (Figure 8.9). The probe should be moved distally along the longitudinal axis of the humerus, until all structures can be identified, and along the transverse plane until the musculocutaneous nerve is located. Nerve identity can be confirmed by electrical stimulation. Nerves may have a round or oval shape and may appear as a honeycomb, since the fascicles are hypoechoic and the surrounding fascia is also hyperechoic. Identification of structures may be difficult after local anesthetic injection due to disruption of the anatomy. Identification of the axillary vein by relieving pressure on the probe is important to prevent accidental intravascular injection. A total of 5–10 mL of local anesthetic around each nerve should provide adequate surgical anesthesia. A single injection of 20 to 30 mL of local anesthetic targeted towards the primary nerve supplying the site of surgery is usually adequate to provide postoperative analgesia.
- Specific side effects and complications: although there are no specific complications for this block, hematoma formation and accidental intraneural or intravascular injection may occur.

## Elbow block

- Indications: hand procedures, supplement incomplete brachial plexus blocks.
- Anatomy: the three nerves that supply the hand and the cutaneous nerves that supply the forearm can be blocked at the elbow. The median nerve lies medial to the brachial artery. The radial nerve lies deep to the brachioradialis muscle and just above the radial head. The ulnar nerve lies within the olecranon groove.
- Technique: the patient is placed in supine position and the arm is supinated. An ultrasound image can be obtained by placing the probe along the transverse plane to obtain a short axis view of the nerves (Figures 8.10, 8.11, and 8.12). Depth of 2 to 3 cm

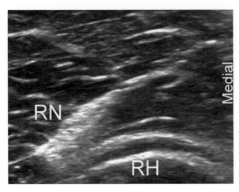

**Figure 8.11.** Elbow block: radial nerve. RH = radial head; RN = radial nerve.

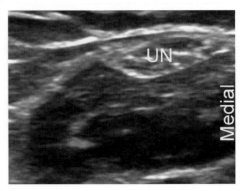

**Figure 8.12.** Elbow block: ulnar nerve. UN = ulnar nerve.

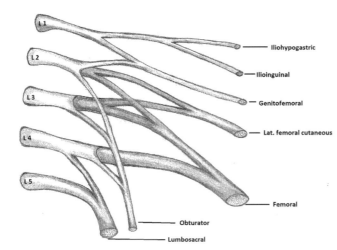

**Figure 8.13.** The lumbar plexus: L1 to L5.

and frequency of 12 to 15 MHz. Injection of 5–10 mL of local anesthetic around each nerve is sufficient for a successful block.

- Specific side effects and complications: the ulnar nerve should be blocked a few centimeters proximal to the olecranon groove. Blocking the nerve in the groove may lead to a compartment syndrome of the nerve.

## Lower extremity blocks

The nerve supply of the lower extremity is provided by two main plexuses, the lumbar and the sacral plexus. The lumbar plexus (Figure 8.13) supplies the anterior portion of the thigh and knee, the medial portion of the leg, and the big toe (saphenous nerve). The sacral plexus supplies the posterior portion of the thigh (posterior cutaneous nerve of the thigh), the posterior aspect of the knee, and the rest of the leg below the knee (Figure 8.14).

L1 gives rise to the iliohypogastric nerve, which receives a branch from T12, and the ilioinguinal nerve. The genitofemoral nerves originate from L1 (femoral branch) and

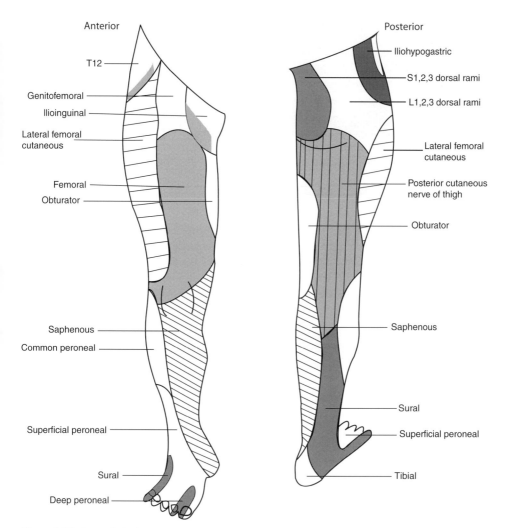

**Figure 8.14.** Lower limb dermatomes.

L2 (genital branch). The lateral femoral cutaneous nerve originates from L2 and L3, and the femoral and obturator nerves receive fibers from L2, L3, and L4.

The lumbar plexus lies deep to the psoas muscle, the L1 nerve root crosses anterior to the muscle while the nerve roots from L2, L3, and L4 run posterior to the psoas muscle. The plexus can be blocked at the nerve root level. However, this approach is not advisable in trauma patients as epidural spread of local anesthetic is common and may have a negative impact on hemodynamic status.

The lumbar plexus lies medial to the psoas muscle next to the sacral bone and is the source of the sciatic nerve, which converges towards the greater sciatic notch, passes deep in the pelvic floor, and emerges midway between the ischial tuberosity and the greater trochanter deep to the gluteus maximus muscle. The nerve passes vertically and caudally in the hamstring compartment and divides into tibial (L4, L5, S1, S2, S3) and common peroneal (L4, L5, S1, S2) nerves at the level of the apex of the popliteal fossa. The tibial nerve

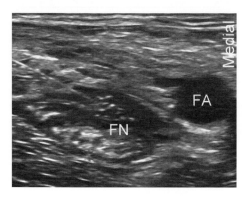

**Figure 8.15.** Femoral nerve block. FA = femoral artery; FN = femoral nerve.

gives rise to the sural nerve that passes laterally around the head of the fibula and supplies the lateral aspect of the leg and foot. The tibial nerve passes deep to the gastrocnemius muscle and supplies the plantar aspect of the foot. The common peroneal nerve divides into superficial and deep peroneal nerves, which supply the dorsum of the foot and the web space between the first and second toes, respectively.

## Femoral nerve block

- Indications: surgeries on the thigh, femur, and knee.
- Anatomy: the femoral nerve passes deep to the fascia iliaca and behind the inguinal ligament as it emerges into the thigh. The fascia iliaca separates the nerve that lies lateral to the vascular sheath containing the femoral artery and vein.
- Technique: with the patient positioned supine and the lower limb in neutral position, the probe is placed on the femoral crease and moved to scan from lateral to medial. A short axis (transverse) view can be obtained with a frequency of 12–15 MHz and a depth setting of 4 cm (Figure 8.15). Visualization of more than one arterial vessel indicates a probe position below the division of the femoral artery into superficial and profunda branches. In such a scenario the probe should be moved more cephalad until only the femoral artery can be seen. If the femoral vein is not visible it is advisable to relieve the pressure on the probe. The fascia iliaca can be identified as a hyperechoic line, which crosses above the femoral nerve and under the femoral artery. The femoral nerve will appear as a wedge-shaped hyperechoic structure below the fascia iliaca and lateral to the femoral artery. Lymph nodes can also appear as hyperechoic structures. These can be differentiated from the femoral nerve by scanning either in a cephalad or caudad direction that will identify the border of the lymph node. The nerve can be approached either out of plane or in plane. Most commonly, an in-plane approach, with needle direction from lateral to medial, is chosen. The out-of-plane approach is used when placing catheters. Visualization of the entire needle is important in order to avoid accidental puncture of the femoral artery and vein. The volume of local anesthetic usually utilized for this block is 25 to 30 mL.

## Lateral femoral cutaneous nerve block

- Indications: following a femoral nerve block failing to cover the lateral aspect of the thigh, procedures on the lateral aspect of the thigh and knee.

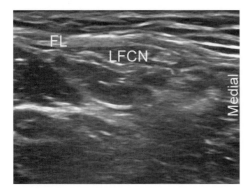

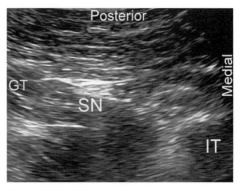

**Figure 8.16.** Lateral femoral cutaneous nerve block. FL = fascia lata; LFCN = lateral femoral cutaneous nerve.

**Figure 8.17.** Sciatic nerve block: gluteal approach. GT = greater trochanter; SN = sciatic nerve; IT = ischial tuberosity.

- Anatomy: the lateral femoral cutaneous nerve originates from L2 and L3 and carries only sensory fibers. The nerve is located inferior and medial to the anterior superior iliac spine and supplies the anterolateral part of the thigh up to the knee.
- Technique: the patient is placed in supine position. The probe is placed on the anterior superior iliac spine, which can be identified as a bony shadow (Figure 8.16). The probe is then moved caudally and medially from the anterior superior iliac spine to locate the fascia lata, which appears as a bright fibrous band. The nerve will be located about 2 cm medial and inferior to the anterior superior iliac spine. Placement of a small amount of local anesthetic medially to the anterior superior iliac spine may allow for easier nerve visualization. Injection of 5 to 10 mL of local anesthetic should be sufficient to assure block success.

## Sciatic nerve blocks

The sciatic nerve can be approached at multiple levels and various angles along its course from the gluteal region to the popliteal fossa. This chapter will only cover two approaches that are commonly performed with ultrasound and may be easily utilized in the trauma population.

### Gluteal approach

- Indications: surgeries involving the posterior aspect of the knee, below the knee, foot and ankle.
- Anatomy: the location of the sciatic nerve in the subgluteal region is very consistent. The sciatic nerve lies approximately midway between the greater trochanter and the ischial tuberosity in the sciatic groove, which is easily palpable in most patients.
- Technique: the patient is positioned in a lateral decubitus position with the side to be blocked upward and the upper thigh and the leg slightly flexed. A curvilinear probe with lower frequency is preferred for this block to allow for better penetration. If a linear probe is utilized, best image quality can be obtained with a frequency of 7 to 8 MHz and a depth of 6 to 8 cm (Figure 8.17). The ischial tuberosity and the greater trochanter can be identified easily since these bony structures will create an acoustic shadow. The sciatic nerve can be visualized as a triangle-shaped structure approximately

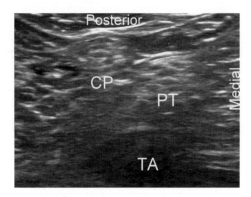

**Figure 8.18.** Sciatic nerve block: popliteal approach. CP = common peroneal nerve; PT = posterior tibial nerve; TA = tibial artery.

midway between the ischial tuberosity and the greater trochanter. The sciatic nerve is located inferior to the gluteus maximus muscle, just lateral to the insertion of the long head of biceps femoris at the ischial tuberosity. The needle can be introduced in plane in a lateral to medial direction. Nerve stimulation can be used in combination with ultrasound to allow for definite target identity confirmation since the insertion of the biceps femoris muscle at the ischial tuberosity may be mistaken for the sciatic nerve. The usual volume of local anesthetic is 25 to 30 mL.

### Lateral popliteal approach

- Indications: foot and ankle surgeries and below-knee amputations.
- Anatomy: the popliteal fossa is formed laterally by the biceps femoris muscle, medially by the semitendinosus and the semimembranosus muscles, and inferiorly by the gastrocnemius muscle. The fossa is filled with fat and contains the sciatic nerve inferior to the tibial artery in the anterolateral aspect of the fossa. The sciatic nerve usually divides into the tibial and the common peroneal nerves at the apex of this fossa, however the level of division is highly variable.
- Technique: this block can be performed with the patient either in supine or prone position. The supine position is frequently preferred in the trauma population since assuming a prone position may cause significant discomfort. If the supine position is chosen, the leg should be positioned in neutral and about 30 degrees flexed in the knee joint. The lower leg should be elevated and supported to create enough space below the popliteal fossa to allow sliding the ultrasound probe under the leg. With a depth setting of 3 to 5 cm and a frequency of 10 MHz, the probe is placed transversely under the popliteal fossa to obtain a short axis view of the sciatic nerve (Figure 8.18). The operator should start scanning at the popliteal crease and continue in a cephalad direction. With this approach the common peroneal nerve and the tibial nerve will appear on the screen as two oval-shaped honeycomb structures, superior to the sciatic artery (the operator needs to remember that this approach will result in an upside-down image since the ultrasound probe is held upside down). The nerves can be confirmed by following their course in a cephalad direction since the common peroneal and tibial nerves will unite together in one sheath to form the sciatic nerve. The block can be performed by introducing the needle in plane at the level of the bifurcation. As an alternative, the

common peroneal nerve and the tibial nerve can be targeted with two separate injections closer to the popliteal crease. The usual volume of local anesthetic utilized for this block is 30 to 35 mL.

# Selection of local anesthetic and catheter placement for peripheral nerve blocks

The selection and concentration of local anesthetic depends largely on what the anesthetic is used for, surgical anesthesia versus postoperative analgesia, the number of nerves being blocked, and the vasculature of the area being blocked.

Local anesthetics with rapid onset and short to medium duration of action, like lidocaine 2% and mepivacaine 1.5%, are frequently used in combination with the long-acting local anesthetic ropivacaine 0.2% or 0.5% for surgical anesthesia, which will last for 5 to 6 hours. Ropivacaine 0.2 to 0.5% is commonly used as a sole anesthetic for post-operative analgesia and usually lasts for 12 to 14 hours.

**Catheter placement indications:**

- Aggressive postoperative physiotherapy
- Moderate to severe pain that lasts more than 24 hours
- Sympathectomy for an ischemic limb due to vasospasm

Low-dose local anesthetic infusion of 0.2% ropivacaine to run at 6–8 cc/hour for brachial plexus catheters and 10–12 cc/hour for lower limb catheters is recommended.

# Local anesthetic toxicity

Toxicity from local anesthetics largely depends on the dose, absorption, and vascularity of the area into which they are injected. Systemic toxic effects primarily involve the central nervous and cardiovascular systems. The clinical signs of toxicity usually manifest in the central nervous system (CNS) before the cardiovascular system. However, CNS symptoms are often subtle or absent and cardiovascular signs may be the only manifestation of severe local anesthetic toxicity. Therefore the diagnosis should be considered in any patient with altered mental status or cardiovascular instability following a regional anesthetic.

CNS signs and symptoms of local anesthetic toxicity include the following:

- Circumoral paresthesias, lightheadedness, dizziness, difficulty focusing, and tinnitus.
- Restlessness and agitation.
- Slurred speech, drowsiness, and unconsciousness.
- Shivering, muscular twitching, tremors, and generalized seizures.
- Respiratory depression and respiratory arrest.

Cardiovascular signs and symptoms of local anesthetic toxicity include the following:

- Bradycardia.
- Hypotension.
- Intractable arrhythmias (ventricular ectopy, multiform ventricular tachycardia, and ventricular fibrillation).
- Cardiovascular collapse and asystole.

Management of systemic local anesthetic toxicity includes stopping local anesthetic administration, airway management, seizure suppression (if needed), and advanced cardiac life support. Lipid emulsion therapy has been shown to be effective in treating the cardiotoxic effects of bupivacaine and lidocaine. The exact mechanism of action of lipid emulsion is not well defined. It has been postulated to work by decreasing circulating amounts of drugs by binding to them, or through a direct "energy source" to the myocardium. The recommended dosing for lipid emulsion is as follows:

- 1.5 mL/kg 20% lipid emulsion intravenous bolus.
- 0.25 mL/kg per minute infusion, continued for at least 10 minutes after circulatory stability is attained.
- If circulatory stability is not attained, consider a second bolus and increasing infusion to 0.5 mL/kg per minute.
- Approximately 10 mL/kg lipid emulsion for 30 minutes is recommended as the upper limit for initial dosing.

## Neuraxial and paravertebral blocks

## Subarachnoid block

Spinal anesthesia is usually not recommended for trauma victims undergoing emergent surgery because there may be problems positioning the patient for the block or determining the etiology of hemodynamic changes. More significantly, the sympathectomy associated with spinal anesthesia may result in catastrophic hypotension and bradycardia in patients who are volume depleted. A spinal anesthetic would be an appropriate option in normovolemic trauma patients undergoing elective surgery for isolated lower limb injuries.

## Epidural block

Although not recommended in trauma victims as the sole anesthetic, this neuraxial block is excellent for postoperative pain management by decreasing overall opiate use, attenuating the surgical stress response, decreasing postoperative ileus, allowing for early mobilization, and decreasing pulmonary complications. Appropriate placement of the epidural catheter and choice of local anesthetic and additive infusion are important for the successful management of pain in these patients.

- Indications include rib fractures, thoracostomy tubes, and thoracic or large abdominal operations. Contraindications include labile hemodynamic status, suspected spine injury, coagulopathy, lack of consent, and altered mental status.
- Anatomic landmarks:
  - C7: the most prominent spinous process in the neck
  - T3: the scapular spine
  - T7: the inferior border of the scapula
  - L1: lower border of the 12th rib
  - L4–5: iliac crests
- Technique:
  - Patient in sitting position with neck and upper back flexion is preferred.
  - Lateral position with flexion of the neck, thighs, and knees is an alternative.

- Midline approach is difficult due to the extreme caudad angles of the spinous processes of T3–T11.
- Paramedian approach is preferred by some over midline approach to circumvent spinous processes.
- Epidural solution for infusion
  - Low-dose local anesthetic infusions are used in patients that are at high risk for postoperative ileus, obstructive sleep apnea, or prolonged nausea and vomiting. However, the use of local anesthetics alone is often limited by hypotension and motor blockade.
  - Opioids act on the mu receptors in the dorsal horn of the spinal cord. Lipophilic opioids (e.g., fentanyl and sufentanyl) diffuse across the dura and arachnoid membranes. Hydrophilic opioids (e.g., morphine, hydromorphone) spread cephalad with passive movement of the cerebrospinal fluid, and act on sites distal to the site of injection. Opioid infusions are not commonly used alone as there are increased side effects like pruritus, nausea and vomiting, respiratory depression, sedation, and postoperative ileus.
  - A combination of local anesthetic and opioid infusion exhibits a synergistic effect and decreases the incidence of side effects.
- Complications include failed block, accidental dural puncture, epidural hematoma, epidural abscess, radicular pain, and injury to the spinal cord.

## Paravertebral block

- Indications: pain management for rib fractures and flail chest, chest wall procedures, and thoracic surgery.
- Anatomy: the paravertebral space is wedge shaped and contains intercostal vessels and nerves, the dorsal ramus of the spinal nerve, and the sympathetic chain. The space is bounded anteriorly by the parietal pleura, posteriorly by the costotransverse ligament, and at the base by the vertebral body. The paravertebral space is contiguous with the epidural space and intercostal spaces medially. It extends from the cervical region to L1 at the origin of the psoas muscle.
- Landmark guided technique: the patient is positioned sitting up or alternatively in the lateral decubitus position with the affected side upward. At the desired level, the spinous process is identified. A point is marked 2.5 cm lateral to the most prominent part of the spinous process. After local anesthetic is injected to anesthetize the skin, a 22 G Tuohy needle is used to identify the transverse process, which is usually encountered at 2 to 4 cm depth. If the transverse process is not encountered on the first needle pass, the needle should be redirected slightly cephalad or caudad. Once the transverse process has been contacted, the needle is walked off the transverse process in a caudad direction not deeper than 1.0–1.5 cm beyond the transverse process. Frequently, a slight click or pop is felt, indicating that the needle has penetrated through the costotransverse ligament. It is important to advance the needle no further than 1.0–1.5 cm beyond the transverse process, since the paravertebral space is located in very close proximity to the transverse process and further needle advancement could result in accidental pleural puncture. A total of 3 to 5 mL of local anesthetic per space is utilized if multiple levels are blocked. A single injection of

15–20 mL of local anesthetic may result in a blockage of up to five dermatomes but carries a higher risk of epidural spread of local anesthetic, when compared to a "low volume – multiple level" technique. In contrast to thoracic or lumbar epidural anesthesia, paravertebral blocks result in fewer hemodynamic side effects due to a lesser degree of sympathetic blockade and are consequently well suited to provide effective pain control in trauma patients with multiple rib fractures and hypovolemia due to other injuries. In addition, there is only minimal impact on bowel or bladder function.

## Key points

- Nerve block anesthesia can be successfully utilized in trauma patients, although careful consideration must be given to hemodynamic instability, coagulation status, preexisting nerve injury, and risk of compartment syndrome.
- Choose blocks that cause minimal hemodynamic changes.
- Missing compartment syndrome is a possibility in trauma patients when administering long-acting nerve blocks.
- Administering intravenous opioids to patients receiving epidural opioids increases the risk of respiratory depression.
- When performing regional nerve block anesthesia:
  - Know the anatomy before starting the block.
  - Choose the proper local anesthetic and keep the total dose below the toxic dose.
  - Identify vascular structures in the region of interest using ultrasound prior to injecting the anesthetic.
  - Do not inject if resistance is felt.
  - Keep the needle tip in view at all times when advancing the needle.
  - Do not inject into the nerve itself.

## Further reading

1. Bhatia A, Lai J, Chan VW, et al. Case report: pneumothorax as a complication of the ultrasound-guided supraclavicular approach for brachial plexus block. *Anesth Analg* 2010;**111**:817–819.

2. Buckenmaier CC, McKnight GM, Winkley JV, et al. Continuous peripheral nerve block for battlefield anesthesia and evacuation. *Reg Anesth Pain Med* 2005;**30**:202–205.

3. Capdevila X, Pirat P, Bringuier S, et al. Continuous peripheral nerve blocks in hospital wards after orthopedic surgery: a multicenter prospective analysis of the quality of postoperative analgesia and complications in 1,416 patients. *Anesthesiology* 2005;**103**:1035–1045.

4. Cometa MA, Esch AT, Boezaart AP. Did continuous femoral and sciatic nerve block obscure the diagnosis or delay the treatment of acute lower leg compartment syndrome? A case report. *Pain Med* 2011;**12**:823–828.

5. Horlocker TT, Wedel DJ, Rowlingson JC, et al. Regional anesthesia in the patient receiving antithrombotic or thrombolytic therapy: American Society of Regional Anesthesia and Pain Medicine Evidence-Based Guidelines (Third Edition). *Reg Anesth Pain Med* 2010;**35**:64–101.

6. Liu SS, Ngeow J, John RS. Evidence basis for ultrasound-guided block

characteristics: onset, quality, and duration. *Reg Anesth Pain Med* 2010;**35**: S26–S35.

7.  Missair A, Gebhard R, Pierre E, et al. Surgery under extreme conditions in the aftermath of the 2010 Haiti earthquake: the importance of regional anesthesia. *Prehosp Disaster Med* 2010;**25**:487–493.

8.  Sites BD, Spence BC, Gallagher JD, et al. Characterizing novice behavior associated with learning ultrasound-guided peripheral regional anesthesia. *Reg Anesth Pain Med* 2007;**32**:107–115.

**Chapter**

**9**

# Monitoring the trauma patient

Richard McNeer and Albert J. Varon

## Introduction

Monitoring of trauma patients during emergency surgery can be especially challenging for the anesthesiologist. Attempts to maintain an adequate depth of anesthesia to prevent awareness and pain can often be compromised by the unfavorable hemodynamic effects of anesthetics in patients experiencing hemorrhagic shock with ongoing bleeding. The functioning of even basic monitors may be problematic in settings of significant hypotension. Once surgical hemostasis is accomplished, resuscitative endpoints may not be clearly established and will vary depending on patient-specific factors and trauma etiology. Excessive fluid resuscitation can lead to adverse consequences that can impact patient morbidity and survival such as pulmonary edema, congestive heart failure, bowel edema, abdominal compartment syndrome, unplanned postoperative open abdomen, and airway edema. The monitoring strategy in trauma patients, as with all surgical patients, follows the American Society of Anesthesiologists (ASA) Standards for basic monitoring – that oxygenation, ventilation, circulation, and temperature should be continually evaluated. This can usually be accomplished using routine non-invasive monitors early in the surgery. However, additional (mostly invasive) monitors are often indicated and implemented in trauma patients. Ultimately, the decision to use a monitor should be based on a number of factors including:

- Accuracy of the generated data
- Potential complications related to generating the data
- Clinical relevance of the data
- Impact of the data on clinical outcome

Generally, a single data point or measurement is less informative than a dataset trend, and trend monitoring can be very useful in assessing therapeutic efficacy and changes in patient status. The strategy used to guide resuscitation may affect patient outcome, and fluid therapy is an important component of this strategy. A relevant question often asked is: will the patient's cardiac output (stroke volume) be increased with a fluid bolus? Available monitors differ in their ability to predict "recruitable" cardiac output. The purpose of this chapter is to discuss the commonly available and practical monitors stratified in terms of basic assumptions and limitations that can affect data interpretation, patient risk, and, when applicable, their role in defining resuscitative endpoints.

*Essentials of Trauma Anesthesia*, ed. A. J. Varon and C. E. Smith. Published by Cambridge University Press.
© Cambridge University Press 2012.

# Non-invasive monitors

*Non-invasive blood pressure monitoring.* The most commonly used monitor for assessing fluid status is the blood pressure. For the most part, the oscillometric method is currently used in automated non-invasive blood pressure monitors. With this method the mean arterial pressure is directly measured, whereas the systolic and diastolic pressures are derived, and these blood pressures correlate reasonably well with invasively measured pressures during normotensive conditions. However, sensitivity in regard to acute blood loss can be poor, and accuracy is diminished at both high and low blood pressure extremes, limiting its usefulness during hemorrhagic shock. Time required to obtain a measurement can be lengthy and may delay detection of significant changes in blood pressure. Additionally, many patients have trauma to the extremities, limiting locations for cuff placement. Valid locations include the forearm, thigh, and calf, as long as cuff size is matched to location circumference. Repeated and frequent cuff inflations can lead to soft tissue and nerve injury. Patient movement and application of oscillations of non-cardiac origin (e.g., from surgeon contact with the cuff) can lead to measurement artifact.

*Pulse oximetry.* Arterial oxyhemoglobin saturation and heart rate can be monitored non-invasively with a pulse oximeter. However, its use in the trauma patient can be problematic. Patients in shock are often hypotensive and peripherally vasoconstricted and frequently have cold extremities, all of which can combine to hinder signal acquisition. Locations for probe placement may be limited due to traumatic injury of fingers and limbs. Response time in detecting hypoxia is increased with distal probe placement, approaching one minute when toes are used. Additionally, current pulse oximeter probes are digit-specific; for example, the Massimo finger probe is calibrated for the index, middle, and ring fingers only. Placement of the probe on a thumb, little finger, toes, ear lobes, lips, nose, and forehead, although sometimes used, may lead to spurious or inaccurate data. Mechanism of injury may include some combustive component (e.g., car fire) that can lead to carboxy-hemoglobinemia with overestimation of the true oxyhemoglobin saturation. Use of multi-wavelength pulse oximeters will eventually allow anesthesiologists to diagnose dyshemoglobinemias non-invasively and prevent misinterpretation of the oxygen saturation signal.

*Capnography.* Presence of end-tidal carbon dioxide ($EtCO_2$) indicates that ventilation and cardiac output are present. This information is crucial, for example, after a difficult intubation and in a patient with hemorrhagic shock.

In surgical patients receiving mechanical ventilation, $EtCO_2$ is used to guide ventilation management, since $EtCO_2$ is a surrogate for arterial $CO_2$ tension ($PaCO_2$). The observation of a small difference (2 to 5 mmHg) between $EtCO_2$ and $PaCO_2$ ($PaCO_2 > EtCO_2$) in normal patients is due to the presence of alveolar dead space. However, this difference may be increased in certain scenarios:

- During general anesthesia.
- In low perfusion states, including hemorrhagic shock.
- After chest trauma (e.g., resulting in increased dead space and ventilation-perfusion inhomogeneity).
- After pulmonary or fat embolism.
- During patient positioning other than supine (e.g., beach chair and lateral decubitus).

Because many of these scenarios occur during management of trauma patients, it is important to correlate $EtCO_2$ with $PaCO_2$, an assessment made feasible since many trauma patients have an indwelling arterial catheter. A recent study showed that when $EtCO_2$ was maintained between 35 and 40 mmHg, trauma patients were underventilated ($PaCO_2 > 40$ mmHg) 80% of the time and *severely* underventilated ($PaCO_2 > 50$ mmHg) 30% of the time. Knowledge of the $EtCO_2$–$PaCO_2$ difference is very useful in managing ventilation of patients with traumatic brain injury (TBI) due to the adverse effects of hypercapnea on intracranial pressure (ICP). The best correlation between $EtCO_2$ and $PaCO_2$ in trauma patients is observed in the setting of isolated TBI, but even this subgroup has been shown to be at risk for hypercapnea if ventilation is guided by $EtCO_2$ alone. The $EtCO_2$–$PaCO_2$ difference may change during the course of surgery. Therefore, it may be prudent to measure the difference at multiple points over time.

*Electrocardiography.* Electrocardiography (ECG) is a standard American Society of Anesthesiologists (ASA) monitor. Abnormalities in ECG may be observed in trauma patients. Severe hemorrhagic shock can be associated with ST segment changes and dysrhythmias as myocardial perfusion and oxygen delivery cease to meet myocardial demand. Resuscitation with blood products can lead to hyperkalemia evidenced by peaked T waves. Patients with TBI can develop marked ECG changes that mimic myocardial ischemia. Blunt and penetrating cardiac injury may occur after chest trauma. Besides non-specific ST segment and T wave abnormalities, the ECG may show the following arrhythmias:

- Sinus tachycardia
- Atrial fibrillation
- Premature ventricular contractions
- Atrioventricular and intraventicular blocks
- Ventricular arrhythmias

Treatment of patients with cardiac injury ranges from continuous ECG monitoring in an intensive care setting, to inotropic and vasopressor support for heart failure, or surgery for tamponade or to repair structural abnormalities (see Chapter 16). A patient sustaining blunt chest trauma who has normal 12-lead ECG has a low probability of having blunt cardiac injury.

Myocardial infarction may also occur in trauma patients with or without chest trauma. The anesthesiologist must be astute and draw on all available information (e.g., patient history, trauma etiology) when suspecting and diagnosing the presence of myocardial ischemia, and continuous ECG monitoring with ST trend analysis and 12-lead analysis may be helpful in this regard.

*Temperature monitoring.* It is essential that temperature be monitored in trauma patients. Sites for measuring temperature include:

- Pulmonary artery (PA)
  - Considered the gold standard for core temperature, but requires placement of a PA catheter for other indications (see section on invasive monitors).
- Nasopharynx
  - Good reflection of core temperature.
- Esophageal
  - Good reflection of core temperature provided there is distal placement.
  - May be inaccurate in the presence of nasogastric tubes attached to wall suction.

- Bladder
  - Many urinary catheters have a built-in temperature probe.
- Axilla
  - Can be used when monitoring other locations is problematic or not possible.

The risk of hypothermia begins at the time of injury and continues during the prehospital period due to altered thermoregulation after shock, environmental exposure, and reduced heat production (see also Chapter 7). Effects of hypothermia on the trauma patient include:

- Leftward shift of the oxyhemoglobin dissociation curve decreasing oxygen delivery.
- Decreased platelet function which may lead to coagulopathy.
- Atrial fibrillation (temperature $< 30\ °C$).
- Ventricular fibrillation (temperature $< 25\ °C$).
- Decreased myocardial response to inotropic agents.
- Decreased metabolism and elimination of medications (e.g., neuromuscular relaxants).
- Decreased efficacy of monitoring (e.g., with the pulse oximeter).

Trauma patients often arrive hypothermic to the operating room (OR), and it is the responsibility of the anesthesiologist to ensure that every possible means of increasing the patient's temperature is implemented. These include:

- Warming of the room.
- Decreasing patient exposure.
- Use of convection air blankets.
- Warming all fluid and blood products (including use of warm irrigation by the surgeon).

*Transesophageal echocardiography* (TEE). This minimally invasive technique can be used as a hemodynamic monitor and as a diagnostic device (e.g., to detect pericardial tamponade) in trauma patients. A systematic approach should be used to identify trauma-related injuries and evaluate causes of hemodynamic instability. TEE examinations in patients with acute hemodynamic disturbances often result in major therapeutic impact (surgical or medical). The key echocardiographic parameters that should be evaluated in trauma patients with hemodynamic instability are:

1. Preload of the right and left ventricle (RV and LV).
2. Global and regional cardiac function.
3. Acute valvular dysfunction.
4. Cardiac and extra-cardiac anatomical or structural lesions that may be responsible for shock.

Chapter 10 is devoted to echocardiography in trauma.

*Awareness monitoring.* Monitoring for awareness is generally indicated in patients at risk of recall of intraoperative events:

- Spinal cord surgery requiring motor or sensory evoked potential measurements (see Chapter 14).
- Cardiac trauma surgery, especially with cardiopulmonary bypass.

It is well known that anesthetics can worsen the hemodynamic status of patients in hemorrhagic shock. In this situation, it is difficult to detect awareness based on clinical assessments of heart rate, which may be already elevated, blood pressure, which may remain low, and patient movement if neuromuscular blocking drugs are utilized. Perhaps for these reasons, trauma patients are at increased risk for experiencing unintended intraoperative awareness. It has been suggested that all trauma patients should be monitored using a bispectral index (BIS) monitor, currently the most commonly used awareness monitor. Touted as an effective monitor to detect and prevent awareness, it processes the electro-encephalogram and presents a number between 0 and 100 that is meant to be a reflection of anesthetic depth. However, recent evidence suggests that efficacy of awareness detection and prevention with BIS in high-risk patients may be no better than when clinical assessment and end-tidal volatile gas concentration are used. Nonetheless, it seems reasonable to draw upon all available data (including data from the BIS monitor) during maintenance of anesthesia in trauma patients, since intraoperative awareness is associated with significant consequences including post-traumatic stress disorder.

*Twitch monitor (nerve stimulator).* Whenever a neuromuscular blocking drug is used, its effects should be monitored in order to determine optimal dosing. This is especially important if the plan is for tracheal extubation at the conclusion of surgery in order to minimize the risk of postoperative residual blockade.

## Invasive monitors

*Arterial catheter.* Placement of an arterial catheter allows invasive measurement of systolic, diastolic, and mean arterial blood pressures. Its use is indicated whenever non-invasive methods for measuring blood pressure fail or are suboptimal, frequent blood draws are expected, and whenever real-time "beat-to-beat" assessment of blood pressure is required. The anesthesiologist must consider certain situations that can lead to inaccurate readings. Resonance can lead to distortion of the arterial waveform and occurs when the natural frequency of the catheter and tubing (preferably greater than 40 Hz) is decreased to such an extent that it coincides with the frequencies making up the physiologic waveform. The waveform is then said to appear to be "ringing" or underdamped. This usually occurs when the tubing connecting the catheter to the transducer is too long. Alternatively, the waveform can be overdamped because of soft tubing or a bubble present in the tubing. The waveform will then appear blunted. The mean arterial pressure (MAP) is the least affected by the dynamic response characteristics of the monitoring system. Accurate pressure readings require that the transducer be "leveled" to the heart. In the absence of these situations that can lead to erroneous readings, the arterial pressure readings are generally very accurate in normotensive (normal flow) patients. However, during hemorrhagic shock, constricted peripheral arterial vessels can reflect "bounce-back" waves back toward the vessel in which the catheter resides. This results in overestimation of the systolic pressure, and in this situation MAP is more accurate. It is important to differentiate between a resonant or underdamped waveform versus the waveform that accompanies severe hemorrhagic shock. This can be accomplished by taking into account all available monitor and vital sign data. Although feasible, it is usually not practical to manually calculate the natural frequency and dampening coefficient of the monitoring system while caring for a trauma patient. How-ever, if after flushing the transducer, more than 2 to 3 oscillation waves are observed before the physiologic waveform is restored, underdamping may be recognized. Useful information that can be obtained from the arterial waveform includes pressure variation with mechanical ventilation (see section below). Insertion and complications of arterial catheterization are discussed in Chapter 5.

*Central venous pressure catheter.* Central venous pressure (CVP) is measured in the superior vena cava or right atrium usually using a central venous or PA catheter. Placement of a central venous catheter can provide much needed central access for infusion of fluids and vasoactive medications (and later for parenteral nutrition). A CVP catheter can also be used to aspirate air in cases of air embolism and to insert cardiac pacemakers and inferior vena cava filters. Measurement of central venous oxygen saturation ($S_{cv}O_2$) can also be done using continuous or intermittent sampling, and is discussed in the section on venous saturation. Useful information that can be obtained by monitoring CVP in trauma patients includes the following:

- Differentiation between pericardial tamponade and hypovolemia in a hypotensive trauma patient.
- Differential diagnosis of increased CVP and hypotension including cardiac tamponade, tension pneumothorax, RV failure, and tricuspid regurgitation.
- Diagnosis of certain arrhythmias (e.g., absence of "a" waves in atrial fibrillation, presence of "a" flutter waves in atrial flutter).
- Diagnosis of valvulopathies (prominent "v" waves in tricuspid regurgitation).

CVP has also been used to assess volume status. In the absence of tricuspid valvulopathy, the CVP correlates with right atrial pressure and RV end-diastolic pressure. However, it is important to keep in mind that the absolute value and trend change of the CVP depends on the interplay between both intravascular volume and RV function, and it is difficult to determine which of these two dependencies are operational. This can confound interpretation and significantly limits the utility of CVP as a resuscitation endpoint. Moreover, ventricular disparity and independence of right and left atrial pressures have been observed in critically ill patients, a fact that may limit the ability of CVP to assess LV function in trauma patients. CVP catheter insertion and complications are discussed in Chapter 5.

*Pulmonary artery catheter.* The use of a PA catheter has declined due to potential for increased risks and the advent of more accurate diagnostic information from less invasive monitors such as echocardiography. Nonetheless, PA catheter monitoring may be indicated when a more accurate hemodynamic assessment is necessary and when this knowledge will help guide resuscitation and therapy. Indications that may apply to trauma patients include:

- Shock despite perceived adequate therapy.
- To assess the effect of a fluid bolus on cardiac function.
- To delineate the cardiovascular component of multiple organ system dysfunction.
- To differentiate non-cardiogenic (ARDS) from cardiogenic pulmonary edema.
- To assess effects of high levels of ventilatory support on cardiovascular status.
- Myocardial infarction complicated by pump failure or pulmonary edema.
- Congestive heart failure unresponsive to simple therapy (to guide preload and vasodilator therapy).

The information obtained from pulmonary artery catheters includes:

- CVP
- PA pressure (systolic, mean, and diastolic)

- PA occlusion pressure (PAOP or "wedge")
- Cardiac output (using thermodilution)
- Continuous mixed venous oximetry ($S_{\bar{v}}O_2$)
- Mixed venous blood gases ($P_{\bar{v}}O_2$ and $P_{\bar{v}}CO_2$) by intermittent sampling

The decision to insert a PA catheter needs to be tempered with the desired benefits (e.g., guidance in management of resuscitation, inotropic/vasopressor, and ventilation therapies) and the potential risks (e.g., arrhythmias such as right bundle branch block, aberrant catheter location, pulmonary artery rupture, infection, and thromboembolism). Additionally, prioritization and time constraints may render insertion of the catheter impractical and interpretation of resulting data superfluous in the patient who is actively exsanguinating, in shock, and in obvious need of resuscitation. This notwithstanding, the PA catheter may be useful once surgical hemostasis has been obtained and when further diagnosis and therapy can be guided, for example, in the intensive care unit or during subsequent surgeries. The use and correct interpretation of PA catheter data require that the anesthesiologist have a good working knowledge of the relevant physiology and of the technical aspects of insertion, calibration of monitors, and artifact troubleshooting. It is important to integrate all data parameters (pressures, cardiac output, and $S_vO_2$) because monitoring of only one parameter (e.g., PAOP) may lead to misinterpretation.

*Pulmonary artery occlusion (wedge) pressure.* The PAOP is obtained by inflating a balloon that has been flow-directed ("floated") to West's zone 3 and measuring the pressure distal to the balloon. The PAOP has been shown to be a reliable index of left atrial pressure (better than PA diastolic pressure) even in the setting of high pulmonary vascular resistance and hypovolemia. The left atrial pressure may reflect LV end-diastolic pressure, LV end-diastolic volume, and end-diastolic muscle fiber stretch (true preload). However, this line of assumptions is not valid if mitral valve disease or premature mitral valve closure is present (e.g., severe aortic regurgitation), or more commonly, if there are changes in LV compliance (e.g., ischemia, diastolic dysfunction, myocardial conduction disturbances, LV hypertrophy).

*Cardiac output.* Cardiac output is commonly measured by the thermodilution technique with a pulmonary artery catheter. In general, a change in heat content of blood is induced at one point in the circulation and the resulting temperature change is measured at a point downstream. Heat content can be induced either by injecting a known volume of fluid at a known temperature, or by transferring a safe level of heat via a thermal filament. PA catheters that use the latter technology are readily available and allow for continuous assessment of cardiac output. In both methods, measurements of temperature with time are obtained at the distal sites, and these data are used by a computer to calculate cardiac output. Numerous factors can lead to a decrease in cardiac output:

- Depleted intravascular volume (absolute or relative)
- Decreased ventricular function
- Tension pneumothorax
- Pericardial tamponade
- Pulmonary embolus

The utility of cardiac output in helping to make a diagnosis depends on simultaneous assessment of other available monitor data and clinical examination.

*Venous saturation.* Oxyhemoglobin saturation measured in blood from the pulmonary artery (via a PA catheter) is referred to as mixed-venous or $S_{\bar{v}}O_2$ (normal is 75%), whereas that measured from the CVP catheter is referred to as superior vena cava saturation ($S_{cv}O_2$). Factors that will decrease venous $O_2$ saturation are:

- Decreased arterial saturation.
- Increased oxygen consumption.
- Decreased cardiac output.
- Anemia (e.g., resulting from blood loss).

Monitoring of $S_{\bar{v}}O_2$ has been used in many clinical scenarios that could occur in trauma patients, including:

- Early detection of myocardial dysfunction.
- Shock.
- Arrhythmias.
- Assessment of efficacy of cardiopulmonary resuscitation (100% mortality when $S_vO_2$ remains less than 40%).

In the specific scenario of hemorrhagic shock, further resuscitation or surgical intervention is advocated when $S_{\bar{v}}O_2$ is less than 65%. Monitoring of $S_{\bar{v}}O_2$ has, therefore, been suggested as a means for determining resuscitative endpoints in trauma patients.

CVP catheters designed to allow continuous oximetric monitoring of blood saturation in the superior vena cava are now available. However, values for $S_{\bar{v}}O_2$ and $S_{cv}O_2$ obtained simultaneously in the same patient do not always correlate. In normal patients, $S_{cv}O_2$ accurately reflects $S_{\bar{v}}O_2$, but in patients experiencing shock, $S_{cv}O_2$ is consistently greater than $S_{\bar{v}}O_2$ by 5–18%. This discrepancy occurs because of a mixture of more desaturated blood from the coronary sinus and redistribution of splenic, mesenteric, and renal blood to the cerebral and coronary circulations during shock. Nonetheless, trend monitoring shows close tracking of both parameters during hemorrhagic shock and in other hemodynamic conditions. Additionally, low $S_{cv}O_2$ implying an even lower $S_{\bar{v}}O_2$ is clinically more important and useful than the fact that absolute values of the two parameters are not equal. Central venous access is commonly obtained in unstable trauma patients. Monitoring of $S_{cv}O_2$, which can be obtained with (simpler and safer) placement of a CVP catheter, should be considered as a viable alternative to monitoring $S_{\bar{v}}O_2$, especially as continuous oximetric CVP catheters have become available. A study in critically ill septic patients reported a mortality benefit in early goal-directed therapy using $S_{cv}O_2$ ($\geq 70\%$) as one of its major endpoints (see reference 7). Whether this outcome benefit applies to trauma patients has yet to be determined. A recent study showed a correlation between changes in $S_{\bar{v}}O_2$ and $S_{cv}O_2$ and changes in cardiac index after volume expansion. Importantly, a change in $S_{cv}O_2$ threshold value of 4% allowed prediction with 86% sensitivity of which critically ill patients would respond to volume resuscitation.

*Dynamic monitors of fluid bolus responsiveness.* An important question that can help guide resuscitation is whether the patient's cardiac output (and associated vital signs) will improve with intravascular volume expansion. Recently, it has been reported that in 50% of critically ill patients, the answer is no. Non-responders are at risk for fluid overload, and may be more prudently managed with inotropic and/or vasopressor therapy. Unfortunately, most of the currently used "static" parameters such as CVP, PAOP, and even LV end-diastolic area measured by TEE are not very effective in predicting the presence of

**Table 9.1.** Comparison of static and dynamic hemodynamic parameters for prediction of responsiveness to fluid bolus: adapted from pooled data (95% confidence intervals) presented in *Crit Care Med* 2009 Vol. 37, No. 9. Higher values for area under curve indicate better prediction

|  | Static | Dynamic | Correlation (r) | Area under curve |
|---|---|---|---|---|
| CVP | Yes | – | .13 | .55 |
| LV end-diastolic area index | Yes | – | – | .64 |
| Global end-diastolic volume index | Yes | – | – | .56 |
| Pulse pressure variation | – | Yes | .78 | .94 |
| Systolic pressure variation | – | Yes | .72 | .86 |
| Stroke volume variation | – | Yes | .72 | .84 |

Abbreviations: CVP = central venous pressure; LV = left ventricular.

recruitable cardiac output (Table 9.1). More effective "dynamic" parameters for assessing volume status and predicting recruitable cardiac output include systolic pressure variation (SPV), pulse pressure variation (PPV), and stroke volume variation (SVV). These parameters are the result of the cyclic variations in LV stroke volume induced by positive pressure ventilation. The presence of an arterial catheter in patients receiving mechanical ventilation facilitates measurement of these parameters in trauma patients.

During mechanical ventilation, the insufflation period is associated with a decrease in RV preload, an increase in RV afterload, and a resultant decrease in RV stroke volume. The RV stroke volume is at a minimum at end inspiration. About two to three heartbeats later, a similar reduction in LV preload and LV stroke volume may occur (usually during expiration). The dynamic methods evaluate the response to reversible variation of preload, and rely on the fact that patients with recruitable cardiac output reside on the ascending portion of the Frank-Starling curve. There are limitations to using recruitable cardiac output monitors:

- Patients cannot be spontaneously breathing
- Tidal volumes should not be less than 8 mL/kg
- The thoracic cage cannot be open
- The patient cannot have arrhythmias

Mechanical ventilation must be used, since spontaneous breathing and pressure support or other modes of ventilation that incorporate spontaneous effort will not allow proper interpretation of data. Fortunately, this does not usually apply to acute trauma patients who are receiving neuromuscular relaxants. A tidal volume of no less than 8 mL/kg is a requirement for dynamic measurements to reflect fluid responsiveness, but this number may not be practical or safe in certain trauma patients. The presence of arrhythmias such as can be observed after cardiac injury may confound interpretation. It is important to keep in mind that recruitable cardiac output monitors do not give information about the shape of a patient's Frank-Starling curve (i.e., ventricular function). However, in the face of unstable vital signs and a determination that a patient resides on the flat portion of the curve (i.e., if variation is not significant), valuable guidance as far as initiating inotropic or vasopressor support may be ascertained.

Although most ORs are not currently equipped with recruitable cardiac output monitors, assessment of recruitable cardiac output can still be performed in the trauma patient. For example, SPV and PPV can be assessed by informally "eyeballing" the arterial waveform on the hemodynamic monitor display. The patient is often described as "cycling" where there is appreciation of wide swings in systolic pressure during mechanical ventilation. Many newer monitor displays allow the anesthesiologist to show the arterial pulse waveform in a grid, and allow placement of graphical user interface cursors to keep track of pressure variations. In this way the SPV and delta up and delta down can be measured more accurately.

Compared to static monitors or indices such as CVP, RV, and LV end-diastolic volume, and echocardiography, the dynamic indices SPV, PPV, and SVV are much better predictors of fluid responsiveness (Table 9.1). Among these dynamic indices, PPV has been shown to have greater diagnostic accuracy than SPV and SVV. The reasons are not clear, however, in the case of SVV, assumptions made when calculating stroke volume may add error to the final assessment. PPV, however, is obtained during sole analysis of the arterial pressure waveform. Implementation of these methods may become more widespread in the OR, especially as new devices with automated algorithms and software analyses are developed and brought to market. Considering that half of critically ill, hemodynamically unstable patients do not respond to fluid resuscitation therapy, the ability to predict the responders and to have clear resuscitation endpoints may help decrease patient morbidity.

*Intracranial pressure monitoring.* TBI is a common occurrence in patients who sustain multiple trauma (see Chapter 13). Intracranial hypertension occurs in approximately 40% of all patients with severe TBI and contributes significantly to poor functional outcome and mortality. Unfortunately, physical findings are often unreliable to ascertain the presence of ICP. The only direct assessment of ICP is obtained by measurement. Measuring ICP permits calculation of cerebral perfusion pressure (CPP), which is defined as the difference between the MAP and ICP. Thus, isolated increases in ICP or decreases in MAP will result in a reduction in CPP. The CPP may be insufficient if ICP increases to more than 20 mmHg. Although in the past, one of the endpoints of central nervous system monitoring was felt to be the control of ICP within safe levels, emphasis has shifted to following CPP itself. Maintaining cerebral blood flow appears to require using an elevated minimal CPP threshold when treating the injured brain. A CPP level of at least 70 mmHg has been suggested.

Severe head injury is the most common indication for ICP monitoring. Patients with a Glasgow Coma Scale (GCS) score $\leq 8$ (see Table 2.3 in Chapter 2) or GCS motor score $\leq 5$ (i.e., not following commands) should be strongly considered for ICP monitoring.

- Patients with a GCS $\leq 8$ who have a normal head computed tomography scan have a very low probability of developing intracranial hypertension if they have fewer than two of the following features:

  - Prior episodes of hypotension
  - Age $> 40$ years
  - Motor posturing
- Although these patients may initially be managed without ICP monitoring, any deterioration should prompt immediate reconsideration of ICP monitoring and re-imaging.

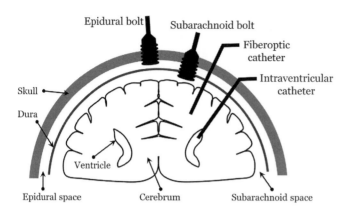

**Figure 9.1.** Methods for measuring intracranial pressure in patients with traumatic brain injury.

Several methods of ICP measurement are available (Figure 9.1). A ventricular catheter connected to a standard strain gauge transducer via fluid-filled lines offers excellent waveform characteristics and permits withdrawal of cerebrospinal fluid (CSF). This catheter, however, may be difficult to insert when cerebral edema or hematoma causes shifting or collapse of the lateral ventricle system. A subarachnoid bolt is easily inserted under any circumstances, although at times may give erroneous readings, depending on its placement relative to the site of injury. Compared to ventricular catheters, the waveforms obtained with a subarachnoid bolt are not as good and CSF drainage is usually not possible. Epidural bolts have a lower risk of complications but are less accurate than ventricular catheters or subarachnoid bolts and do not permit withdrawal of CSF. Non-fluid-coupled systems utilizing fiberoptic or catheter-tip strain gauge technology can be placed into ventricular, subdural, or parenchymal sites. These devices appear to offer advantages over conventional ICP monitors, especially in their ability to measure brain parenchymal pressures. Complications of ICP devices include:

- Infection
- Hemorrhage
- Malfunction
- Obstruction
- Malposition
- Bacterial colonization (risk increases significantly after five days of implantation, but significant intracranial infections are uncommon).

## Serum markers of tissue perfusion and oxygen debt

*Lactate.* Tissue hypoperfusion that results from hemorrhagic shock can be indirectly assessed by measuring the serum lactate level and base deficit. As oxygen delivery falls below the threshold needed for oxidative phosphorylation to occur, cells begin to convert glucose to pyruvate and then to lactate (anaerobic glycolysis). The degree of global (whole body) oxygen debt is therefore indirectly related to lactate levels. Hyperlactemia has been studied with regard to outcome. Initial lactate levels above 4 mmol/L are associated with higher mortality. Both the degree and duration of hyperlactemia are associated with higher morbidity and mortality. Meanwhile, a greater than 5% decrease in lactate levels within the first hour of fluid resuscitation is associated with a very favorable prognosis. The time for hyperlactemia to resolve to 2 mmol/L or less is inversely related to survival.

*Base deficit.* The base deficit gives an approximation of global tissue acidosis and the primary mediator of tissue acidosis is lactate. Base deficit can be used to assess the severity of hemorrhagic shock:

- Severe: −15 or less
- Moderate: −6 to −14
- Mild: −5 or greater

Base deficit can be used to guide fluid resuscitation, and trend monitoring can give valuable feedback regarding resuscitation efficacy. 65% of patients who have a worsening base deficit despite resuscitative efforts may still be hemorrhaging.

The degree of correlation between lactate and base deficit is not clear, as some studies show a strong correlation while others show a poor correlation, with lactate identified as more reliable than base deficit. Combined monitoring of both lactate and base deficit levels may be more effective than either value alone in allowing prediction of oxygen debt and outcome. Interpretation of base deficit values is problematic in trauma patients who have received sodium bicarbonate, as base deficit will be overestimated (appear less severe) due to the addition of iatrogenic metabolic alkalosis. In such instances, lactate may be a more reliable parameter to monitor.

## Monitoring of trauma patients when monitors fail

Trauma patients can be so unstable that implementation of even the most basic monitors may be problematic.

- Attempts to apply or maintain ECG leads on diaphoretic or burned skin can be difficult.
- Pulse oximetry may not yield an accurate reading because of shock, hypotension, peripheral vasoconstriction, and hypothermia.
- Oscillometric blood pressure readings will be inaccurate or not register at all.
- It may be difficult to place an arterial catheter in the setting of hypotension and peripheral vasoconstriction.
- Placement of a central venous catheter may be difficult during emergency surgery for bleeding and in patients who are volume contracted.

This scenario is not uncommon, and when monitors are not effective, the patient should be examined for the presence of a pulse. If the patient is pulseless, advanced life support measures should be initiated, including chest compressions. The presence of a pulse allows estimation of the systolic blood pressure:

- Radial pulse indicates a minimum of 80 mmHg.
- Femoral pulse indicates a minimum of 70 mmHg.
- Carotid pulse indicates a minimum of 60 mmHg.

However, one study has suggested that these pressures may be overestimates. It can be difficult to palpate a pulse in the obese hypotensive trauma patient despite the pulse being present (false negative). For all of these reasons, one very useful but often overlooked monitor for perfusion is capnography, which is present in every OR and easily implemented in any patient that is able to be ventilated. The presence of $EtCO_2$ indicates that pulmonary blood flow (right-sided cardiac output) is present. Trend monitoring of $EtCO_2$ can be invaluable in assessing resuscitative therapy in the absence of other traditional or invasive monitors. The anesthesiologist must rely on all sources of clinical information and consider the surgical context when dealing with an acute decrease in $EtCO_2$. (i.e., decreased cardiac output versus other causes such as air embolism or ventilator circuit leak). Additionally, ventilation-perfusion inhomogeneity, dead space processes, and $CO_2$ retention can evolve over time, potentially confounding interpretation of $EtCO_2$ trend monitoring. Nonetheless, as a last resort, $EtCO_2$ monitoring can be used momentarily to guide fluid and pressor therapy and assess adequacy of chest compressions or cardiac massage until more accurate invasive monitors can be implemented.

## Key points

- Effective monitoring of trauma patients should draw on all available data that can result from clinical assessment, the use of standard and invasive monitors, and serum markers of tissue perfusion.
- The decision to use invasive monitoring should be based on weighing the risks with the utility of the obtained data to guide fluid resuscitation and pharmacologic therapy.
- Intra-arterial catheters are frequently used in trauma patients and allow invasive blood pressure monitoring, intermittent blood draws, and assessment of volume status.
- Though not frequently used, $S_{\bar{v}}O2$ may be a useful resuscitation endpoint: further fluid resuscitation or surgical intervention may be indicated when $S_{\bar{v}}O_2 < 65\%$
- Dynamic monitors may become more common in the OR allowing assessment of recruitable cardiac output and reasonable prediction of patient response to fluid bolus.
- Monitoring of ICP may be indicated in patients suspected of having severe TBI.
- Serum markers such as lactate and base deficit allow monitoring of oxygen debt and hypoperfusion during resuscitation and may allow prediction of outcome.

## Further reading

1. Bendjelid K. System arterial pressure and fluid responsiveness: not only a swing story. *Crit Care Med* 2011;**39**:1579–1580.

2. Cavallaro F, Sandroni C, Antonelli M. Functional hemodynamic monitoring and dynamic indices of fluid responsiveness. *Minerva Anestesiol* 2008;**74**:123–135.

3. Giraud R, Siegenthaler N, Gayet-Ageron A, et al. ScvO2 as a marker to define fluid responsiveness. *J Trauma* 2011;**70**:802–807.

4. Marik PE, Cavallazzi R, Vasu T, Hirani A. Dynamic changes in arterial waveform derived variables and fluid responsiveness in mechanically ventilated patients: a systematic review of the literature. *Crit Care Med* 2009;**37**:2642–2647.

5. Napolitano LM. Resuscitative endpoints in trauma. *Transfus Altern Transfus Med* 2005;**6**:6–14.

6. Rivers EP, Ander DS, Powell D. Central venous oxygen saturation monitoring in the critically ill patient. *Curr Opin Crit Care* 2001;**7**:204–211.

7. Rivers EP, Nguyen B, Havstad S, et al. Early goal-directed therapy in the treatment of severe sepsis and septic shock. *N Engl J Med* 2001;**345**:1368–1377.

8. Shepherd SJ, Pearse RM. Role of central and mixed venous oxygen saturation measurement in perioperative care. *Anesthesiology* 2009;**111**:649–656.

9. Varon A. Arterial, central venous, and pulmonary artery catheters.

In: Civetta JM, Taylor RW, Kirby RR, eds. *Critical Care*, 3rd edition. Philadelphia, PA: Lippincott-Raven Publishers; 1997.

10. Varon AJ, Kirton OC, Civetta JM. Physiologic monitoring of the surgical patient. In: Schwartz SI, ed. *Principles of*

*Surgery*, 7th edition. New York, NY: McGraw-Hill; 1999.

11. Wilson M, Davis DP, Coimbra R. Diagnosis and monitoring of hemorrhagic shock during the initial resuscitation of multiple trauma patients: a review. *J Emerg Med* 2003;**24**:413–422.

Chapter

# 10

# Echocardiography in trauma

Ashraf Fayad and Michael Woo

## Introduction

Since the introduction of transesophageal echocardiography (TEE) as a monitor in the cardiac operating rooms (ORs) there have been changes, modifications, and expansion of the technology, as well as its clinical applications and indications. The introduction of innovations such as multi-plane and multi-frequency probes, Doppler techniques, and portable echocardiography machines has facilitated a broader range of clinical applications for echocardiography. In the cardiac OR, TEE is well established not only as a monitor for hemodynamic status, but also as an essential diagnostic tool. Following upon these advances, its introduction as a hemodynamic monitor in the management of high-risk patients presenting for non-cardiac surgery, including trauma patients, is a natural progression.

Echocardiography is a readily available monitor to evaluate biventricular function, volume status, and valvular function, and to detect cardiac emergencies such as tamponade and aortic disruption. Echocardiographic hemodynamic assessment is superior to the information derived from the pulmonary artery (PA) catheter, and is a sensitive tool with incremental clinical value over other monitors.

The benefits of limited ultrasound exams like focused assessment with sonography for trauma (FAST) are well described in emergency departments (EDs). A focused echocardiography examination is often sufficient to exclude major cardiovascular emergencies. In addition, echocardiography is a useful, sensitive, and low-cost procedure to evaluate patients with blunt thoracic trauma. Trauma patients may require an immediate surgical intervention and may sustain hemodynamic instability in the OR. Echocardiography, in particular the TEE modality, is an ideal monitoring tool to guide the perioperative management of the hypotensive patient who requires continuous resuscitation with fluid administration, blood transfusion, vasopressors, and inotropes in order to optimize organ perfusion. The purpose of this chapter is to highlight the clinical applications of echocardiography as a diagnostic and a monitoring tool in managing trauma patients undergoing non-cardiac surgical procedures.

## Indications for echocardiography in trauma patients requiring non-cardiac surgery

Transthoracic echocardiography (TTE) should be considered as an initial test to diagnose cardiac emergencies in trauma patients with hemodynamic instability. It should also be

*Essentials of Trauma Anesthesia*, ed. A. J. Varon and C. E. Smith. Published by Cambridge University Press.
© Cambridge University Press 2012.

**Table 10.1.** Indications for use of perioperative transesophageal echocardiography in trauma patients excluding cardiac surgical procedures

**Category I indications:**

– Intraoperative evaluation of acute, persistent, and life-threatening hemodynamics in which patients have not responded to treatment

– Preoperative use in unstable patients with suspected thoracic aortic dissection or disruption who need to be evaluated quickly

– Perioperative use in unstable patients with unexplained hemodynamic disturbance, suspected acute valve lesions, or any cardiac emergency

**Category II indications:**

– Perioperative use in trauma patients with increased risk of myocardial ischemia or infarction

– Perioperative use in patients with increased risk of hemodynamic disturbance

– Preoperative assessment of patients with suspected acute thoracic aortic dissection or disruption

– Intraoperative use during repair of descending thoracic aortic dissections

**Category III indications:**

– Intraoperative monitoring for emboli during orthopedic procedures

– Intraoperative assessment of repair of thoracic aortic injuries

– Intraoperative evaluation of pleuropulmonary diseases

– Right ventricular function assessment during major pulmonary resection

considered in patients with chest trauma. If a trauma patient is susceptible for hemodynamic instability and requires urgent surgery, TEE should be considered as an intraoperative monitor to guide hemodynamic management. Indications for perioperative TEE are classified into three evidence-based categories by the American Society of Anesthesiologists (ASA) and the Society of Cardiovascular Anesthesiologists (SCA). Category I indications are supported by the strongest evidence and expert opinion. Category II indications are supported by weak evidence and expert consensus. Category III indications have little current scientific or expert support; lack of evidence for category III indications is often owing to the absence of relevant studies rather than to existing evidence of ineffectiveness. In general, the commonest indication for echocardiography in trauma patients is to determine the cause of hypotension (Table 10.1). Awareness of the clinical indications to perform echocardiography exams may allow clinicians to perform TEE or TTE in a logical manner based on the mechanism of injury and perioperative course. In the 2010 practice guidelines update for perioperative TEE, the consultants and ASA members concluded the following:

- Agree that TEE should be used for non-cardiac surgical patients when the patient has known or suspected cardiovascular pathology that might result in hemodynamic, pulmonary, or neurologic compromise.
- Strongly agree that TEE should be used during unexplained persistent hypotension.
- Agree that TEE should be used when persistent unexplained hypoxemia occurs.
- Strongly agree that TEE should be used when life-threatening hypotension is anticipated.
- Agree that TEE should be used during major abdominal or thoracic trauma.

**Table 10.2.** Contraindications to the performance of TEE

| Medical conditions |
| --- |
| – Esophageal or mouth trauma |
| – Patient with unprotected airway |
| – Active upper gastrointestinal bleeding |
| – Patient's refusal |
| – Esophageal stricture or history of dysphagia |
| – Post-esophageal or gastric surgery |
| – Esophageal or gastric tumor |
| – Other esophageal/gastric diseases (e.g., Mallory-Weiss tear, scleroderma) |

- Are equivocal regarding the use of TEE during endovascular aortic procedures.
- Disagree with the assertion that TEE should be used during orthopedic surgery.

## Contraindications for TEE

TEE examination is considered a safe and relatively non-invasive procedure. However, proper patient assessment is warranted to exclude any contraindications to TEE probe placement. The overall rate of TEE-related morbidity ranges from 0.2 to 1.2%. Conditions that are considered contraindications to TEE probe insertion are listed in Table 10.2.

In patients with contraindications to TEE insertion or for whom there has been an unsuccessful attempt at probe insertion, TTE as an alternative echocardiography modality may be considered.

## Clinical applications of echocardiography in trauma patients

Clinical applications of echocardiography can be divided into diagnostic and monitoring applications.

### Diagnostic applications

The initial diagnostic advantage of echocardiography in trauma patients involves the TTE modality rather than the TEE. However, TEE could be the best diagnostic modality in detecting thoracic aortic dissection and the extension of cardiac trauma lesions. TTE has been used as part of the FAST examination since the 1970s in Germany and Japan. FAST is a non-invasive bedside ultrasound examination performed in trauma patients to identify pneumohemothorax, pericardial effusion, and intra-abdominal hemorrhage. It became more widespread in the United States and the United Kingdom in the 1980s and has evolved rapidly with the advent of affordable high-quality portable ultrasound machines. Point-of-care ultrasonography or FAST is now part of the Advanced Trauma Life Support (ATLS) protocols by the American College of Surgeons. It has evolved from simply identifying free fluid to the non-invasive assessment of shock and guiding therapy accordingly. Point-of-care ultrasonography is also becoming an integral part of many trauma units in North America. Many trauma centers that adopted this technology have developed different protocols including the Rapid Ultrasound for Shock and Hypotension (RUSH)

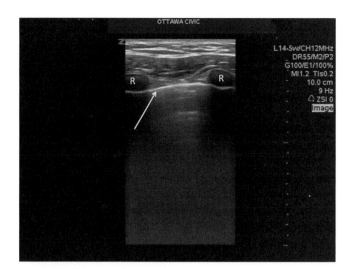

**Figure 10.1.** Rib shadows (R) above and below. The pleura is seen as a white line (arrow) and lung granular appearance below.

and Abdominal Cardiac Evaluation with Sonography in Shock (ACES) to improve diagnostic certainty and guide patient management.

The following conditions may be diagnosed with the initial echocardiography scan to exclude life-threatening conditions such as hemopneumothorax, cardiac tamponade, aortic dissection, hypovolemia, myocardial contusion, and valvular regurgitation.

## Pneumothorax

The FAST exam has expanded to include assessment for pneumothorax. It was first described in 1986 and it is best referred to as the extended FAST or eFAST. The eFAST enables the clinician to rule out a pneumothorax with a sensitivity of 90.9% and a specificity of 98.2% compared with chest X-ray (CXR) sensitivity of 50.2% and specificity of 99.4%. The presence of subcutaneous emphysema may obscure the ultrasound images and make interpretation unreliable.

A low or high frequency transducer is applied to the chest, usually in the mid-clavicular line at the third to fourth intercostal space in the longitudinal plane with the marker pointed towards the head of the patient. The clinician needs to identify the presence of lung sliding and/or comet tails in a dynamic fashion at the pleural line where the visceral and parietal pleura meet (Figure 10.1). Once the pleural space is identified and examined, motion (M) mode imaging modality is useful in confirming the presence or the absence of a pneumothorax. In the absence of pneumothorax, M mode generates a distinct pattern called the seashore sign (Figure 10.2). If one of these sonographic signs is present, then pneumothorax can be ruled out in most cases. Trauma patients with pleural adhesion, pulmonary contusion, lung fibrosis, pulmonary bullous diseases, and acute respiratory distress syndrome (ARDS) may not show the lung sliding signs.

## Hemothorax

Ultrasound is a sensitive and specific diagnostic modality in detecting hemothorax. The fluid/blood level is easily detected as an echogenic (black) area with ultrasound techniques. Ultrasonography detects volumes of $\geq$ 20 mL, versus 200 mL on CXR. Hemothorax in trauma patients can be identified with point-of-care ultrasonography during the initial contact with the patient in the ED. Once diagnosed, a clinical decision is made on whether a

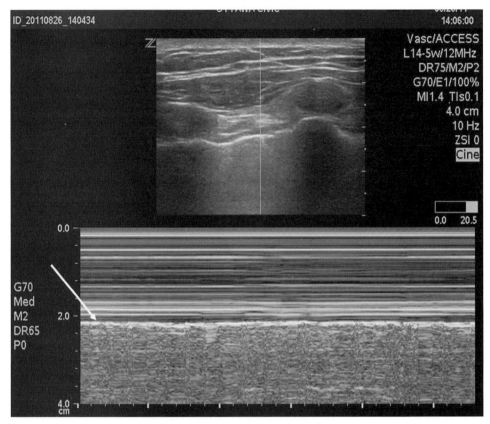

**Figure 10.2.** M-mode image demonstrates a linear, laminar pattern in the tissue superficial to the pleural line (arrow) and a granular or "sandy" appearance below the pleural line (seashore sign).

chest tube insertion is required or observation and follow-up (see Chapter 16). Ultrasonography is used to assist safe insertion of the chest tube away from any solid organ or lungs and ensure its correct position. If the patient is to undergo emergency surgery, TEE can be used to observe the hemothorax for any expansion and guide intraoperative management.

The low frequency transducer is placed in a longitudinal plane in the mid-axillary line at the level of the xiphoid with the marker pointed towards the head of the patient. At this point, the diaphragm can be visualized with the solid organs (liver/spleen) below the diaphragm. Hemothorax is diagnosed as presence of a black area above the diaphragm in the most dependent area. If TEE is utilized, the hemothorax is visualized as an echo-free space posterior to the descending thoracic aorta (Figure 10.3).

### Pericardial effusion and cardiac tamponade

Pericardial effusion is visualized on echocardiography as an echo-free space in the pericardial sac. Early recognition of this life-threatening condition with TTE at the initial contact in a hypotensive trauma patient facilitates proper intervention (see Chapter 16). TTE enables the clinician to perform pericardiocentesis under ultrasound guidance using the subcostal or apical view to temporize the situation as a preparation for the definitive surgical treatment in the OR.

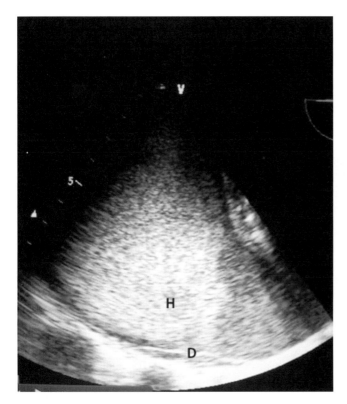

**Figure 10.3.** Transesophageal echocardiography (TEE) image of right hemothorax. Blood (hemothorax) collected at the costo-phrenic angle (H) and lower right chest above the diaphragm (D).

**Table 10.3.** Size of pericardial effusion

| Size | Width | Amount of fluid |
|------|-------|-----------------|
| Small | <1 cm, localized | < 100 mL |
| Moderate | 1–2 cm, circumferential | 100–500 mL |
| Large | >2 cm, circumferential | > 500 mL |

The volume of pericardial fluid can be estimated based on the width of the pericardial sac as in Table 10.3.

Pericardial tamponade is a clinical diagnosis that occurs when the pericardial effusion pressure exceeds the intracardiac pressure. In a patient with chest trauma, cardiac tamponade is suspected when there is persistent hypotension, tachycardia, pulsus paradoxus, and distended jugular veins. The sonographic features of cardiac tamponade include the following:

- Presence of pericardial effusion.
- Right atrial systolic collapse.
- Right ventricular (RV) diastolic collapse.

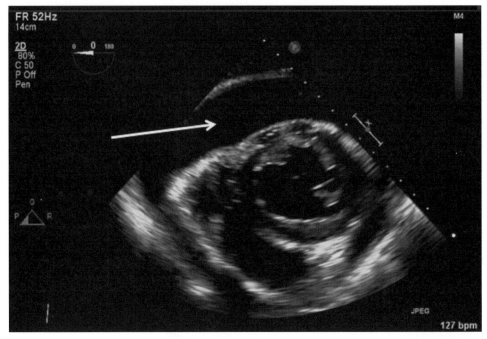

**Figure 10.4.** Transgastric short axis transesophageal echocardiography (TEE) view of the left ventricle shows significant pericardial effusion (arrow).

- Inferior vena cava (IVC) plethora: dilated IVC without the usual partial collapse during inspiration in spontaneously breathing patients.
- Respiratory variation in RV and left ventricular (LV) dimensions: an exaggeration of the normal RV and LV variations during respiratory cycle in spontaneously breathing patients (normally, during inspiration, there is an increase in the RV volume and dimension and a reduction in the LV volume and dimension).
- Respiratory variation in pulmonic and tricuspid flow velocities (Doppler waves): a significant increase in the tricuspid and pulmonic peak velocities during inspiration.

In patients with cardiac tamponade receiving positive pressure ventilation, the echocardiographic signs related to respiratory variation may be reversed.

With TTE, pericardial effusion is best viewed through the subxiphoid approach using a low frequency phased array transducer. The probe is placed just below the xiphoid, turned cephalic and positioned almost parallel to the abdomen in a supine position patient. Other images that can be acquired include the parasternal long axis and the apical four chamber views. If TEE is used, midesophageal and transgastric views are obtained to diagnose pericardial effusion (Figure 10.4). Direct visualization of the needle to aspirate the pericardial effusion, if required, can be achieved using TEE transgastric views.

### Aortic dissection

Blunt chest trauma is a common cause of aortic injury in previously healthy subjects. Aortic dissection is a life-threatening condition that requires rapid diagnosis and treatment (see Chapter 16). Depending on patient factors, operator skill, and location of injury, traumatic

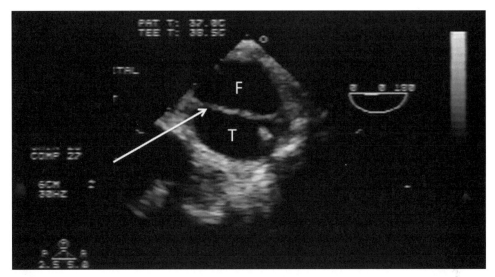

**Figure 10.5.** Transesophageal echocardiography (TEE) short axis image of the descending thoracic aorta with aortic dissection. The intimal flap (arrow) divides the aorta into false lumen (F) and true lumen (T).

aortic dissections may be visualized by TTE using the suprasternal approach. However, TEE has the advantage of being closer to the aorta and a more accurate diagnosis can be made. The sensitivity of TEE to diagnose thoracic aortic dissection approaches 100%. Diagnosis of aortic dissection is based on the identification of the intimal flap that divides the aorta into false and true lumens (Figure 10.5). Color flow Doppler (CFD) is used to identify the entry and exit site between the two lumens. The echocardiography exam is further used to detect aortic insufficiency (AI) and any involvement of the coronary artery ostia as a result of the dissection. Clinical presentation of significant blunt trauma to the chest that is associated with back pain is suggestive of aortic dissection and should prompt the initiation of a TEE exam in hemodynamically stable patients. The portability of the echocardiography machine and the short scan time required to detect aortic dissection are great advantages of TEE over other imaging techniques. Early surgical intervention may be required and TEE may be utilized to guide stent deployment for endovascular repair or assess the results of open surgical repair. Computed tomographic (CT) scan is also evolving as one of the best imaging modalities, with sensitivity approaching 100% to detect aortic dissection. It provides the ability to image the entire aorta, including abdominal aorta and aortic arch. However, scanning may require a longer time to perform and information regarding aortic valve involvement may be lacking. Echocardiography skills, if available, represent a reliable and practical diagnostic tool of thoracic aorta dissection in the perioperative setting.

### Hypovolemia, myocardial contusion (injury to the cardiac myocardium), and valvular regurgitation

The initial TTE scanning in unstable patients is used to determine other potential cardiac causes of hypotension including hypovolemia, regional wall motion abnormalities (RWMA), reduced myocardial contractility, and valvular lesions.

Echocardiography is superior to other diagnostic tools to detect hypovolemia. Rapid TTE parasternal or apical scanning can easily identify hypovolemia. If the TEE modality is

**Table 10.4.** Correlation between IVC diameter and CVP

| Size (cm) | Collapsibility with inspiration | CVP (mmHg) |
|---|---|---|
| Small < 1.5 | 100% | 0–5 |
| Normal 1.5–2.5 | 50% | 5–10 |
| Dilated > 2.5 | 50% | 15–20 |
| Dilated > 2.5 | 0%. With dilated hepatic veins | > 20 |

employed, transgastric views of the LV cavity are preferred to estimate volume status and monitor the response to fluid therapy. Assessment of IVC diameter provides a good indication of the patient's volume status and an estimation of central venous pressure (CVP) (Table 10.4).

With myocardial contusion, the RV and right atrium (RA) are more commonly affected than the LV and left atrium (LA). Rapid TTE scanning of the LV provides a rough idea of LV systolic function. Detection of RWMA at the initial TTE scanning may be obvious. However, in a controlled environment like the OR, recognition of RWMA is easier.

The presence of acute severe valvular regurgitation or insufficiency in patients who sustained chest trauma may result in hemodynamic instability. Early recognition of the lesion by echocardiography facilitates appropriate patient management and surgical intervention.

Trauma patients at risk of hemodynamic instability due to hypovolemia, focal and global ventricular dysfunction, or valvular insufficiency may require surgical intervention for non-cardiac injuries. Utilization of echocardiography as a perioperative monitoring tool may be of value in these situations.

## Monitoring applications

For patients who require emergency or urgent surgical procedures, echocardiography may be used as a monitoring tool to guide perioperative management. The monitoring applications of echocardiography can be divided into general and specific. The specific applications are related to either certain surgical procedures (e.g., endovascular thoracic aortic aneurysm repair) or presence of specific cardiac lesions.

### Volume status

Preload and volume status assessment are crucial elements for successful hemodynamic management. The amount of intravenous (IV) fluid administration in trauma patients may present a challenge to ED and perioperative physicians. Both hypovolemia and excessive fluid therapy result in higher morbidity in surgical patients. Based on injury severity, trauma patients may show undesirable fluid shifts and bleeding that make the need for precise fluid resuscitation an important component of their care. Invasive and non-invasive hemodynamic monitors are used to provide guidance for the IV fluid administration in trauma patients undergoing surgical procedures (see Chapter 9). There is developing evidence to demonstrate the benefits of goal-directed fluid therapy to improve outcomes during major surgery. Further, blood pressure restoration by means of vasopressors in hypovolemic patients may lead to a reduction in organ blood flow and metabolic acidosis.

Echocardiography represents an accurate and practical tool to guide goal-directed fluid therapy. Echocardiography can rapidly estimate the LV volume by examining changes in LV size. The LV transgastric short axis (SAX) mid-papillary view is the most commonly used view to estimate LV volume. Obliteration of the LV cavity during systole indicates severe hypovolemia. In addition, respiratory variation of the IVC diameter measured in the transgastric view is another indicator of the volume status. The correlation between IVC diameter and the estimated CVP is shown in Table 10.4. The superior vena cava diameter is also useful in assessing preload.

## Ventricular function

Reduction in ventricular function is not uncommon in trauma patients. It may be a result of myocardial contusion, metabolic acidosis, myocardial hypoperfusion, or other pathology. Echocardiography is a real-time monitor for both RV and LV function. Ventricular dysfunction may present in the form of acute systolic or diastolic dysfunction or both. Echocardiography can be used to identify diastolic or systolic failure in hemodynamically unstable patients, and can determine if it involves either or both ventricles. Hemodynamic instability due to acute systolic dysfunction occurs in a significant percentage of trauma patients undergoing emergency or urgent surgery. A quick "eyeball method" by a trained echocardiographer can rapidly determine the LV systolic function and estimation of the LV ejection fraction is easily obtained. If LV systolic dysfunction is diagnosed, titration of inotropes can be started and ventricular response can be closely monitored by echocardiography. An increase in the afterload produced by administering vasopressors to restore blood pressure can significantly reduce LV contractility and unmask LV dysfunction.

When trauma patients become hemodynamically unstable despite normal preload and contractility, diastolic dysfunction may be considered. Diastolic parameters can be examined using Doppler techniques such as transmitral flow, pulmonary venous flow, and tissue Doppler. Acute diastolic dysfunction of the LV during aortic cross clamping has been reported and resulted in hemodynamic instability. RV dysfunction has also been reported to cause significant hemodynamic instability. Pulmonary embolism, pneumothorax, hemothorax, pericardial effusion, hypoxia, or acidosis may result in acute RV failure. Echocardiographic signs of RV failure include the following:

- Hypokinesis
- Abnormal septal shape and motion
- Loss of the RV triangle shape
- Reduced tricuspid annular plane systolic excursion

If treatment is initiated to reduce RV afterload, echocardiography can be used to determine if the treatment is effective or dose adjustment is required.

## Myocardial ischemia and RWMAs

Patients who sustain major trauma may be at risk of myocardial ischemia and infarction. Early detection and treatment of myocardial ischemia could be crucial for patient management. Echocardiography is a well-recognized sensitive monitor for perioperative myocardial ischemia detection. Analysis of LV segmental function is based on assessment of wall motion and thickening during systole. During the echocardiography study, the LV is divided into 16 segments as recommended by the American Society of Echocardiography to allow accurate examination of the LV walls and documentation of any abnormal wall motion or wall thickening. It also allows identification of affected coronary artery territories. The transgastric mid-papillary SAX view of the LV can detect RWMAs of each major coronary artery territory and is therefore a popular view among echocardiographers for monitoring RWMAs. A standard grading scale for describing regional wall motion is normal (0), hypokinetic (1), akinetic (2), or dyskinetic (3). With evolving technology, speckle-tracking echocardiography (STE) may provide a means of more accurately quantifying wall movement and assessing LV global and regional function. By analyzing speckle motion, STE can assess LV motion in multiple planes (longitudinal, radial, torsion, twist) and measure myocardial tissue velocity, strain, and strain rate independently of cardiac translation and beam angle. Once a new RWMA is detected, treatment can be started and monitored by echocardiography. If RWMA is persistent and not responding to treatment, it may indicate myocardial infarction. Detection of new-onset mitral regurgitation (MR) or an increase in the degree of preexisting MR may represent early echocardiographic features of myocardial ischemia.

### Valvular lesions

Acute valvular regurgitation may occur as a result of direct chest trauma in a patient requiring urgent or emergency non-cardiac surgery. In this case, the TEE is not focused only on identifying the pathology, but rather on monitoring the hemodynamics, adequacy of cardiac output (CO) and forward stroke volume, and the amount of regurgitant volume. Measures should be taken to maximize CO and minimize the regurgitant volume. Acute hemodynamic instability caused by severe regurgitation of the mitral and aortic valves has been reported. New development of severe MR in the perioperative period may occur due to myocardial ischemia or infarction and result in cardiogenic shock. The response to medical treatment can be closely monitored by TEE.

### Assessment of CO and hemodynamic monitoring

Perioperative goal-directed fluid management and optimization of the preload is easily achieved by continuous TEE LV monitoring. Perioperative management in severely compromised patients or patients in shock is a challenging task and requires a reliable monitoring tool to ensure adequate CO. Monitoring the changes in CO in response to clinical interventions remains a key component of hemodynamic management in trauma patients. With the ability to measure CO and assess the response to therapy, echocardiography is becoming the monitor of choice particularly with the declining usage of PA catheters. Left-sided CO can be measured utilizing a combined 2D (LV outflow tract diameter) and CFD (aortic valve) technique. Although more technically challenging, right-sided CO can similarly be estimated by measuring the pulmonary valve velocity time integral and the 2D RV outflow diameter.

### Intracardiac and intrapulmonary shunting

Shunting due to trauma to the chest has been reported. Also, trauma patients with existent shunting may present for urgent surgical procedures. Persistent hypotension, hypoxia, and acidosis precipitate right to left shunt and result in hemodynamic instability or refractory hypoxemia. Urgent cardiac surgery to repair the defect may be required. However, patients with shunting may sustain other non-cardiac injuries and require urgent non-cardiac procedures. Echocardiography is used to identify the shunt and monitor the results of measures taken to minimize it. CFD and agitated saline contrast are mainly used for both diagnosis and monitoring of the shunt fraction. In the non-trauma setting, atrial septal defect (ASD) or patent foramen ovale (PFO) are the most common causes of shunting. Right to left shunting may also occur in the presence of pulmonary arteriovenous fistulas. The presence of an ASD or PFO may increase the risk of paradoxical embolization or hypoxemia particularly during trauma procedures. In trauma patients, the risk of hypoxemia is increased in the setting of increased right-sided pressures, acidosis, systemic hypotension, and hypoventilation.

### Pulmonary emboli; air and fat emboli monitoring

Multiple factors may lead to coagulopathy and thromboembolic events in trauma patients. Pulmonary embolism (PE) may lead to hemodynamic instability, morbidity, and mortality. Echocardiography is a specific and reliable tool compared to other perioperative monitors like precordial Doppler and end-tidal carbon dioxide in the diagnosis of intraoperative PE. Intraoperative TEE may permit direct visualization of PE in transit, or secondary signs of high RV afterload. The use of intraoperative TEE to monitor air and fat embolism in both neurosurgery and orthopedic surgery has been described.

## Performance of the perioperative echocardiography exam

Performance of the perioperative echocardiography exam as a baseline assessment follows the same steps as the comprehensive intraoperative TEE exam recommended by the ASE/SCA task force. However, in hemodynamically unstable patients, echocardiography should focus primarily on examining ventricular function and preload conditions.

The following six questions need to be answered:

1. What is the volume status? Is the heart full or empty?
2. Are the LV and RV contracting adequately?
3. Are there RWMAs?
4. Is there a significant valvular lesion?
5. Is there significant pericardial effusion?
6. Is there a significant hemothorax or pneumothorax?

A focused examination to assess the hemodynamics may be achieved with a limited number of views. The clinician should be familiar with the nomenclature and terminology used during the echocardiography exam.

The TTE examination, if performed, should include the standard three window views (see Figure 10.6):

- Parasternal view (long axis [LAX] and SAX)
- Apical window (4/5 chamber views, LAX two-chamber, LAX three-chamber)
- Subcostal window (LAX and SAX)

Once the patient is stabilized, a full comprehensive TEE exam can be performed, including assessment of the aorta. The TEE comprehensive exam consists of 20 cross-sectional views. Those views apply for 2D echocardiography techniques. Because of the patient's position, anatomic variations, pathology, and comorbidity, not all views can be obtained in all subjects. CFD, spectral Doppler, M-mode, and others are used as required. The sequences of obtaining the views may vary from one examiner to the other.

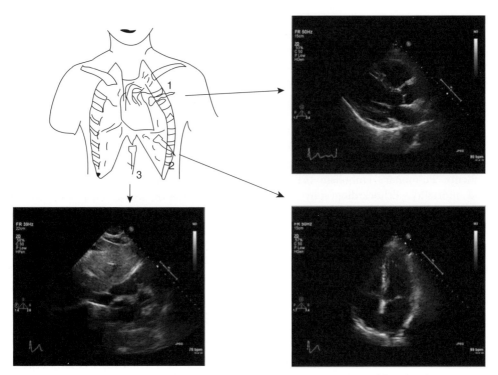

**Figure 10.6.** Focused echocardiography exam. (1) Parasternal long axis view. (2) Apical four-chamber view. (3) Subcostal view.

An echocardiography report should be produced for all studies. The perioperative echocardiography exam report should be marked as such with its indication. A summary of the case and hemodynamic management may be added to the report with the supporting images.

## Conclusions

Initial echocardiographic scanning and continuation of perioperative echocardiography utilization in trauma patients offer a unique means of real-time cardiovascular assessment with a wide variety of clinical applications. Echocardiography should be considered as the diagnostic tool of choice in trauma patients with hemodynamic instability or chest trauma. It should also be considered as the hemodynamic monitor of choice in trauma patients undergoing urgent surgery and at risk of perioperative hemodynamic instability. Trauma centers should exert efforts to ensure that echocardiography technology is readily available in the surgical suites to provide evaluation of unexplained hemodynamic instability and to evaluate cardiac emergencies. Training is required to perform echocardiography, as misinterpretation of an echocardiographic study can have catastrophic implications on hemodynamic goal-directed patient management.

Echocardiography in EDs and ORs is relatively novel, and it is anticipated to have a rapidly expanding role in the management of trauma patients and patients with hemodynamic instability undergoing non-cardiac procedures. Residency training programs should consider adopting training in echocardiography as part of the postgraduate curricula.

# Key points

- Echocardiography is a valuable diagnostic and monitoring tool in trauma patients.
- Echocardiography provides a real-time cardiovascular assessment and facilitates management.
- FAST, FOCUS, and limited echocardiographic exams offer early detection of life-threatening pathology and may alter patient management.
- Echocardiography should be considered as the hemodynamic monitor of choice in trauma patients undergoing emergency surgery and at risk of perioperative hemodynamic instability.
- Proper training in echocardiography is required to utilize this technology.

## Further reading

1. Atkinson PR, McAuley DJ, Kendall RJ, et al. Abdominal and Cardiac Evaluation with Sonography in Shock (ACES): an approach by emergency physicians for the use of ultrasound in patients with undifferentiated hypotension. *Emerg Med J* 2009;**26**:87–91.

2. Boulanger BR, Brenneman FD, McLellan BA, et al. A prospective study of emergent abdominal sonography after blunt trauma. *J Trauma* 1995;**39**:325–330.

3. Darmon PL, Hillel Z, Mogtader A, Mindich B, Thys D. Cardiac output by transesophageal echocardiography using continuous-wave Doppler across the aortic valve. *Anesthesiology* 1994;**80**:796–805.

4. Fayad A, Yang H, Nathan H, Bryson GL, Cina CS. Acute diastolic dysfunction in thoracoabdominal aortic aneurysm surgery. *Can J Anaesth* 2006;**53**:168–173.

5. Jamet B, Chabert JP, Metz D, Elaerts J. [Acute aortic insufficiency]. *Ann Cardiol Angeiol (Paris)* 2000;**49**:183–186.

6. Jhanji S, Vivian-Smith A, Lucena-Amaro S, et al. Haemodynamic optimisation improves tissue microvascular flow and oxygenation after major surgery: a randomised controlled trial. *Crit Care* 2010;**14**:R151.

7. Hiratzka LF, Bakris GL, Beckman JA, et al. 2010 ACCF/AHA/AATS/ACR/ASA/SCA/ SCAI/SIR/STS/SVM guidelines for the diagnosis and management of patients with Thoracic Aortic Disease: a report of the American College of Cardiology Foundation/American Heart Association Task Force on Practice Guidelines, American Association for Thoracic Surgery, American College of Radiology, American Stroke Association, Society of Cardiovascular Anesthesiologists, Society for Cardiovascular Angiography and Interventions, Society of Interventional Radiology, Society of Thoracic Surgeons, and Society for Vascular Medicine. *Circulation* 2010;**121**:266–369.

8. Mueller X, Stauffer JC, Jaussi A, Goy JJ, Kappenberger L. Subjective visual echocardiographic estimate of left ventricular ejection fraction as an alternative to conventional echocardiographic methods: comparison with contrast angiography. *Clin Cardiol* 1991;**14**:898–902.

9. Osterwalder JJ. Update FAST. *Praxix (Bern 1994)* 2010;**99**:1545–1549.

10. Perera P, Mailhot T, Riley D, Mandavia D. The RUSH exam: Rapid Ultrasound in SHock in the evaluation of the critically ill. *Emerg Med Clin North Am* 2010;**28**:29–56.

11. Practice guidelines for perioperative transesophageal echocardiography. A report by the American Society of Anesthesiologists and the Society of Cardiovascular Anesthesiologists Task Force on Transesophageal Echocardiography. *Anesthesiology* 1996;**84**:986–1006.

12. Practice guidelines for perioperative transesophageal echocardiography. An updated report by the American Society of Anesthesiologists and the Society of Cardiovascular Anesthesiologists Task Force on Transesophageal Echocardiography. *Anesthesiology* 2010;**112**:1084–1096.

13. Shanewise JS, Cheung AT, Aronson S, et al. ASE/SCA guidelines for performing a comprehensive intraoperative multiplane transesophageal echocardiography examination: recommendations of the American Society of Echocardiography Council for Intraoperative Echocardiography and the Society of Cardiovascular Anesthesiologists Task Force for Certification in Perioperative Transesophageal Echocardiography. *Anesth Analg* 1999;**89**:870–884.

# Postoperative care of the trauma patient

Brandon A. Van Noord, Scott Margraf, and Jeb Kucik

Given the significant physiologic responses that often accompany severe trauma, postoperative trauma care must be an organized and coherent team effort. While the postanesthesia care unit (PACU) may be utilized for patients deemed stable enough for extubation following surgery, care will often take place in the intensive care unit (ICU). The trauma anesthesiologist must be as facile in the PACU and ICU environments as in the operating room (OR). Adequate monitoring and prevention of complications are the keys to postoperative management. If the patient is awake and alert, a more detailed medical history should be obtained to elucidate injury mechanism. A tertiary survey must be performed to rule out occult injuries. Important postoperative considerations, organized by organ system, will be discussed in this chapter.

## Neurologic considerations

Delayed emergence should be investigated if a patient fails to regain a normal level of consciousness within an hour following general anesthesia. Whenever possible, proper investigation should begin with a thorough history. Preoperative mental status should be reviewed, keeping in mind that intoxication or preexisting dysfunction are possible etiologies.

Of note, lingering sedation may be attributable to the residual effects of intraoperative medication. Opiates result in dose-dependent bradypnea. In such cases, naloxone may be used cautiously and titrated to optimal effect. Naloxone use in patients who are hypovolemic, hypotensive, or have previously experienced severe pain or stress may result in catecholamine-mediated arrhythmias, vasoconstriction, and pulmonary edema from systemic-to-pulmonary vascular fluid shifts. When using bolus administration, vigilance for re-narcotization must be maintained. Benzodiazepines can be reversed with flumazenil (0.2 mg to 1 mg given at 0.2 mg/min). To avoid unintended re-sedation, doses may need to be repeated every 20 minutes, but no more than 3 mg should be given in any one hour. Prolonged weakness, secondary to residual neuromuscular block, inadequate reversal or neuromuscular disease, including ICU-acquired weakness, or phase II block from succinylcholine (e.g., plasma cholinesterase deficiency), may masquerade as persistent sedation and can be evaluated with a peripheral nerve stimulator using train-of-four monitoring.

If the patient's perioperative record and neuromuscular blockade monitoring fail to explain the decreased level of consciousness, or appropriate rescue medications are unsuccessful, the potential for untoward intraoperative events should be investigated. Neurologic complications such as postictal state, stroke, anoxic brain injury, or traumatic brain injury are possible after trauma and should be investigated with electroencephalogram or brain computed tomography imaging, and appropriate consultation. Additional etiologies for postoperative neurological deficit include metabolic abnormalities (adrenal gland, electrolyte, or glucose), respiratory failure, hypothermia, and systemic inflammatory response syndrome (SIRS).

While delirium may affect all ages, it most often occurs in children and the elderly. Supportive measures, such as verbal orientation, or having family members present at the bedside, are typically effective. Pain and anxiety are classical causes of agitation and confusion, and underscore the importance of early postoperative analgesia as well as global evaluation for sources of discomfort unrelated to the surgical site (e.g., urinary urgency, gastric distension, nausea, corneal abrasions, infiltrated intravenous [IV] sites, or positioning problems). Though postoperative sequelae may not be elicited in the aged until months following surgery, and while these may be related to normal aging, elderly patients frequently suffer cognitive deficits postoperatively (see also Chapter 21). Finally, increased metabolic demands, coupled with the constant sensory input and the repetitive procedures of a modern ICU, may quickly contribute to ICU-acquired delirium. Whenever possible, sleep hygiene and sedation should be optimized to ensure adequate rest.

## Postoperative pain

In the postoperative period, analgesia is best provided using multi-modal therapies to provide synergistic pain control while minimizing opiate-related side effects. Analgesic therapy may include the following:

- Hydromorphone is usually the preferred opiate, as it causes less histamine release than morphine and does not produce an active metabolite. Peak effect typically occurs after 10–20 minutes with 4–6 hour duration.
- For awake, cooperative patients, patient-controlled analgesia (PCA) is superior to medication delivered on either fixed or as needed schedules. PCA empowers patients, decreases the amount of time spent in pain, and improves pain control. However, care must be taken while programming the device to prevent over- or under-dosing.
- Ketorolac is currently the only parenteral non-steroidal anti-inflammatory drug (NSAID) currently available in the United States. Potential adverse effects include nephrotoxicity, gastric ulceration, and bleeding. Therefore, special care should be taken in elderly and hypovolemic patients and use should not exceed five days. Unlike opioids, there is a therapeutic ceiling beyond which increasing NSAID dose results in no additional pain relief.
- The maximum recommended daily dose of acetaminophen has recently been changed from 4000 to 3000 mg and special care should be taken when administering to patients with hepatic dysfunction. A parenteral formulation has recently been approved.
- Ketamine is a dissociative anesthetic that antagonizes the N-methyl-D-aspartate (NMDA) receptor. Low doses decrease opiate requirements and prevent opiate-induced hyperalgesia. Of the same class of drugs as phencyclidine (PCP), high-dose administration of ketamine may induce hallucinations.
- Regional anesthesia is infrequently used in the ICU due to infection and coagulopathy concerns. An exception may be warranted in patients with multiple rib fractures since thoracic epidural analgesia decreases mortality compared with IV analgesia (see Chapter 16).

# Pulmonary considerations

Occult pulmonary injuries may go unrecognized and untreated in the OR; pulmonary dysfunction may also develop during convalescence.

- Dead space or wasted ventilation occurs when lung parenchyma is inadequately perfused. An immobile patient with traumatic injury is at high risk for pulmonary embolization secondary to venous stasis and endothelial injury. While fat embolization can occur with any major fracture, it is most common following pelvic and long-bone fractures.

- Intrapulmonary shunt results from inadequate ventilation and commonly occurs following trauma.

  - Postoperative atelectasis frequently occurs due to bronchial obstruction from edema, secretions, or blood.

  - Perioperative airway obstruction (e.g., laryngospasm) can result in postobstructive ("negative pressure") pulmonary edema due to decreased interstitial hydrostatic pressure.

  - Head injury resulting in increased intracranial pressure can lead to neurogenic pulmonary edema. While the etiology is poorly understood, it may result from massive sympathetic discharge.

  - Patients with preexisting cardiovascular disease and high pulmonary artery pressures are predisposed to cardiogenic pulmonary edema. This often occurs within an hour of surgery completion.

  - Inflammation from trauma, massive transfusion, disseminated intravascular coagulation, sepsis, and aspiration may all increase capillary permeability and result in fluid translocation from pulmonary capillaries to the alveoli via the interstitial space. Subsequent pulmonary edema decreases forced vital capacity.

  - Acute respiratory distress syndrome (ARDS), acute respiratory failure without evidence of left heart failure, is defined by an arterial oxygen tension to inspired oxygen concentration ratio ($PaO_2/FiO_2$) < 200. The chest radiograph will demonstrate bilateral infiltrates. Acute lung injury (ALI), a less-severe form, is defined by $PaO_2/FiO_2$ < 300. For example, an $FiO_2$ of 45% in ARDS and 30% in ALI would be required to maintain a $PaO_2$ of 90 mmHg. Treatment involves ventilatory support and addressing underlying etiology. Euvolemia or slight hypervolemia should also be maintained. Permissive hypercapnia may be necessary to facilitate the lung protective ventilation strategies discussed below.

# Ventilatory support

In the severely injured patient, or when staged damage control surgery is planned, patients may remain tracheally intubated. Additionally, tracheal intubation and mechanical ventilation may be initiated in the ICU for airway protection, or when hypoxemia persists despite administering maximal $FiO_2$ non-invasively.

## Level of support

Unless the work of breathing is exceedingly high or there is extreme difficulty in achieving adequate gas exchange, partial ventilatory support (e.g., assist control, synchronized intermittent mandatory ventilation, and pressure support), in which mechanically delivered breaths are triggered by the patient, is preferred over full ventilatory support (e.g., volume control and pressure control) during trauma convalescence. Partial support decreases sedation and neuromuscular relaxation requirements, and maintains a respiratory pattern that more closely approximates normal physiology. Spontaneous respiration improves ventilation/perfusion mismatching and cardiac output. The following are initial recommended settings:

- Tidal volumes 6–8 mL/kg to prevent alveolar overdistension.
- Positive end-expiratory pressure (PEEP) higher than the lower inflection point on the pressure-volume curve to preserve intrinsic physiologic PEEP and prevent atelectatic trauma.
- Plateau pressure < 35 mmHg to prevent barotrauma.
- If respiratory rate and inspiratory:expiratory ratio adjustment does not achieve the above goals, hypercapnia may be tolerated.
- Though oxygen toxicity is unlikely in adults, $FiO_2$ should gradually be decreased as tolerated.

Although mechanical ventilation is often life-saving, complications are possible and include:

- Atelectasis primarily occurs due to alveolar compression in the supine position. PEEP, frequent turning, suctioning, chest physiotherapy, recruitment maneuvers, and intermittent prone positioning can all be used to treat or prevent atelectasis. High $FiO_2$ may paradoxically contribute to hypoxemia through the mechanism of absorption atelectasis.
- Ventilator-associated lung injury may occur from alveolar overdistension and from repeated opening and closing of the alveoli (atelectrauma).
- Oxygen toxicity results in free radical induced pulmonary damage. Unless limited by other considerations such as head injury, most practitioners seek a target $PaO_2$ of 80 mmHg.
- Positive pressure ventilation increases intrathoracic pressure and decreases venous return. High intrathoracic pressures transmitted to the pulmonary vasculature result in increased pulmonary vascular resistance. Downstream physiologic effects include increased right ventricular (RV) afterload, decreased RV ejection fraction, and decreased left ventricular (LV) filling. These effects can be mitigated through intravascular volume loading, although special care must be taken in patients with congestive heart failure or chronic renal failure.
- Appropriate preventive measures have decreased the incidence of ventilator-associated pneumonia (see Infection and sepsis section below).
- Subglottic stenosis risk increases after 10–14 days of intubation.

## Cardiovascular considerations

Following massive trauma, hypotension is most likely due to hemorrhagic shock. Source control (i.e., surgical correction of the bleeding) should be addressed in addition to assessment of the adequacy of resuscitation. Other possible shock etiologies are obstructive (pericardial tamponade or tension pneumothorax), cardiogenic (blunt cardiac injury, arrhythmia, or myocardial infarction), distributive (SIRS/sepsis), and neurogenic (high spinal cord injury).

Arrhythmias in trauma patients often occur secondary to nociception and increased catecholamine discharge, blunt cardiac injury, drug ingestion, hypoxemia, hypercarbia, electrolyte disturbances, or myocardial ischemia. When treating sinus tachycardia, the underlying etiology should be elucidated before beginning empiric treatment. Current Advanced Cardiac Life Support (ACLS) guidelines should be followed.

Traumatic insult or underlying coronary artery disease (CAD) may result in myocardial infarction. When postoperative coronary perfusion pressure (aortic diastolic blood pressure – LV end-diastolic pressure) is decreased by vasodilation from re-warming or inflammatory mediators, vasopressors may be needed. As symptomatic angina is rare in the PACU due to lingering anesthetic effects, hypotension or ventricular arrhythmias (e.g., premature ventricular contractions, ventricular tachycardia) may be the only presenting signs of myocardial infarction. Furthermore, 10 to 30% of electrocardiograms (ECGs) may be non-diagnostic. Consequently, a high index of suspicion for cardiac ischemic events should be maintained in patients with cardiovascular risk factors. In patients at increased risk for myocardial infarction and suspicious hemodynamic changes, early, non-invasive interventions (morphine, oxygen, nitrates, aspirin, beta-blockers) should be undertaken. As lytic therapy following trauma may result in significant hemorrhage, cardiology consultation, in close communication with the surgical team, is advised.

Hypertension following trauma is most commonly due to pain. Other etiologies include preexisting primary hypertension, bladder distension, increased intracranial pressure, and hypoxemia. The anesthetic record should be reviewed for vasopressor administration and to aid fluid status assessment.

## Fluid and electrolyte considerations

As volume status is indirectly measured, multiple resuscitation endpoints including central venous pressure (CVP), arterial blood gas, lactate, pulse pressure, stroke volume variation, and central or mixed venous oxygen saturation ($S_{CV}O_2$ and $S_{\overline{V}}O_2$, respectively) should be considered in the evaluation (see Chapter 9).

Overarching goals in trauma care are volume resuscitation and correction of hypothermia, coagulopathy, and acidosis. As under-resuscitation results in organ dysfunction, the goal of fluid resuscitation is normovolemia or slight hypervolemia. There is evidence that early, over-aggressive resuscitation resulting in increased blood pressure may increase hemorrhage and mortality secondary to immature clot disruption. In patients without head injury or preexisting hypertension, initial systolic blood pressure targets of 70 to 80 mmHg are acceptable. Therefore, when hypotensive resuscitation technique is employed during initial management (see Chapters 4 and 6), continued resuscitation in the ICU may be necessary.

Organ perfusion is more important than specific fluid selection. In patients with traumatic brain injury, normal saline (NS) or hypertonic saline are preferred as these solutions decrease cerebral edema. Lactated Ringer's solution is otherwise preferred, as excess NS may produce hyperchloremic metabolic acidosis. While albumin increases colloid osmotic pressure, this theoretic advantage is lost if capillary integrity is compromised by massive trauma or inflammation.

Acid-base disturbances are common in the critically injured patient, and may include the following:

- Respiratory acidosis is most commonly caused by hypoventilation secondary to oversedation. Metabolic compensation through increased bicarbonate production usually requires more than 24 hours. Prolonged or excessive sedation, respiratory depression, and carbon dioxide ($CO_2$) retention can create a negative spiral of "narcosis" by decreasing medullary respiratory center responsiveness to elevated $CO_2$. Treatment involves minimizing sedation and supporting ventilation.

- Lactic acidosis results from anaerobic metabolism in hypoxic tissues, and is a common cause of high anion gap metabolic acidosis following trauma. If the anion gap is normal, then a likely cause is bicarbonate dilution with acidic NS (pH 5.0). Improved cardiac output and global perfusion should improve lactic acidosis. Sodium bicarbonate may be administered cautiously in cases of severe acidosis, preferably in mechanically ventilated patients as carbonic anhydrase converts bicarbonate to $CO_2$, possibly worsening acidosis.
- Respiratory alkalosis, from hyperventilation, may result from pain, anxiety, or excessive mechanical ventilation. Lowering minute ventilation, either through ventilator manipulation or treating any underlying pain or anxiety, should ameliorate the abnormality.
- Metabolic alkalosis is a common disturbance in the surgical ICU. Treatment includes hydration and correcting hypochloremia and hypokalemia.

Electrolyte disturbances may also be encountered in critically ill trauma patients, and may include the following:

- Traumatic head injury can affect the pituitary and increase antidiuretic hormone secretion, leading to free water retention, and decrease serum osmolality. As hyponatremia progresses, cerebral edema may lead to agitation, visual disturbances, unconsciousness, and grand mal seizures. Treatment includes free water restriction and furosemide. While hypertonic saline may be used in extreme cases (i.e., when neurological symptoms are present), serum sodium should be checked often and increased by less than 0.5 mEq/L/hr to avoid central pontine myelinolysis. Head trauma less commonly results in central diabetes insipidus. The resulting hypernatremia is treated with desmopressin.
- Hypokalemia is frequently seen following head and spinal cord injury. While the exact pathophysiology is unknown, epinephrine release leading to beta-2 mediated intracellular translocation has been hypothesized. Potassium is typically replaced at $\leq 20$ mEq/hr unless paralysis or ventricular arrhythmias are present.
- Hyperkalemia can occur due to acidosis, ischemia-reperfusion injuries, rhabdomyolysis, burns, and drugs such as succinylcholine, beta-blockers, angiotensin-converting enzyme inhibitors, digitalis, and potassium-sparing diuretics. Management includes calcium gluconate or chloride to stabilize the cell membrane; insulin and glucose, bicarbonate, and beta-2 agonists to drive potassium into the cell; and kayexalate, furosemide, and hemodialysis to decrease total body potassium.
- Hypocalcemia is expected after massive transfusion as the citrate anticoagulant present in many banked blood products chelates calcium. Packed red blood cells contain the preservative ADSOL (adenine, dextrose, sorbitol, sodium chloride, and mannitol), which does not cause hypocalcemia.

## Renal considerations

Acute kidney injury (AKI) is a common feature among trauma patients requiring critical care.

**Table 11.1.** Risk, Injury, Failure, Loss, and End-stage kidney disease (RIFLE) classification

| Category | GFR decrease | Serum creatinine increase | Urine output |
|---|---|---|---|
| Risk | > 25% | x1.5 | < 0.5 cc/kg/hr × 6 hr |
| Injury | > 50% | x2 | < 0.5 cc/kg/hr × 12 hr |
| Failure | > 75% | x3 | < 0.3 cc/kg/hr × 24 hr or anuria × 12 hr |
| Loss | Persistent ARF = complete loss of kidney function > 4 weeks | | |
| ESKD | End-stage kidney disease (> 3 months) | | |

Abbreviations: GFR = glomerular filtration rate; ARF = acute renal failure; ESKD = end-stage kidney disease.

- Prerenal causes of AKI include hypovolemia, cardiogenic shock, and abdominal compartment syndrome (e.g., after pelvic fracture or retroperitoneal bleed).
- Renal causes include hemoglobinuria and myoglobinuria (e.g., after crush injury, electric shock, or massive transfusion) and contrast agents.
- Postrenal causes include urethral or ureteral injury or obstruction (e.g., retroperitoneal hematoma).

Sepsis can precipitate AKI either through prerenal (hypotension) or renal (acute tubular necrosis) mechanisms. In the trauma population, the etiology of AKI is usually multi-factorial. In patients with AKI, tracking based on the Risk, Injury, Failure, Loss, and End-stage kidney disease (RIFLE) criteria is recommended (Table 11.1). The three less severe categories (Risk, Injury, Failure) are highly sensitive while the two more severe (Loss, End-stage kidney disease) are highly specific.

Management should focus on ameliorating underlying causes, maintaining perfusion, and avoiding nephrotoxins. Low-dose dopamine and fenoldopam can increase renal blood flow. In conjunction with furosemide, these agents have been used to treat renal dysfunction. However, none of these drugs have been shown to reduce dialysis-need or mortality in critically ill patients with early acute tubular necrosis.

# Nutrition

Adequate nutrition is crucial for optimal wound healing and should be tailored to patient injuries and comorbidities. Staged damage control surgery with frequent travel to the OR, as well as recurrent cancellations in a busy OR schedule, have the potential to significantly impair delivery of required nutrients. Postoperative enteral nutrition is considered the preferred route of nutritional support, unless contraindicated by ileus, bowel obstruction or perforation, enterocutaneous fistula, massive gastrointestinal bleed, or severe diarrhea. Although total parenteral nutrition is associated with more complications and higher costs, it should be considered when enteral nutrition is not possible. When using total parenteral nutrition, low-dose enteral nutrition ("trickle feeds") should be considered to maintain gastrointestinal mucosal integrity and normal flora. While hyperglycemia is associated with deleterious effects, the risk of hypoglycemia from aggressive blood sugar control may outweigh any possible benefits in trauma patients.

# Hematologic concerns

Coagulopathy independently predicts functional recovery, mortality, and length of ICU stay following trauma. Traumatic coagulopathy is a multi-factorial consequence of:

- Coagulation factor consumption and loss.
- Factor dysfunction secondary to acidosis or hypothermia.
- Factor dilution following conventional resuscitation.
- Hemorrhagic shock and decreased perfusion contribute to acidosis (secondary to anaerobic metabolism) and hypothermia (secondary to decreased muscle metabolism).

Coagulopathy resulting from acidosis, hypothermia, and hemorrhagic plasma loss perpetuates bleeding in an interrelated "lethal triad." Recent evidence shows that tissue injury and low-flow states lead to decreased fibrinogen utilization, systemic anticoagulation, and increased fibrinolysis that is modulated by the C-protein pathway (see more detailed trauma coagulopathy discussion in chapter 6).

Ironically, stabilized trauma patients are at high risk for developing deep venous thrombosis (DVT) secondary to endothelial injury sustained during the primary insult and venous stasis from prolonged immobility. Patients with spinal cord injury are at especially high risk for DVT. Common preventive measures include low molecular weight heparin, elastic stockings, and sequential compression devices. Inferior vena cava filters are utilized when there are contraindications to anticoagulation, or when there is progression of a thrombus or new emboli while on anticoagulation.

# Infection and sepsis

Shock, mechanical ventilation, prolonged hospitalization, indwelling catheters, and AKI are common following major trauma. Thus, infection is a significant concern. Antibiotics must be selected according to suspected infection site and culture and sensitivity reports. Given the tenuous state of many trauma patients and the fact that nosocomial infections are frequently caused by antibiotic-resistant organisms, extreme vigilance and adherence to proper infection precautions are of paramount importance.

Systemic inflammatory response syndrome (SIRS) results from widespread activation of the immune system and can be precipitated by non-infectious causes such as trauma or surgery. Sepsis (SIRS plus evidence of infection) is a disease spectrum ranging from mild inflammation to multi-organ failure. Appropriate fluid management, source control, and broad-spectrum antibiotics subsequently tailored to culture results are treatment pillars. Pathophysiologic consequences of sepsis are related to inflammatory-mediated changes in epithelial permeability, leading to intravascular hypovolemia, microvascular thrombi, and hypoxia. Tachycardia and hypotension result from vasodilation, hypovolemia, and myocardial depression. Increased alveolar capillary permeability can lead to hypoxia, hyperventilation, and ALI/ARDS. Hypovolemia can produce prerenal AKI, while inflammation can initiate acute tubular necrosis.

- SIRS inclusion criteria are satisfied when two or more of the following conditions are met:

  - Temperature $> 38°C$ or $< 36°C$
  - Respiratory rate $> 20$ breaths/min
  - Arterial $CO_2$ ($PaCO_2$) $< 32$ mmHg

- Heart rate > 90 beats/min
- White blood cells > 12,000 or < 4,000 (> 10% bands)
- Early goal-directed therapy seeks to optimize fluid management:
  - CVP > 8 mmHg or > 12 mmHg if mechanically ventilated (maintain using crystalloid bolus)
  - Mean arterial pressure (MAP) 65–90 mmHg (maintain using vasopressors)
  - Urine output > 0.5 mL/kg/hr
  - $S_{cv}O_2$ > 70%

While catheter-associated bloodstream infections are associated with increased mortality, they are largely preventable through proper aseptic technique. Catheters impregnated with heparin, chlorhexidine, or minocycline have lower infection rates. Subclavian central lines have the lowest infection rates of central lines, while femoral lines have the greatest rates. Although scheduled line changes are not recommended, central line catheters should be removed as soon as they are no longer needed.

Strategies to prevent ventilator-associated pneumonia (VAP) focus on minimizing aspiration and decreasing colonization of the airway by gastrointestinal tract pathogens. Since tracheal tubes negate the vocal cords' ability to protect the lungs from oral flora, allowing microaspirations even around fully inflated cuffs, the mere presence of a tracheal tube in any patient should prompt formulation of a removal plan. While there is evidence that early tracheostomy (within the first week) decreases pneumonia and length of mechanical ventilation, a clear survival benefit remains elusive. Other, more common, prophylactic strategies include elevating the head of the bed 30 degrees, limiting the use of prophylactic antibiotics and shortening the course of empiric antibiotics, removing nasopharyngeal tubes, intermittent suctioning of the oropharynx and tracheal tube, and extubation as soon as possible. Controversial measures include topical oral antibiotics, selective gastrointestinal tract decontamination, and use of antibiotic-coated tracheal tubes. Empiric monotherapy with imipenem, doripenem, or meropenem is appropriate with mild to moderate infection. If severe VAP occurs in patients with multiple comorbidities or recent antibiotic administration, combination therapy with the addition of fluoroquinolone or aminoglycoside is appropriate. Suspected methicillin-resistant *Staphylococcus aureus* infection should be treated with linezolid or vancomycin. Empiric antibiotic therapy should be adjusted once culture results are available.

Catheter-associated urinary tract infections are a potential source of severe gram-negative infection. Like catheter-associated bloodstream infections, catheter-associated urinary tract infections are largely preventable through proper sterile technique. Closed drainage systems, secured to the leg to prevent traction, should be used. Urinary catheters should be removed as soon as feasible. Empiric fluoroquinolone or third-or fourth-generation cephalosporin treatment should be modified once culture results are obtained.

Antibiotic therapy should be a carefully weighted decision, as *Clostridium difficile*-associated diarrhea is a complication of almost all antibiotics (clindamycin, cephalosporins, and ampicillin most commonly). If watery or bloody diarrhea develops after antibiotic treatment, enzyme-linked immunosorbent assay for *C. difficile* toxin should be ordered, the causative antibiotic should be stopped, if possible, and metronidazole or oral vancomycin should be initiated.

As a consequence of a successful vaccination program, tetanus is almost non-existent in the United States. Recently, there have been no deaths reported attributable to tetanus in the

United States in trauma patients who received the primary childhood immunization. Therefore, tetanus toxoid has been recommended in adults only if it has been more than 10 years since the patient's last immunization. Since tetanus toxoid administration provides protection against a subsequent injury and not the current injury, there is no urgency for the administration of the toxoid in the acute setting. On the other hand, patients with traumatic wounds without a complete primary immunization history or known booster within the last 10 years should receive tetanus immunoglobulin.

## Hypothermia

After trauma, a patient may be hypothermic for many reasons including impaired thermo-regulation and decreased heat production. Volatile anesthetics and propofol decrease systemic vascular resistance, causing body heat to redistribute from the core to the periphery, and may also decrease the hypothalamic temperature set point for vasoconstriction and shivering to roughly 34.5°C. Neuromuscular blocking drugs further decrease metabolic heat generation. Large surgical exposures generate high radiative and conductive heat losses. Passive insulation or forced air warmers should be used wherever possible and every effort should be made to warm intravenous fluids prior to administration.

While preliminary evidence suggests a neurologic advantage to hypothermia following circulatory arrest, a temperature of less than 36°C may increase length of stay and lead to adverse effects:

- Vasoconstriction decreases oxygen and immune cell delivery, contributing to wound infection.
- Hypothermia directly impairs collagen deposition, hindering wound healing and facilitating contamination spread.
- Decreased thromboxane A3 release decreases platelet activation and aggregation, promoting coagulopathy.
- As many enzymes are temperature sensitive, hypothermia prolongs drug duration.
- Shivering may cause increased heart rate, cardiac output, oxygen consumption, and $CO_2$ production. Increased oxygen consumption is especially deleterious in patients who are already hypoxic due to injuries.
- Severe hypothermia can cause atrial or ventricular irritability or unconsciousness.

Hypothermia treatment includes external warming with warmed blankets and forced-air warming devices, and internal warming with warm intravenous fluids. Small doses of meperidine may help reduce shivering.

## Key points

- After massive trauma, patients commonly present with acidosis, hypothermia, and coagulopathy. Prevention and treatment of these interrelated factors depends on control of hemorrhage, adequate resuscitation, active re-warming, and early treatment of coagulopathy.
- Continued ICU resuscitation is often required due to the increasing prevalence of hypotensive resuscitation and damage control surgery.
- Acute respiratory distress syndrome (ARDS) is defined by $PaO_2/FiO_2 < 200$ and absence of LV failure. Acute lung injury (ALI) is a less severe form, with $PaO_2/FiO_2 < 300$. Massive trauma is a major risk factor for ARDS/ALI.

- To employ lung protective ventilation, tidal volumes of 6–8 mL/kg and plateau pressures $< 35$ mmHg are utilized. PEEP should be used and $FiO_2$ minimized (while still maintaining $SpO_2 > 92\%$). Permissive hypercapnia may be necessary to achieve these objectives.
- Acid-base disturbances are common in the critically injured patient, and may include respiratory acidosis, lactic acidosis from anaerobic metabolism in hypoxic tissues, respiratory alkalosis, and metabolic alkalosis.
- In the trauma population, the etiology of AKI is usually multi-factorial. In patients with AKI, tracking based on the Risk, Injury, Failure, Loss, and End-stage kidney disease (RIFLE) criteria is recommended.
- Systemic inflammatory response syndrome (SIRS) is precipitated by widespread activation of the immune system, and is defined by at least two of the following: temperature $> 38°C$ or $< 36°C$, respiratory rate $> 20$, $PaCO_2 < 32$, white blood cells $> 12,000$ or $< 4,000$, and heart rate $> 90$. SIRS pathophysiology causes increased epithelial permeability and microvascular thrombi and hypoxia.
- Early goal-directed therapy optimizes fluid management in SIRS. Objectives should include CVP $> 8$ mmHg ($> 12$ if mechanically ventilated), MAP 65–90 mmHg, urine output $> 0.5$ mL/kg/hr, and $S_{cv}O_2 > 70\%$.

## Further reading

1. Amato MB, Barbas CS, Medeiros DM, et al. Effect of a protective-ventilation strategy on mortality in the acute respiratory distress syndrome. *N Engl J Med* 1998;**338**:347–354.

2. Barash P, Cullen B, Stoelting R, Cahalan M. *Clinical Anesthesia*. Philadelphia, PA: Wolters Kluwer/Lippincott Williams & Wilkins; 2009.

3. Berlot G, Delooz H, Gullo A. *Trauma Operative Procedures*. Milan: Springer-Verlag; 1999.

4. Brohi K, Cohen MJ, Ganter MT, et al. Acute traumatic coagulopathy: initiated by hypoperfusion: modulated through the protein C pathway? *Ann Surg* 2007; **245**:812–818.

5. Demetriades D, Asensio J. *Trauma Management*. Georgetown, TX: Landes Bioscience; 2000.

6. Rivers E, Nguyen B, Havstad M, et al. Early goal-directed therapy in the treatment of severe sepsis and septic shock. *N Engl J Med* 2001;**345**:1368–1377.

7. Venkataraman R, Kellum J. Defining acute renal failure: the RIFLE criteria. *J Intensive Care Med* 2007;**22**:187–193.

**Chapter**

# 12

# Chemical and radiologic exposures in trauma

Joseph H. McIsaac, III and Jeb Kucik

## Introduction

Ethanol and recreational drugs are by far the most common chemical exposures associated with trauma. This chapter, however, covers other possibly associated exposures: toxic industrial chemicals, chemical weapons, and radiation.

Limited exposures occur commonly in the industrial setting. The Bhopal disaster of 1984, mustard use during the Iran–Iraq War, and the 2011 Fukushima earthquake, tsunami, and nuclear disaster are examples of large-scale combined trauma/toxic exposure. Indeed, chemical weapons of World War I such as phosgene, chlorine, and cyanide are common industrial chemicals which are still used in vast quantities and are capable of producing mass casualties.

Combined trauma-exposure management begins with Advanced Trauma Life Support (ATLS) guidelines, balanced by the need for caregiver personal protective equipment (PPE) and rapid decontamination. After resuscitation, toxidrome treatment and advanced management commence. No specific antidotes exist for most chemical exposures; supportive care through emergency, operative, and critical care phases is key.

Common toxic injury patterns include:

- Inhalational injury
- Chemical burns
- Metabolic poisoning

Frequently, two or more types are present. When combined with conventional trauma, they synergistically increase morbidity and mortality.

## Resources for agent identification and management

- The US Department of Health and Human Services' Chemical Hazards Emergency Medical Management (CHEMM) website (http://chemm.nlm.nih.gov/index.html)

    - Allows "first responders, first receivers, other healthcare providers, and planners to plan for, respond to, recover from, and mitigate the effects of mass-casualty incidents involving chemicals."
    - Has tools for rapid toxidrome (i.e., clinical syndromes) identification, patient management, and planning.
- The Radiation Emergency Medical Management website (www.remm.nlm.gov/index.html)

    - Focuses on radiation events.

---

*Essentials of Trauma Anesthesia*, ed. A. J. Varon and C. E. Smith. Published by Cambridge University Press.
© Cambridge University Press 2012.

# CHEMICAL TERRORISM AGENTS AND BIOLIGICAL TOXINS

| Agents | Symptom Onset | Symptoms | Signs | Clinical Diagnostic Tests | Decon-tamination | Exposure route and treatment | Differential diagnostic considerations |
|---|---|---|---|---|---|---|---|
| Nerve agents | Vapor: seconds Liquid: minutes to hours | **Moderate exposure:** Muscle cramping, runny nose, difficulty breathing, eye pain, dimming of vision, sweating, diarrhea **High exposure:** Loss of consciousness, flaccid paralysis, seizures **Delayed Onset:** The onset of symptoms may be delayed up to 18 hours, especially with local exposures | Pinpoint pupils (miosis); often absent without conjunctival exposure to vapor. Excessive lacrimation Pulmonary secretions Wheezing Muscle twitching & rippling under the skin (fasciculations) Sweating Hypersalivation Diarrhea seizures, apnea | Red blood cell or serum cholinesterase (whole blood) **Treatment based on signs and symptoms;** Use lab tests only for later confirmation Collect urine for later confirmation and dose estimation | Rapid disrobing, Water wash with soap and shampoo | **Inhalation & dermal absorption** Atropine 2–6 mg IV or IM 2-PAMCl 600–1800 mg injection or 1.0 g infusion over 20–30 minutes Additional atropine 2 mg q 3–5 min to decreased secretions. One additional 2-PAMCl 600mg injection or 1.0 g infusion over 20–30 minutes at 1 hr if necessary Diazepam or lorazepam to prevent seizures in patients with severe enough exposure to require 6 mg of atropine at on time Ventilation support | Pesticide poisoning from organophosphorous agents and carbamates cause virtually identical syndromes |
| Cyanide | Seconds to minutes | **Moderate exposure:** Dizziness, nausea, headache, eye irritation **High exposure:** Loss of consciousness | **Moderate exposure:** non-specific findings, gasping, flushing, (typically not cyanosis) **High exposure** Marrow suppression with lymphocytopenia | Cyanide (blood) or thiocyanate (blood or urine) levels in lab: increased arteriovenous oxygen difference **Treatment based on signs and symptoms;** Use lab tests only for later confirmation | Clothing removal | **Inhalation & dermal absorption** Oxygen (face mask) Amyl nitrite Sodium nitrite (300mg IV) and sodium thiosulfate (12.5g IV) | Similar CNS illness results from: Carbon monoxide (from gas or diesel engine exhaust fumes in closed spaces) $H_2S$ (sewer, waste industrial sources) Sulfur mustard symptoms of pain usually delayed; Lewisite symptoms usually immediate |
| Blister Agents (Sulfur mustard) | 2–48 hours | Burning itching, or red skin Mucosal irritation (prominent tearing, and burning and redness of eyes) Shortness of breath Nausea and vomiting | Skin erythema Blistering Conjunctivitis and lid swelling Upper airways sloughing Pulmonary edema | Often smell of garlic, horseradish, and mustard on body Oily droplets on skin form ambient sources NO specific diagnostic tests | Clothing removal Large amounts of water | **Inhalation & dermal absorption, & oral ingestion** Thermal burn type treatment Supportive care For Lewisite and Lewisite/ Mustard mixtures: British Anti-Lewisite (BAL or dimercaprol) | Diffuse skin exposure with irritants, such as caustics, sodium hydroxides, ammonium, etc., may cause similar syndromes. Sodium hydroxide (NaOH) form trucking accidents |
| Pulmonary agents (phosgene etc.) | 1–24 (rarely up to 72) hours | Shortness of breath Chest tightness Wheezing Mucosal and dermal irritation and redness | Pulmonary (non-cardiogenic) edema with some mucosal irritation (signs after symptoms) | NO tests available by source assessment may help identify exposure characteristics (majority of trucking incidents generating exposures to humans have labels on vehicle) | None usually needed | **Inhalation** Supportive care Specific treatment depends on agents Consider steroids | Inhalation exposures are the single most common form of industrial agent exposure (eg: phogene, chlorine) Mucosal irritation, airways reactions, and deep lung effects depend on the specific agent |
| Ricin (castor bean toxin) | 18–24 hours | **Ingestion:** Nausea, diarrhea, vomiting, fever, abdominal pain **Inhalation:** chest tightness, coughing, weakness, nausea, fever | Clusters of acute lung or GI injury; circulatory collapse and shock | ELISA (from commercial laboratories) using respiratory secretions, serum, and direct tissue | Clothing removal Water rinse | **Inhalation & Ingestion** Supportive care For ingestion: charcoal lavage | Tularemia, plague, and Q fever may cause similar syndromes, as may CW agents such as staphylococcal enterotoxin B and phosgene |
| T-2 mycotoxin | 2–4hours | Dermal & mucosal irritation; blistering, necrosis Blurred vision, eye irritation Nausea, vomiting, and diarrhea Ataxia Coughing and dyspnea | Mucosal erythema and hemorrhage Red skin, blistering Tearing, salivation Pulmonary edema Seizures and coma | ELISA from commercial laboratories Gas chromatography/Mass spectroscopy in specialized laboratories | Clothing removal Water rinse | **Inhalation & dermal contact** Supportive care For ingestion: charcoal lavage Possibly high dose steroids | Pulmonary toxins ($O_3$, $NO_2$, phosgene, $NH_3$) may cause similar syndromes though with less mucosal irritation. |

**Figure 12.1.** Chemical terrorism agents and biological toxins.

- Wireless Information System for Emergency Responders (WISER, http://wiser.nlm.nih.gov)
  - Available for download to mobile devices.
- CHEMTREC® (www.chemtrec.com/)
  - Commercial service focused on industrial and transportation accidents involving chemicals.
- A chemical-induced illness pocket card ("Chem card") can be downloaded at www.healthquality.va.gov/biochem/bio_poc_chem.pdf (Figure 12.1).

## Decontamination and personal protective equipment (PPE)

Decontamination begins as soon as possible, preferably during the prehospital phase. Simply removing clothing can dramatically reduce both patient and caregiver exposure. Large volumes of water (with or without detergent) remove more persistent agents. Water should be avoided when flammable metals (e.g., lithium, sodium, potassium) are suspected; in such cases, mineral oil is used until debridement is possible. Adsorbents (e.g., sand, cat litter) are also effective for most agents.

- Topical decontamination of military agents can be accomplished using Reactive Decontamination Skin Lotion (www.rsdecon.com/).
- First responders should wear PPE Level C or higher when treating contaminated patients (www.remm.nlm.gov/osha_epa_ppe.htm).
- Level A or B is indicated for unknown agents or high concentrations of any substance.
- Decontamination at the hospital is indicated for persistent agents or when field decontamination was incomplete.

Life-saving medical treatment takes precedence over decontamination. The "ABCs" should be managed throughout the decontamination process. Level C PPE respiratory protection includes hooded National Institute for Occupational Safety and Health (NIOSH)-certified powered air-purifying respirators (PAPR) with assigned protection factors of $\geq 1000$ and appropriate chemical/radiological filters. These respirators should be used by hospital personnel receiving contaminated victims. Operating room (OR) procedures can be performed wearing PAPR when needed. Double gloving with at least one nitrile glove is recommended when dealing with chemical exposure victims.

Several studies demonstrate the difficulty of performing manual medical procedures (intubation, venipuncture) while wearing PPE. Maneuvers requiring less fine motor skill (e.g., laryngeal mask airway or intraosseous needle placement) should be considered, especially in mass casualties.

## Inhalational injuries

Acute inhalation injuries are frequently a consequence of industrial or household accidents. Agents released into confined spaces result in relatively high concentrations. Larger releases may result from bulk stored agents at industrial sites or during transportation accidents.

Several mechanisms of toxicity exist:

- Acute asphyxiants (e.g., carbon dioxide, argon, methane, nitrogen) simply displace oxygen and prevent its uptake, resulting in hypoxemia, anaerobic metabolism, and metabolic acidosis.

- Water-soluble agents (e.g., chlorine, ammonia) at low concentrations cause upper airway mucosal injury, while higher concentrations penetrate deeper into the airway and may induce bronchospasm and mucosal sloughing.
- Less soluble agents cause injury to lung parenchyma, resulting in necrosis or pulmonary edema.
- Pulmonary edema is also common with nitrogen oxides, isocyanate, and phosgene.
- Different inhalational injury mechanisms are commonly superimposed. Survivors often develop chronic obstructive pulmonary disease.

Mainstays of acute asphyxiant therapy are supportive oxygenation, ventilation, and bronchodilators. Positive end-expiratory pressure (PEEP) helps reduce pulmonary edema, while diuretics are of limited value, and steroids have been shown to be ineffective. Serial chest X-rays, arterial blood gases, and pulmonary function tests allow clinicians to follow closely the disease course. Once the acute phase subsides, therapy follows conventional critical care management guidelines.

# Chemical burns

Chemical injuries cause 3% of burn admissions but 30% of burn deaths (see also Chapter 19). Degree of injury frequently parallels exposure time. Tissue destruction occurs due to saponification of fats by alkali, coagulative necrosis by acids, and protein denaturation by organic materials and reactive metals. Chemical warfare agents produce both local and systemic toxicity. The extent of chemical injury is frequently underestimated. Decontamination should occur as soon as possible at the scene and emergency department to limit the extent of injury; the incidence of full thickness burns increases fivefold when irrigation is not initiated within 10 minutes.

- General decontamination procedures include clothing removal and flushing with water or adsorbents; water is contraindicated in case of reactive metals or phenol injury.
- Management includes ATLS followed by burn center admission. The "ABCs" should generally not be delayed due to the presence of chemicals.
- Caregivers should wear PPE.
- The advanced life support for acute toxic injury (TOXALS) protocol, introduced by Baker in 1996, is one method for managing acute chemical injury.

Identification of the chemical agent allows for more specific treatment and prognostication. Material Safety Data Sheets and chemical placards on transport vehicles should be noted. Firefighters are often excellent sources of chemical information in the prehospital setting. Poison control centers, CHEMM, WISER, and CHEMTREC are also useful. Consultation with or transfer to a burn center should be considered.

Hydrogen fluoride binds calcium, penetrating deeply into tissues and bone. Patients with skin involvement should receive topical calcium gluconate and monitoring for hypocalcemia. Hand injuries are treated with fasciotomy and intra-arterial calcium gluconate infusions. Injury is often more extensive than initially thought. Burn center and surgical consultation is always indicated.

Mustard (bis-(2-chloroethyl) sulfide) binds to deoxyribonucleic acid (DNA), interrupting rapidly dividing cells such as epithelium and resulting in inflammation, pain, and blistering. Moist areas (e.g., eyes, genitals) are easily affected, while pulmonary and systemic effects are also possible. After decontamination, treatment is largely supportive. Irrigation, topical antibiotics, and systemic analgesics reduce symptoms and scarring. Small skin blisters can be left intact, while large bullae should be unroofed, irrigated, and treated with a topical antibiotic in the same manner as a thermal burn. Fluid loss into blisters may be significant, necessitating volume resuscitation. Pulmonary mucosal injury is managed supportively. Large mustard exposures depress bone marrow within 3–5 days; resuscitative surgery should occur before immune compromise occurs or after the white count rebounds. Gut sterilization can be considered if leukopenia develops.

Lewisite (2-chlorovinyl dichloroarsine) is similar to mustard, but immediate pain is the prominent symptom. There are no immunologic effects. Treatment includes early dimercaprol application and supportive care.

## Metabolic poisons

Hydrogen cyanide (HCN), hydrogen sulfide ($H_2S$), and carbon monoxide (CO) are classic inhaled metabolic poisons. They act at the cellular level, inhibiting oxygen binding or utilization. Supplemental or hyperbaric oxygen are therapeutic mainstays for CO. Sodium nitrite and sodium thiosulfate are indicated for HCN toxicity, while only sodium nitrite treats $H_2S$.

Heavy metals like lead (Pb) respond to chelation therapy. Calcium disodium ethylenediaminetetraacetic acid (EDTA) and dimercaptosuccinic acid (DMSA) are effective.

Nerve agents such as tabun (GA), sarin (GB), soman (GD), and VX, are another metabolic toxin class. Organophosphate toxidromes may also occur from pesticide exposures. Both types of agents bind and inhibit cholinesterase, resulting in excess acetylcholine and overstimulation of nicotinic and muscarinic receptors resulting in miosis, lacrimation, salivation, bronchospasm, dyspnea, vomiting, incontinence, seizures, central apnea, and respiratory paralysis. Patients require respiratory support and treatment with atropine and an oxime (pralidoxime, obidoxime, HI-6). Seizures are treated with benzodiazepines or propofol. Heavy exposures require substantial critical care resources. Caregivers should wear Level C PPE until patients are fully decontaminated to avoid exposure.

Delayed onset of succinylcholine and vecuronium action has been reported in nerve agent-exposed swine. Prolongation of muscle relaxant effect may also occur. All nerve agent-exposed patients should be considered to have a "full stomach." Etomidate and ketamine are appropriate induction hypnotics in these patients. While propofol and thiopental are also acceptable, they may result in profound cardiac depression, bradycardia, and vasodilation. Opioids may be used, however, morphine may exacerbate bronchospasm. Fentanyl and morphine may also induce bradycardia, while remifentanil action may be prolonged by nerve agent-inhibition of non-specific tissue esterases.

Multiple other toxins exist. Some biologic agents (e.g., botulinum) are treated with early administration of antitoxin. Others, such as ricin, are treated supportively. The CHEMM website can guide casualty care.

## Radiation injuries

A person exposed to ionizing radiation is said to be irradiated. External irradiation does not make a person radioactive; thus, this patient poses no threat to healthcare providers. Contamination occurs when radioactive material comes to rest on a person or item; it poses a threat until it is removed. However, unlike chemical or biological agents, there is no

**Table 12.1.** Weighting factors ($W_R$) associated with various types of ionizing radiation. (Adapted from the National Council on Radiation Protection and Measurements Report No. 116, 1993.)

| Type of ionizing radiation | $W_R$ |
|---|---|
| Alpha particle | 20 |
| Beta particle, X-ray, and gamma ray | 1 |
| Neutron | 5–20 (depends on inherent energy level) |

documentation of a healthcare provider ever receiving radiation injury while caring for a contaminated patient. Internal contamination occurs when radioactive material is ingested, inhaled, or inspissated in wounds. Internal contamination may be confined to the lungs or gastrointestinal tract, or distributed throughout the body. Therefore, decontamination may require irrigation of oral and nasal passages, expectorants, emetics, gastric or pulmonary lavage, or medications that block absorption or incorporation of radioactive contaminants.

Radiological effects decrease with decreased time of exposure, increased distance from the source, and increased shielding. First responders should wear protective gear and rotate team members in order to minimize potential exposure and heat stress. Personal dosimeters should be considered.

Radiation may be particles (alpha, beta, neutrons) or electromagnetic waves (X-rays, gamma rays). Alpha particles are positively charged equivalents of helium nuclei (two neutrons, two protons) that quickly interact with nearby electrons and have a very short range. They tend to be dangerous only if inhaled, ingested, or absorbed from wounds. Beta particles are in essence free electrons. They have a larger range than alpha particles, can be stopped by thin solids (e.g., an aluminum sheet), and can cause eye damage or pruritus, paresthesias, and erythema if allowed to stay on the skin for long periods. Just like alpha particles, internal contamination with beta particles can be harmful. Neutrons are emitted from atomic fission, and are only encountered after a nuclear detonation. Their penetrance is significant, and they easily cause considerable damage to DNA. Gamma and X-rays are neutral energy packages that travel at the speed of light. They penetrate deep tissues; dense materials (e.g., lead, concrete) can block them.

Humans receive cosmic or terrestrial radiation every day. Increased doses are received during an airplane flight or a radiologic study.

- Absorbed radiation is typically measured in radiation absorbed dose (rad) or in Grays (Gy), where 100 rad = 1 Gy = 1 joule/kilogram.
- Expression in terms of *equivalent doses* accounts for different biological effects of various radiation types.
- The Roentgen-equivalent man (rem) and the Sievert (Sv) reflect absorbed dose (rad or Gy) multiplied by a weighting factor ($W_R$), where 100 rem = 1 Sv.

For example, gamma and X-rays have a $W_R$ of 1, while alpha particles have a $W_R$ of 20. (Table 12.1). Therefore, for an absorbed dose of 100 rad of undifferentiated radiation,

100 rad (gamma) × 1 ($W_R$ for gamma) = 100 rem or 1 Sv
100 rad (alpha) × 20 ($W_R$ for alpha) = 2000 rem or 20 Sv

**Table 12.2.** Approximation of relative hazard given exposure. (Adapted from the American College of Radiology, Disaster Preparedness for Radiology Professionals Response to Radiological Terrorism, 2006.)

| Radiation dose | Effects |
| --- | --- |
| < 0.010 Sv (1 rem) | No acute effects; minimal increased risk of cancer development |
| 0.1 Sv (10 rem) | No acute effects; 0.5% additional cancer risk |
| 1 Sv (100 rem) | Possible nausea, vomiting, and bone marrow depression; 5% additional cancer risk |
| > 2 Sv (200 rem) | Nausea, vomiting, development of Acute Radiation Syndrome |

Abbreviation. Sv: Sievert, rem: Roentgen-equivalent man.

Thus, *type* of exposure markedly affects biological results.

- Acute radiation syndrome (or radiation sickness) occurs hours to weeks after a rapid whole-body exposure.
- When sufficient radiation doses reach internal organs, DNA can be irreversibly damaged, with rapidly dividing cell lines (marrow, gastrointestinal mucosa) suffering most acutely.
- Different dose ranges produce different manifestations including hematopoietic, gastrointestinal, and cardiovascular/central nervous system subtypes.
- Each syndrome tends to progress through prodromal, latent, and manifest illness stages, culminating in either death or recovery.
- Higher doses predictably cause higher morbidity, as well as a faster transit through stages of illness (Table 12.2).

"$LD_{50/60}$" describes the dose that will kill 50% of an exposed population within 60 days. $LD_{50/60}$ is decreased (i.e., increased death with decreased dose) in extremes of age, chronic malnutrition or comorbidity, trauma, or infection. When combined with burns, trauma, infection, or chemical exposure, a radiation injury that would have otherwise been survivable will have significantly greater morbidity. A generally accepted $LD_{50/60}$ for untreated radiation injury is 3–4 Gy; optimal medical treatment can increase survival in most patients receiving $LD_{50/60}$ of 6 Gy, or less.

Radiological injuries present difficulties even in a single patient; incomplete information on the radiological incident, variations in the time course of non-specific findings, and patient anxiety or psychosomatic illness will confound diagnosis and prognosis. Large patient loads will present after an industrial or terrorist incident, making clinical judgment, rigorous triage, rapid laboratory analysis, and conservation of resources crucial in deciding which patients will receive treatment and which will not recover despite the best care possible. Tables 12.3 and 12.4 can be used to predict dose, and therefore, prognosis, on the basis of clinical findings.

The hematopoietic syndrome occurs at radiation doses above 0.7 Gy, affecting erythropoiesis, myelopoiesis, and thrombopoiesis. Lymphocyte counts fall precipitously with higher doses, and serial absolute lymphocyte counts help predict outcome. Red cell levels may return to normal quickly, while lymphocyte and platelet levels may remain low, imparting an increased risk of infection, bleeding, and poor wound healing. Prodromal nausea, vomiting, anorexia, and malaise may last days. During a latent stage of one to six weeks, the victim appears to improve despite continuing hematopoietic stem cell depletion.

**Table 12.3.** Using presence, onset, and duration of vomiting to estimate absorbed dose. (Adapted from Dickerson W. Acute Radiation Syndrome, Medical Effects of Ionizing Radiation Course, Armed Forces Radiobiology Research Institute, December 14, 2006.)

| Estimated dose (Gy) | Time of onset (hours) | Duration (hours) |
|---|---|---|
| 0.5–2 | 2–24 or longer | < 24 |
| 2–3 | 2–6 | 12–24 |
| 3–5 | 1–2 | 24 |
| > 5 | < 1 | 48 |

Abbreviation. Gy: Grays, where 100 rad = 1 Gy = 1 joule/kg.

**Table 12.4.** Likely outcomes with optimum care after sustaining a radiation injury. (Adapted from the *Textbook of Military Medicine*, Part I, Volume 2, Medical Consequences of Nuclear Warfare, 1989.)

| Dose range (Gy) | Prognosis |
|---|---|
| 0.5–1.0 | Excellent |
| 1.0–2.0 | Probable survival (>90%) |
| 2.0–3.5 | Likely survival (>75%) |
| 3.5–5.5 | Death likely in 3–6 weeks |
| 5.5–7.5 | Death likely in 2–3 weeks |
| 7.5–10.0 | Death in 1–3 weeks |
| 10.0–20.0 | Death in 5–12 days |
| > 20.0 | Death in 2–5 days |

Abbreviation. Gy: Grays, where 100 rad = 1 Gy = 1 joule/kg.

Ensuing frank illness may last months, yielding immunosuppression, neutropenic fevers, malaise, hemorrhage, and infection. Recovery may occur if sufficient stem cells regenerate.

The gastrointestinal syndrome can occur when radiation damages the rapidly growing endothelial cells of the small intestine, causing mucosal sloughing, loss of neural control, submucosal edema, malabsorption, fluid loss, and electrolyte abnormalities. Within a few hours of a radiation dose of 6–10 Gy, the victim develops profound nausea, vomiting, cramping, diarrhea, fatigue, tachycardia, and hypotension lasting a few days. A latent stage of roughly one week is then followed by the return of symptoms, along with immunosuppression and anemia from a superimposed hematopoietic syndrome. Transmigration of intestinal flora can lead to sepsis, shock, and death, generally within two or three weeks. Survival data for the gastrointestinal syndrome is scant; death from hemorrhage or infection is likely despite optimal care. Clinicians thus face therapeutic and ethical dilemmas, and must judge whether limited resources might be better used on those with better chances of recovery. In any event, palliative measures such as antiemetics and narcotics are indicated.

The cardiovascular/central nervous system syndrome develops after doses exceeding 20 Gy. Profound, intractable symptoms occur within minutes, including dysesthesias, mental status changes, seizures, nausea, vomiting, bloody diarrhea, hypotension, autonomic dysregulation, coma, and cardiovascular collapse. Death occurs regardless of treatment, generally within three days. When history, physical, and radiation readings confirm such an overwhelming dose, the patient should be categorized as expectant and given comfort measures, particularly in the setting of multiple casualties.

## Patient care approaches

Patients with potentially survivable radiation injuries may not develop symptoms for three to four weeks, more than enough time for any traumatic cause of mortality to take its toll. As in any emergency response, providers must address life-threatening injuries first, while not becoming casualties themselves.

- Standard ATLS protocol should be used to secure the airway, ventilate, and control hemorrhage, with decontamination following as soon as practicable.
- Once triage, stabilization, and decontamination take place, patients are admitted for longitudinal care and monitoring.
- Radiation dose can be estimated based on the size and type of exposure (nuclear, radiological dispersal device, orphan source), whether there was an explosion yielding embedded sources, the radionuclide involved (e.g., cesium, iodine, cobalt), time course of radiation-related symptoms, distance from the source, exposure duration, and whether any shielding was present.
- Continuous radiological surveys and laboratory analysis can help estimate exposure.
- Patients that have received a critically high dose and are unlikely to survive should receive comfort and spiritual support.
- Expert consultation is available from the Centers for Disease Control (800-CDC-INFO), the Radiation Emergency Assistance Center/Training Site (865–576–3131), or the Armed Forces Radiobiology Research Institute (301–295–0530).

Severe internal contamination can cause acute radiation syndrome, while prolonged low-grade internal exposure can lead to distribution throughout the body, profound damage to organs, and cancer induction. Absorption is markedly faster through mucous membranes and lungs than through intact skin. If the eyes are affected, they should be rinsed gently but copiously. If significant lung exposure has occurred, bronchoscopic lavage may be of benefit. Radioactive contamination of the gastrointestinal tract is treated similarly to oral poisoning. Recently swallowed contamination can be lavaged by means of an orogastric or nasogatric tube. Laxatives can speed transit of gastrointestinal contamination, decreasing exposure time. Osmotic laxatives such as polyethylene glycol or magnesium citrate are more effective than bulk laxatives such as psyllium, but may cause increased abdominal discomfort, obscuring clinical findings. Activated charcoal selectively binds chromium, while alginates, barium sulfate, and aluminum-based antacids (e.g., Maalox®, Gaviscon®) can bind strontium-90. The ion exchange resin Prussian blue (ferric ferrocyanide, Radio-gardase®) binds cesium-137 and thallium. Adult dosing for Prussian blue is 3 g three times a day, while a pediatric dose is 1 g three times a day.

Blocking and diluting agents (e.g., potassium iodide, potassium perchlorate) saturate target organs, crowding out harmful radionuclides. Mobilizing agents (e.g., oral ammonium chloride plus intravenous calcium gluconate) increase metabolism of ingested contaminants, hastening their elimination. Chelating agents (e.g., deferoxamine, calcium diethylenetriaminepentaacetic acid [Ca-DTPA]) form complexes with metallic ions, removing them from circulation. Each should begin as soon as possible, guided by daily dose assessments and urinary levels.

Laboratory monitoring can reveal marked lymphocyte depletion soon after injury. Complete blood counts with white cell differential, taken every 6 hours for 48 hours, aid in determining dose and prognosis. Urinalyses help determine baseline renal function and track the degree of radionuclide-induced kidney damage. Urine human chorionic gonadotropin measurement is appropriate in all women of childbearing age. Pregnant victims should be counseled by an obstetrician regarding potential teratogenesis. Fetal sensitivity to radiation is highest three to seven weeks post-conception.

Opportunistic infections pose extreme risk in irradiated, neutropenic patients. A fine line must be maintained between intervention and infection control; invasive procedures, including line placement and surgery, should be avoided if possible, particularly during the neutrophil nadir two days post-exposure. If wounds must be left open, topical antibiotics should be considered. Hygiene and nosocomial risk minimization must be enforced. Stable patients can be discharged before the neutrophil nadir, with outpatient follow-up performed away from the hospital's nosocomial risk. Positive pressure isolation rooms will benefit inpatients. If fever develops during the neutropenic phase, empiric antibiotics should be started, tailored to the hospital's bacterial susceptibility profile and culture results. Prophylaxis should start when the absolute neutrophil count falls to $0.5 \times 10^9$ cells/L, continuing until the count rebounds above $1.0 \times 10^9$. Empiric 21-day intravenous regimens include quinolones (ciprofloxacin, levofloxacin) for gram-negative infection, possibly supplemented by penicillin, amoxicillin, piperacillin, or vancomycin for gram-positive coverage. A third- or fourth-generation cephalosporin (ceftriaxone, cefepime), imipenem, or an aminoglycoside (gentamicin, amikacin) may be substituted for the quinolone if needed. If afebrile, antibiotics should end after seven days. Oropharyngeal mucositis or known/suspected Herpes simplex virus infection should prompt addition of acyclovir. If clostridial enterocolitis develops, a 500 mg dose of metronidazole three times a day for one to two weeks should begin. Fluconazole should be used for fungal infections.

If immune compromise and gastrointestinal symptoms develop, gut decontamination should be considered. Normal gut flora may be affected by radiation, causing overgrowth of *Enterobacteriaceae*, possible transmigration, and sepsis. Effective options include oral ciprofloxacin, polymyxin B, or trimethoprim-sulfamethoxizole. Though rarely used due to gastrointestinal side effects, oral neomycin is also effective. Immunization status should be addressed after acute phase treatments. Revaccination against *Streptococcus pneumoniae*, *Neisseria meningitidis*, and *Haemophilus influenzae* B should be given for positive serologies or functional hyposplenism, guided by CDC and Infectious Disease Society of America (IDSA) protocols. Live vaccines should be deferred for two years (Table 12.5).

Nutritional demands must be tempered by possible bowel mucosa injury. Similarly to burns, trauma, or infection, radiation induces hypermetabolic stress. Increased needs are satisfied enterally or parenterally. Regular diets are avoided initially, replaced by soft elemental diets that minimize mechanical, acidic, and enzymatic damage to remaining mucosa, decrease bacterial growth, and encourage normal function. Enteral glutamine may aid in mucosal rehabilitation. If bowel function is impaired (e.g., malabsorption, obstruction) or mucosal breakdown is likely, parenteral nutrition should be used, necessitating central access and infective risk. Dietary consultation *en masse* for similar patients may help in a mass casualty (Table 12.6).

**Table 12.5.** Infection control and treatment

| Modality | Treatment | Comments |
|---|---|---|
| Infection control measures | | Strict contact and droplet precautions<br>Proper hand washing<br>Positive pressure room<br>Minimize invasive procedures<br>Early discharge if appropriate |
| Antibiotics | • Quinolone (ciprofloxacin, levofloxacin)<br>or<br>• 3rd/4th generation cephalosporin<br>or<br>• Imipenem<br>or<br>• Aminoglycoside (gentamicin, amikacin)<br>and<br>• Gram-positive coverage (penicillin, amoxicillin, vancomycin) | Broad-spectrum, prophylactic antibiotics during the neutropenic period, continue until ANC recovers |
| | • Acyclovir<br>• Fluconazole<br>• Topical antibiotics<br>• Flagyl 500 mg PO q8 x7–14 days<br>• Consider gut prophylaxis | If HSV positive or suspected<br>If fungal infection present<br>For open wounds in neutropenic phase<br>To treat *C. difficile* if it occurs<br>For risk of translocation of intestinal bacteria |
| Vaccines | • *Streptococcus pneumoniae*<br>• *Neisseria meningitidis*<br>• *Haemophilus influenzae B* | As hyposplenism or serology dictates (see CDC and IDSA guidelines)<br>No live vaccines for 2 years |

Abbreviations: CDC = Centers for Disease Control; IDSA = Infectious Disease Society of America; HSV = Herpes simplex virus.

**Table 12.6.** Nutritional support

| Route | Characteristics |
|---|---|
| Enteral | Provides adequate calories<br>Promotes mucosal growth and patency<br>Hastens return of normal bowel function<br>Decreases acidic and enzymatic damage<br>Prevents overgrowth of abnormal flora<br>Risk of mechanical wall stress |
| Parenteral | Can provide adequate calories (if total parenteral nutrition)<br>Viable option if gut not functioning<br>Minute design of intake possible<br>Infective risk of central line<br>Risks villous atrophy and bacterial transmigration |

**Table 12.7.** Cytokine therapy

| Drug | Dosage |
|------|--------|
| G-CSF (Filgrastim) | • 5–10 mcg/kg SQ/IV qD or<br>• 200–400 mcg/m$^2$/day |
| GM-CSF (Sargramostim) | • 2.5–5.0 mcg/kg SQ/IV qD or<br>• 100–250 mcg/m$^2$/day |
| PEG G-CSF (Pegfilgrastim) | • 6mg SQ q week |

Abbreviations: G-CSF = Granulocyte colony-stimulating factor; GM-CSF = Granulocyte-macrophage colony-stimulating factor.

Cytokines (Table 12.7) are potent inducers of inflammation and hematopoiesis. Subcutaneous or intravenous granulocyte colony-stimulating factor (Filgrastim) or granulocyte-macrophage colony-stimulating factor (Sargramostim) given after a 3 Gy dose can augment cell production and minimize neutropenia. Lower thresholds (2 Gy) are used in extremes of age (< 12, > 60). Cytokines such as stem cell factor, thrombopoietin, and interleukins (IL-1 through IL-16) are investigational.

## Surgical treatment and anesthetic management

Coexisting trauma is likely in patients that are close to an explosion or that survive secondary (flying object striking patient) or tertiary (shock wave throws patient against fixed object) blast trauma, requiring general, orthopedic, plastic, vascular, or neurosurgical intervention. Anesthetic plans assume a full stomach necessitating rapid sequence induction, definitive airway control, close hemodynamic management including invasive monitors, and fluid and blood component therapy. When decontamination is suboptimal, anesthesiologists should wear PPE as indicated by a radiation safety officer. Whenever possible, intravascular lines should be started in uncontaminated parts of the body. Resources may be limited, including surgical instruments, anesthesia machines, ventilators, monitors, drugs, endotracheal tubes, fluids, blood, medical gases, and even electricity. Likewise, personnel, including anesthesiologists, non-physician anesthetists, surgeons and surgical technicians, and OR and recovery nurses, will also represent precious commodities. Maximum use of ancillary personnel, including technicians, medical students, volunteers, and the walking wounded, is critical.

Interventions performed outside the OR with minimal anesthetic requirement will do the most good for the most patients. Properly employed light sedation, hypnotics, and regional anesthesia that maintain spontaneous ventilation will help alleviate shortages. The decision to go to the OR must be tempered by the relative likelihood of surgical success, the needs of other patients, and equipment availability. Supplies may need to be washed and reused. In extreme cases, two or more surgeries may be performed in the same suite with a single anesthesia provider caring for them simultaneously.

Wounds are assumed to be contaminated. Higher priority is given to wounds than to intact skin due to possible bloodborne spread of radionuclides. The aggressiveness of debridement should be tempered by bleeding, comorbidities, number of wounds, amount of inspissated material, relative radiotoxicity of the species involved, and competing OR demands.

Radiation-induced lymphopenia can cause immunosuppression, delayed wound healing, increased rates of infection, and failure of primary closure. If possible, definitive treatment should be undertaken within 36 hours of injury, before the white cell count decreases significantly. Surgical protocols that require multiple OR trips may be catastrophic for these patients, who may benefit more from wide excision, amputation, and early primary closure with sufficient margins of healthy, non-irradiated tissue. Hyperbaric oxygen therapy may be beneficial. Primary closure of wounds still containing radioactive material will yield infection and dehiscence.

Wounds should be draped with impermeable material to limit contamination spread. If sufficient PPE is not available, runoff and dressings should go into a shielded container. Radiation safety personnel should periodically inspect ORs. Radiation readings should guide focused debridement. Grossly contaminated wounds may require serial returns to the OR before primary or graft-assisted closure. Once normal radiation levels are reached, the wound can be treated normally.

Long-range health concerns after radiation exposure come in two varieties:

- Deterministic effects, wherein a definitive (often linear) causal relationship exists between exposure and sequelae.

  - Disease *severity* increases with dose. Examples include cutaneous injury, cataract formation, sterility, leukopenia, and decreased immunity.

- Stochastic effects, in which a causal relationship cannot be proven but where exposure increases the likelihood of development.

  - Disease *probability* (e.g., cancer) increases with dose suffered.
  - Disease severity may be attenuated by host and environmental factors.

- Survivors of radiation injuries remain at risk for multiple health problems for years to come, and should have close health surveillance.

- Women of childbearing age and men at risk for radiation-induced sterility should be offered genetic counseling, while exposed pregnant women should receive obstetrical advice.

- Support groups exist for patients who suffer radiation-associated diseases. Social services should help patients find support long before discharge.

## Key points

- Mass casualties lead to unavoidable shortages. Efficient use of personnel (including technicians, students, volunteers, and walking wounded) and supplies (including alternate anesthetic techniques, wash and reuse of equipment) is critical. Anesthesiologists may need to care for multiple patients simultaneously.

- Decontamination limits exposure, but should not delay resuscitation. Caregivers should wear PPE until decontamination is performed.

- Most chemical exposures require supportive care only. Some chemical injuries have specific treatments. The CHEMM website is an excellent resource for first responders/first receivers.

- Irradiation is exposure to radiation, and does not make the patient a threat to healthcare providers. Contamination occurs when radioactive material comes to rest on or inside a patient; it poses a threat until removed.
- Radiological damage decreases with shorter exposure time, increased distance from the source, and increased shielding.
- Acute radiation syndrome occurs after exposure of more than 1 Gy. The hematopoietic syndrome affects bone marrow, leading to immunosuppression, neutropenic fevers, hemorrhage, and infection. The gastrointestinal syndrome causes mucosal sloughing, malabsorption, and possible transmigration of gut flora. Death from hemorrhage or infection is likely despite care. The cardiovascular/central nervous system syndrome results in mental status changes, seizures, hypotension, autonomic dysregulation, and cardiovascular collapse within minutes. It is uniformly fatal.

# Further reading

1. Armed Forces Radiobiology Research Institute. *Medical Management of Radiological Casualties Handbook*, 2nd edition. Bethesda, MD: AFRRI; 2003.

2. Baker DJ, The pre-hospital management of injury following mass toxic release; a comparison of military and civilian approaches. *Resuscitation* 1999;**42**:155–159.

3. Centers for Disease Control and Prevention. Acute Radiation Syndrome: A Fact Sheet for Physicians. www.bt.cdc.gov/radiation/arsphysicianfactsheet.asp. Accessed October 22, 2006.

4. Hamilton MG, Conley JD, Grychowski K, Lundy PM. Anaesthetic Management Problems in Combined Chemical/Trauma Casualties, http://ftp.rta.nato.int/public/PubFullText/RTO/TR/RTO-TR-HFM-041/TR-HFM-041–1999-Files/Brussels%20CD-ROM/Brussels/OP%20Poisoning%20Anticonvulsant/Hamilton.pdf, 1999. Accessed August 12, 2011.

5. Jarrett DG, Sedlak RG, Dickerson WE. *Current Status of Treatment of Radiation Injury in the United States*. Published in the proceedings of the NATO Human Factors and Medicine (HFM) Panel Research Task Group (RTG) 099 Meeting, "Radiation Bioeffects and Countermeasures," Bethesda, MD, June 21–23, 2005. www.afrri.usuhs.mil/www/outreach/pdf/jarrett_NATO_2005.pdf. Accessed October 23, 2006.

6. National Council on Radiation Protection and Measurements. Report No. 65, *Management of Persons Accidentally Contaminated with Radionuclides*, 7th edition. Bethesda, MD: NCRP; 1997.

7. Pellmar TC, Ledney GD. *Combined Injury: Radiation in Combination with Trauma, Infectious Disease, or Chemical Exposures*. Published in the proceedings of the NATO Human Factors and Medicine (HFM) Panel Research Task Group (RTG) 099 Meeting, "Radiation Bioeffects and Countermeasures," Bethesda, MD, June 21–23, 2005. www.afrri.usuhs.mil/www/outreach/pdf/pellmar_NATO_2005.pdf. Accessed October 23, 2006.

8. Seth R, Chester D, Moiemen N. A review of chemical burns. *Trauma* 2007;**9**:81–94.

9. Tucci MA, Camporesi EM. Risks and effects of radiation terrorism. *Semin Anesth Perioperat Med Pain* 2003;**22**:268–277.

10. Vijayan VK. Toxic trauma affecting the lungs with special reference to the Bhopal disaster. *Pulmon* 2006;**8**:44–50.

11. Weinbroum AA, Rudick V, Paret G, Kluger Y, Ben Abraham R. Anaesthesia and critical care considerations in nerve agent warfare trauma casualties. *Resuscitation* 2000;**47**:113–123.

Chapter

# 13

# Anesthetic considerations for adult traumatic brain injury

Armagan Dagal, Deepak Sharma, and Monica S. Vavilala

Traumatic brain injury (TBI) is an acquired insult to the brain due to an external mechanical force and can lead to transient or long-term impairment of cognitive, physical, and psychosocial functions. Anesthesiologists are most often involved in the care of patients with moderate to severe TBI for a variety of procedures including but not limited to initial evaluation and resuscitation, diagnostic imaging, surgical intervention, and intensive care unit (ICU) management.

## Epidemiology

- The global incidence rate of TBI is estimated at 200 per 100,000 people per year.
- About 1.7 million cases of TBI occur in the United States every year leading to 275,000 hospitalizations and 52,000 deaths. Of those who die, 50% do so within the first two hours of their injury.
- TBI is responsible for approximately one-third of all injury-related deaths.
- It is estimated that approximately 5.3 million people live with TBI-induced disability in the United States.
- TBI results in an estimated $84 billion in direct and indirect costs.
- Males have four times higher incidence of TBI than females.
- Falls (35.2%) are the leading cause of TBI followed by motor vehicle traffic crashes (17.3%), struck by/against events (16.5%), assaults (10%), and unknown/other (21%) causes.
- Motor vehicle crash is the leading cause of TBI-related death. Rates are highest for ages 20 to 24 years.
- Persons aged 75 years and older have the highest death rate after TBI, primarily because of falls.

## Pathophysiology

TBI has been described in two distinct epochs: primary and secondary. Primary injury is the result of the initial, mechanical forces on the brain tissue and skull, resulting in skull fracture, brain contusion and/or intracranial hematoma as a result of shearing and compression of neuronal, glial, and vascular tissue. Axonal tissue is more vulnerable to TBI than vascular tissue. Thus, focal injuries are usually superimposed upon more diffuse neuronal injury. The consequences of the initial TBI include physical disruption of cell membranes and infrastructure, and disturbance of ionic homeostasis secondary to increased membrane permeability. This in turn

**Table 13.1.** Marshall's classification of traumatic brain injury

| Category | Definition |
|---|---|
| Diffuse injury I | No visible intracranial pathology on CT scan |
| Diffuse injury II | Cisterns are present with midline shift < 5 mm and/or lesion densities present<br>No high- or mixed-density lesion > 25 mL, may include bone fragments and foreign bodies |
| Diffuse injury III | Cisterns compressed or absent with midline shift 0–5 mm<br>No high- or mixed-density lesion > 25 mL |
| Diffuse injury IV | Midline shift > 5 mm<br>No high- or mixed-density lesion >25 mL |
| Evacuated mass lesion | Any lesion surgically evacuated |
| Non-evacuated mass lesion | High- or mixed-density lesion >25 mL, not surgically evacuated |

Abbreviation: CT = computed tomography.

may lead to astrocytic and neuronal swelling, relative hypoperfusion, perturbation of cellular calcium homeostasis, increased free radical generation and lipid peroxidation, mitochondrial dysfunction, inflammation, apoptosis, and diffuse axonal injury. The Marshall classification is frequently utilized for classifying TBI based on computed tomographic (CT) characteristics (Table 13.1). Secondary injury is described as the consequence of progressive pathological insults, such as ischemia, reperfusion, and hypoxia starting immediately after the initial TBI. Systemic insults such as hypotension (systolic blood pressure, SBP < 90 mmHg), hypoxemia ($PaO_2$ < 60 mmHg), hypoglycemia, hyperglycemia, hypocarbia, and hypercarbia are major causes of secondary injury. The early management of TBI is, therefore, directed towards minimizing secondary insults. Although delayed brain ischemia appears to be the major common pathway of secondary brain damage, reperfusion hyperemia may also occur.

## Preoperative considerations

In any trauma patient, priority must first be given to general evaluation and stabilization, with particular attention to the airway, breathing, and circulation during the primary survey. A baseline neurological assessment should be performed using the Glasgow Coma Scale (GCS) score (Table 13.2). TBI is classified severe if GCS score is ≤ 8 and is associated with higher morbidity and mortality. It is classified moderate if GCS score is 9–12 and mild if GCS score is 13–15. Secondary surveys will identify other injuries.

Knowledge of the mechanism of injury is important for prognostication as well as for anticipation of associated injuries. Penetrating injuries have a worse outcome than blunt trauma. Females may fare less well. Pedestrians and cyclists do worse than vehicle occupants in motor vehicle accidents, and ejection from the vehicle leads to a higher risk of TBI.

Surgical procedures for TBI include craniotomy for the evacuation of epidural, subdural, or intracerebral hematomas, and decompressive craniectomy for the treatment of intracranial hypertension (ICH) refractory to medical treatment. Anesthesia providers should actively look for manifestations of increased intracranial pressure (ICP) including

**Table 13.2.** Glasgow Coma Scale score*

|  |  | Score |
|---|---|---|
| Best eye response | Spontaneous | 4 |
|  | To speech | 3 |
|  | To pain | 2 |
|  | None | 1 |
| Best verbal response | Oriented | 5 |
|  | Disoriented | 4 |
|  | Inappropriate words | 3 |
|  | Incomprehensible sounds | 2 |
|  | None | 1 |
| Best motor response | Obeys verbal orders | 6 |
|  | Localize pain | 5 |
|  | Flexion (withdrawal) to pain | 4 |
|  | Flexion (decortication) to pain | 3 |
|  | Extension (decerebration) to pain | 2 |
|  | None (flaccid) | 1 |

* Total Glasgow Coma Scale score (range 3–15) is summation of best eye + verbal + motor response scores.

Cushing's triad of hypertension, bradycardia, and irregular respiration. Patients with high preoperative ICPs are at risk of cerebral ischemia and hypotension following evacuation of intracranial hematoma. Issues related to urgent or emergent craniotomy include the need for adequate vascular access, the availability of blood products, and the ability for rapid resuscitation. The management of patients with TBI can be challenging and complicated by associated extracranial injuries and coexisting hypovolemic and neurogenic shock.

The pre-anesthetic evaluation should comprise:

- Airway and cervical spine assessment.
- Assessment of oxygenation with ventilation.
- Assessment of blood pressure, heart rate, and rhythm.
- Assessment of neurological status.
- Assessment of associated extracranial injuries.
- Review of available medical, surgical, and anesthetic history, allergies and current medications including anticoagulant use (e.g., clopidogrel, aspirin, or warfarin) or herbal supplements.
- Relevant laboratory data (hematocrit, coagulation profile, glucose, electrolytes).
- Planning of the postoperative management and discharge destination (e.g., ICU).

Medically unstable conditions warranting further evaluation are rare since craniotomy for TBI is typically urgent or emergent, hence delaying surgery is seldom indicated. However, a number of TBI patients suffer from associated injuries and may require extracranial surgery. The decision of which surgery should be performed first depends on several factors including the severity of TBI, severity of associated injuries, and patient stability. If polytrauma patients with possible TBI are stable during initial evaluation, abdominal and head CT may be performed prior to management of extracranial injury. Patients with possible TBI who are hemodynamically unstable and have abdominal trauma typically require emergency laparotomy. Intraoperative ICP monitoring may be initiated prior to a head CT if coagulation parameters are normal and the index of suspicion for TBI is high. In this case, head CT is obtained after extracranial surgery. Some patients may require simultaneous emergency craniotomy and laparotomy.

Coexisting conditions may impact the surgical and postoperative course. For elderly patients who sustain falls, particular attention should be paid to pre-injury cardiac, pulmonary, and endocrine status since congestive heart failure, hypertension, chronic obstructive pulmonary disease, and type II diabetes mellitus are common in this population. These coexisting conditions may result in perioperative complications such as congestive heart failure, pulmonary edema, or hyperglycemia.

- Antihypertensive drugs: Diuretics can cause electrolyte imbalance resulting in arrhythmias. Patients receiving beta-blockers prior to surgery may experience bradycardia and fail to increase their heart rate in response to acute blood loss. Calcium channel blockers and angiotensin-converting enzyme inhibitors or angiotensin II antagonists may cause hypotension, especially when combined with beta-blockers and diuretics.
- Antiplatelet and anticoagulant drugs: Patients who receive antiplatelet or anticoagulant drugs may have an increased risk of bleeding and transfusion. Transfusion of platelet or other coagulation products may be required. Rapid reversal of anticoagulants may be achieved by administration of vitamin K therapy with fresh frozen plasma, prothrombin complex concentrates, or recombinant factor VIIa (rFVIIa).
- Herbals: Garlic, ginseng, ginger, and gingko may interfere with platelet function, particularly when combined with non-steroidal anti-inflammatory drugs or warfarin, and increase the risk of bleeding.
- Oral hypoglycemic drugs: Patients who receive oral hypoglycemic drugs may develop perioperative hypoglycemia.

## Laboratory investigations

Preoperative tests may be ordered selectively for guiding or optimizing perioperative management on the basis of the patient's clinical characteristics and the urgency of the surgical procedure. However, these investigations should not delay the start of surgical management. For rapid assessment, prothrombin time, fibrinogen, platelet count, and hematocrit obtained together, as an "emergency hemorrhage panel", may facilitate timely transfusion therapy. Preoperative hyperglycemia may portend intraoperative hyperglycemia and poor outcome, and glucose levels should be obtained prior to surgery and hourly during surgery. Patients with TBI may have electrolyte disturbances and the treatment for these should be initiated while the patient proceeds to surgery.

## Intraoperative management

There are no formal intraoperative guidelines for the management of TBI. Intraoperative TBI care is largely based on physiological optimization and may be guided by the recommendations from the Brain Trauma Foundation (Table 13.3).

**Table 13.3.** Brain Trauma Foundation recommendations for severe TBI

| | |
|---|---|
| Blood pressure | Monitor and avoid hypotension (SBP < 90 mmHg) |
| Oxygenation | Monitor and avoid hypoxia ($PaO_2$ < 60 mmHg or oxygen saturation < 90%) |
| Hyperosmolar therapy | Mannitol is preferred choice and effective in reducing ICP |
| $PaCO_2$ | Prophylactic hyperventilation ($PaCO_2$ $\leq$ 25 mmHg) is not recommended Hyperventilation is recommended as a temporizing measure for the reduction of elevated ICP |
| Temperature | Prophylactic hypothermia is not significantly associated with decreased all-cause mortality Hypothermia may have higher chances of reducing mortality when cooling is maintained for more than 48 hours |
| ICP | ICP monitoring is recommended when there is a risk of ICH. Ventricular catheter with external pressure transducer is the preferred choice. Parenchymal transducers are an alternative when ventricular ICP is not obtained or if there is an obstruction in the fluid couple. Treat when ICP is > 20 mmHg |
| CPP | Treat with fluid and vasopressors to maintain CPP between 50–70 mmHg |
| Brain oxygenation | $SjvO_2$ and brain tissue oxygen monitoring are recommended in addition to standard ICP monitors. Treat when $SjvO_2$ < 50% or brain tissue oxygen tension < 15 mmHg |
| Glucose control | Hyperglycemia is associated with worsened outcome |
| Thromboprophylaxis | Intermittent pneumatic compression stockings and low-dose heparin or low molecular weight heparin are recommended for deep vein thrombosis prophylaxis |
| Antiseizure prophylaxis | Anticonvulsants are indicated to decrease the incidence of early post-traumatic seizures (within seven days of injury). Anticonvulsants are not recommended for late post-traumatic seizure prophylaxis |
| Steroids | Not recommended due to potential deleterious effects. Steroids do not improve outcome or lower ICP |

Abbreviations: CPP = cerebral perfusion pressure; ICH = intracranial hypertension; ICP = intracranial pressure; $PaCO_2$ = arterial carbon dioxide tension; $PaO_2$ = arterial oxygen tension; SBP = systolic blood pressure; $SjvO_2$ = jugular venous oxygen saturation; TBI = traumatic brain injury.

A minimum of two large-bore, peripheral, intravenous catheters should be placed, preferably in the upper extremities. General anesthesia with tracheal intubation is required for control of oxygenation and ventilation (see Chapter 7). Some patients with TBI requiring emergency craniotomy may be intubated when they arrive in the operating room. In these patients, adequate positioning of the tracheal tube must be confirmed. In patients who are not already intubated, expedient tracheal intubation is often necessary based on the patient's clinical condition. Airway management can be challenging because of several factors, including:

- Urgent/emergent nature of the procedure
- Potential for aspiration

- Potential instability of the cervical spine
- Potentially complicated airway (airway injury, blood, skull base fracture)
- Elevated ICP
- Uncooperative or combative patient
- Existing impaired oxygenation, ventilation, or hemodynamic status

The choice of intubation technique is determined by urgency, personnel experience, and available resources (see Chapter 3). In general, rapid sequence induction (RSI) and intubation with manual in-line immobilization is recommended. If the cervical collar is in place, the anterior portion is removed to allow greater mouth opening and facilitate laryngoscopy. Cervical collars have not been shown to significantly reduce neck movement by themselves and may, in fact, make intubation more difficult. Since the injured brain has minimal tolerance to hypoxia, hypercarbia, and increased ICP, it is important to have a variety of emergency airway equipment immediately available, including indirect laryngoscopy (e.g., Glidescope), gum elastic bougie, laryngeal mask airway, and emergency surgical airway equipment. Nasotracheal intubation should be avoided in patients with base of skull fractures, severe facial fractures, or bleeding diathesis.

## Oxygenation and ventilation

Hypoxia, hypercarbia, and hypocarbia should be avoided as they cause secondary injuries after TBI. Oxygenation should be monitored and maintained at $PaO_2 > 60$ mmHg or oxygen saturation > 90%. Hyperventilation causes cerebral vasoconstriction and can result in ischemia. The current guidelines for managing TBI indicate that prophylactic hyperventilation ($PaCO_2 \leq 25$ mmHg) is not recommended and hyperventilation should be avoided during the first 24 hours after TBI when cerebral blood flow (CBF) is often critically reduced. Hyperventilation is recommended as a temporizing measure for the reduction of elevated ICP and may be utilized briefly during emergent evacuation of expanding intracranial hematoma.

## Anesthetic technique

Anesthetic agents, including sedative/hypnotic agents used to facilitate intubation, can affect cerebral physiology in multiple ways. Choice of induction agent depends on hemodynamic status. Thiopental and propofol are indirect cerebral vasoconstrictors, reducing cerebral metabolic rate for oxygen ($CMRO_2$) coupled with a corresponding reduction of CBF. Both autoregulation and $CO_2$ reactivity are preserved. However, propofol and thiopental can cause cardiovascular depression and venodilation leading to hypotension, especially in the presence of uncorrected hypovolemia. Etomidate decreases the cerebral metabolic rate, CBF, and ICP. At the same time, because of minimal cardiovascular effects, cerebral perfusion pressure (CPP) is well maintained. However, etomidate has been shown to inhibit adrenal hormone synthesis with persisting low cortisol levels for approximately 12–24 hours after administration and may necessitate vasopressor use. The effect of single induction dose of etomidate on TBI outcome is not clear. Ketamine is a weak non-competitive N-methyl-D-aspartate (NMDA) antagonist that has sympathomimetic properties. Its cerebral effects are complex and are partly dependent on the action of other concurrently administered drugs. Ketamine causes limited cardiovascular changes but increases CBF and ICP. Therefore, it is generally not recommended for TBI patients.

The effects of anesthetic technique (inhalation versus total intravenous anesthesia) on TBI outcome have not conclusively revealed superiority of one technique over another. However, in general, low-dose volatile agents preserve cerebral hemodynamics compared to high-dose volatile agents. The cerebral effects of inhaled anesthetic agents appear to be twofold; at low doses, they preserve flow metabolism coupling whereas at doses $> 1$ minimum alveolar concentration (MAC), direct cerebral vasodilation may cause cerebral hyperemia and increased ICP. With the exception of sevoflurane, which appears to preserve cerebral autoregulation at all clinically relevant doses, other inhalational agents impair cerebral autoregulation in a dose-dependent manner. Nitrous oxide is generally avoided due to increased $CMRO_2$ and increased ICP from cerebral vasodilatation. Preexisting pneumocephalus may be aggravated by the use of nitrous oxide.

Neuromuscular relaxants have little or no effect on CBF and ICP. Succinylcholine and rocuronium are both suitable options for muscle relaxation during RSI (see Chapter 7). Succinylcholine may contribute to increased ICP, which can be blunted by administration of an adequate dose of an induction agent. While the clinical significance of the effect of succinylcholine on ICP is questionable, increases in ICP secondary to hypoxia and hypercarbia are well documented and much more likely to be clinically important. Coughing and bucking during intubation can also cause a large increase in ICP. Hence, in patients with TBI, clinicians should not avoid using succinylcholine when difficulty in airway management is anticipated.

In general, opioids are safe to use in patients with TBI whose trachea is intubated. However, opioids may cause hypercarbia and ICP elevation if the airway is not secure. There is no evidence of direct opiate-mediated cerebral vasodilatory action in the presence of controlled ventilation. However, in patients with decreased intracranial compliance, opioid-induced systemic hypotension can also lead to secondary increase in ICP from compensatory vasodilatation.

## Intraoperative monitoring

In additional to standard American Society of Anesthesiology (ASA) monitors, arterial catheterization is recommended for beat-to-beat blood pressure monitoring and for blood gas analysis, glucose, and blood electrolyte sampling during surgery. Central venous catheterization may be useful for resuscitation and when vasopressors are administered but should not delay surgical decompression, as vascular access may be obtained using femoral or intraosseous catheters, should peripheral intravenous access prove to be difficult. Ultrasound guidance should be used to facilitate internal jugular vein cannulation, thereby reducing the need for Trendelenburg positioning, which may increase ICP.

In general, ICP monitoring is recommended in all salvageable patients with severe TBI (GCS $\leq 8$) and an abnormal CT scan (hematomas, contusions, swelling, herniation, or compressed basal cistern), and in patients with severe TBI with a normal CT scan if two or more of the following features are noted at the admission: age $> 40$ years, unilateral or bilateral motor posturing, or SBP $< 90$ mmHg. For patients with TBI undergoing extracranial surgeries, intraoperative ICP monitoring is desirable to optimize cerebral physiology and avoid secondary increases in ICP. However, intraoperative placement of ICP monitors is not desirable if coagulopathy is present (see also Chapter 9).

Despite their increasing application in intensive care units, advanced neuromonitoring techniques have not gained widespread acceptance for intraoperative management of patients undergoing urgent/emergent surgical decompression. Jugular venous oximetry may be performed in select patients as it allows assessment of the global oxygenation status of the brain as well as adequacy of CBF. Normal $SjvO_2$ ranges between 55 and 75%. The ischemic threshold has been reported to be an $SjvO_2 < 50\%$ for at least 10 minutes. In TBI, $SjvO_2$ is most commonly used for the detection of reduced cerebral perfusion and titration of hyperventilation in patients with increased ICP. Both transcranial Doppler ultrasonography and brain tissue oxygenation monitoring have been used to optimize CBF and cerebral oxygenation.

## Hemodynamic management

Blood pressure and CPP are often low after TBI. Several studies have documented worsened outcome in TBI patients who have experienced episodes of hypotension (SBP < 90 mmHg) after TBI. Thus, continuous monitoring and optimization of blood pressure and CPP are a fundamental part of TBI management. The Brain Trauma Foundation currently recommends CPP of 50–70 mmHg in patients with TBI. It is worth noting that there is a lack of intraoperative data and it is unclear as to what the optimal intraoperative hemodynamic goals should be. However, cerebral autoregulation may be impaired after TBI and this is important because when blood pressure is low-normal, cerebral ischemia may result; whereas in the presence of normal-high blood pressures, cerebral hyperemia may ensue. Therefore, cerebral autoregulation is one important mediator of CBF and outcome after TBI.

## Fluid management

Isotonic crystalloid solution is preferable in TBI for fluid replacement. Glucose-containing solutions should be avoided. The role of colloids is controversial. According to the Saline versus Albumin Fluid Evaluation (SAFE) study, resuscitation with albumin is associated with higher mortality rate and unfavorable outcome in TBI patients. A multi-center, clinical randomized controlled trial to determine whether out-of-hospital administration of hypertonic fluids would improve neurologic outcome following severe TBI has been terminated early due to presumed futility. The investigators concluded that initial fluid resuscitation of patients with severe TBI with either hypertonic saline/dextran or hypertonic saline (HTS) was not superior to 0.9% saline with respect to six-month neurologic outcome or survival.

Osmotherapeutics have been shown to decrease ICP and improve cerebral perfusion pressure. Mannitol is the first-line osmotic agent for the treatment of ICH in TBI. The recommended dose of mannitol is 0.25 to 1 g/kg body weight administered over 20 minutes. Its use prior to ICP monitoring should be restricted to patients with signs of transtentorial herniation or progressive neurological deterioration only due to intracranial pathology. However, due to osmotic diuresis, mannitol administration may result in hypovolemia and hypotension, reverse osmotic shift as a result of excessive administration leading to worsening cerebral edema and secondary brain injury, as well as acute kidney injury. In addition, when compared to HTS, mannitol appears to disturb blood coagulation more. There is limited evidence regarding the benefit and favorable side effect profile of HTS over mannitol administration in TBI. However, HTS has been shown to have beneficial vasoregulatory, immunomodulatory, and neurochemical effects on the injured brain while improving brain tissue oxygenation and hemodynamics (higher CPP and cardiac output) when used as a second-tier therapy after mannitol administration for elevated ICP. Current Brain Trauma Foundation Guidelines indicate that mannitol is an effective osmotic agent to treat high ICP.

## Anemia

Evidence suggests that both anemia and packed red blood cell (PRBC) transfusion are associated with poor neurological outcome in TBI. While anemia is associated with increased in-hospital mortality, lower hospital discharge GCS score, and lower discharge Glasgow outcome score, RBC transfusion is associated with acute lung injury, longer intensive care unit and hospital stay, and mortality in TBI.

Mechanisms proposed for anemia-induced brain injury include tissue hypoxia, reactive oxygen species, disruption of blood-brain barrier function, vascular thrombosis, and anemic cerebral hyperemia. However, a number of cerebro-protective physiological mechanisms become effective with anemia which include aortic chemoreceptor activation, increased sympathetic activity leading to increased heart rate, stroke volume and cardiac index, reduced systemic vascular resistance, and enhanced oxygen extraction. Moreover, a number of cellular mechanisms of cerebral protection become effective in acute anemia. These include Hypoxia Inducible Factor, increased nitric oxide synthase and nitric oxide in the brain (nNOS/NO), erythropoietin and vascular endothelial growth factor-mediated angiogenesis, and vascular repair.

The overall effects of anemia on the brain, therefore, depend on the relative balance between these competing protective and harmful factors of anemia and PRBC transfusion. It is unclear whether the transfusion trigger in patients with TBI should be any different from other critically ill patients and whether the injured brain is more susceptible to the deleterious effects of anemia. The optimal hemoglobin level in TBI patients is unclear, but there is no benefit of a liberal transfusion strategy in moderate to severe TBI patients.

Monitoring modalities such as brain tissue oxygen tension, near infrared spectroscopy, and jugular bulb catheter sampling can be used to monitor the regional or global oxygenation, and may help to determine transfusion needs. Their effectiveness in patient outcome, however, remains to be proven. The anesthesiologist should individualize the decision for transfusion during craniotomy based on preexisting comorbidities and ongoing blood loss, and after weighing risks versus benefits.

## Coagulopathy

Coagulopathy is a common problem after TBI. Coagulation disorders can cause secondary brain injury from ongoing intracranial bleeding and worsen outcome. TBI is associated with the release of tissue thromboplastin that activates the extrinsic coagulation pathway. The activation of clotting cascades may lead to the formation of intravascular fibrin and the consumption of procoagulants and platelets, which results in disseminated intravascular coagulation (DIC) (Table 13.4).

At present, there is no standard guideline for treatment of coagulopathy in TBI. The management of DIC includes platelets and blood component replacement. However, plasma, platelet concentrates, heparin, antithrombin III, procoagulant drugs such as rFVIIa, and antifibrinolytic agents such as tranexamic acid have been tested using different protocols to correct coagulopathy in patients with TBI, though not all studies returned with significant benefit on outcome, and there is no strong evidence supporting the benefit of FVIIa in TBI patients.

**Table 13.4.** International Society of Thrombosis and Homeostasis diagnostic criteria for DIC

| Category | Value | Score |
|---|---|---|
| Platelet count ($10^3$/mm$^3$) | > 100 | 0 |
| | 50–100 | 1 |
| | < 50 | 2 |
| D-dimer (nmol/L) | < 1 | 0 |
| | 1–5 | 1 |
| | > 5 | 2 |
| PT (sec) | < 3 | 0 |
| | 3–6 | 1 |
| | > 6 | 2 |
| Fibrinogen (g/dl) | >1 | 0 |
| | < 1 | 1 |
| DIC score | ≥ 5 points | DIC |
| | < 5 points | Suggestive (but not confirmative) for non-overt DIC |

Abbreviations: PT = prothrombin time; DIC = disseminated intravascular coagulation.

# Glucose control

Hyperglycemia is a stress response after TBI and is associated with increased morbidity and mortality. Blood glucose levels are known to increase during anesthesia even in patients who do not have preexisting diabetes mellitus. Approximately 15% of adults and 23% of children undergoing emergent/urgent craniotomy for TBI have intraoperative hyperglycemia. Risk factors for intraoperative hyperglycemia include age < 4 years or > 65 years, severe TBI (GCS < 9), presence of subdural hematoma on CT scan, and preoperative hyperglycemia. Intraoperative hyperglycemia is associated with increased mortality after TBI. However, the benefit of tight glucose control is unproven. Tight control may in fact lead to hypoglycemia, which may be detrimental for the injured brain. In the absence of strong evidence for tight control, it is recommended to maintain intraoperative glucose values < 180 mg/dL. More importantly, however, glucose should be monitored at least at hourly intervals during general anesthesia. Development and clinical implementation of continuous or frequent glucose monitoring devices and "closed-loop" glycemic control systems coupled with algorithm-driven treatment protocols may reduce both extremes of hypoglycemia and hyperglycemia.

# Therapeutic hypothermia

Proposed mechanisms by which hypothermia protects the brain include reduction in brain metabolic rate, attenuation of blood-brain barrier permeability, reduction of the critical threshold for oxygen delivery, calcium antagonism, blockade of excitotoxic mechanisms, preservation of protein synthesis, reduction of intracellular acidosis, modulation of the inflammatory response, decrease in edema formation, suppression of free radicals and antioxidants, and modulation of apoptotic cell death. Furthermore, hypothermia lowers the cerebral metabolic rate by 6–7% for every 1°C decrease in core temperature, which consequently improves oxygen supply to the areas of ischemic brain and decreases ICP. However, multi-center phase III trials have failed to demonstrate a benefit of hypothermia in TBI. One randomized, multi-center clinical trial (NABIS: H II) of very early mild hypothermia maintained for 48 hours was terminated early due to no significant difference in outcome in patients treated with hypothermia compared with those treated with normothermia. Current Brain Trauma Foundation guidelines cite prophylactic hypothermia as a level III treatment option (degree of clinical certainty not established) that may confer better outcomes when target temperature is maintained for $\geq$ 48 hours. Intraoperative hypothermia may be undesirable in the presence of ongoing coagulopathy. It is important to note that hyperthermia is detrimental to the injured brain and should be prevented.

## Decompressive craniectomy

Persistent uncontrolled ICH results in poor outcomes following TBI. Up to 15% of severe TBI patients with ICH do not respond to maximum medical management and may need second tier therapies including decompressive craniectomy. In addition, decompressive craniectomy may improve compliance, CBF, and brain oxygenation. Recently published results from the Australian multi-center DECRA study reported on 155 adults with severe diffuse TBI and refractory ICH. According to the study, early bifronto-temporoparietal decompressive craniectomy lowers ICP and the length of stay in the ICU, but leads to more unfavorable outcomes. Rates of death were found to be similar in both the craniectomy group (19%) and the standard-care group (18%) at six months. Another randomized trial on decompressive craniectomy, the United Kingdom initiated RESCUEicp study, is currently ongoing.

## Emergence from anesthesia

The management of emergence in the TBI patient may be dictated by multiple factors:

- TBI severity
- Preoperative level of consciousness
- Associated injuries
- Brain conditions at the end of the surgical procedure
- Intraoperative complications
- Need for ongoing resuscitation

The decision to extubate the trachea in the operating room in TBI patients must be individualized. During emergence, blood pressure and $PaCO_2$ control are important as hypertension and hypercarbia may be deleterious and may warrant aggressive blood pressure control. Patients planned for delayed tracheal extubation because of aforementioned factors should be taken directly to the ICU. Multi-modal monitoring, ICP control, brain protective strategies, and optimization of CPP are fundamental objectives for the ICU team. Adequate analgesia and sedation reduce anxiety, agitation, and pain as they can increase ICP. Commonly used sedatives include propofol, midazolam, and dexmedetomidine. Adequate analgesia can be provided with continuous intravenous infusion of short-acting opioids such as remifentanil or fentanyl. Coughing, straining, and hypertension during transportation may lead to intracranial bleeding and elevation of ICP;

neuromuscular relaxants help to prevent this. Hypertension can be treated with labetalol or esmolol, and supplemental barbiturates or short-acting benzodiazepines such as midazolam can be given for sedation. In many centers, it is considered prudent to obtain an immediate postoperative CT scan to rule out remediable surgical complications. Patients with severe TBI are often transported with the head of bed elevated to prevent ICP increase.

## Key points

- Careful pre-anesthesia evaluation including mechanism of injury and neurological assessment, Brain Trauma Foundation guided physiologic optimization, and multi-modal cerebral monitoring are the current cornerstones of severe TBI management.
- Data on the impact of anesthetic technique (inhalation versus total intravenous anesthesia) on TBI outcome have not conclusively revealed superiority of one technique over another.
- Prophylactic hyperventilation ($PaCO_2 \leq 25$ mmHg) is not recommended and hyperventilation should be avoided during the first 24 hours after severe TBI. Low and high blood pressures may result in cerebral ischemia and cerebral hyperemia, respectively, and should be avoided. Currently, maintaining a CPP between 50–70 mmHg is recommended in severe TBI.
- Isotonic crystalloid solutions are preferable to hypotonic solutions. The role of colloids is controversial. The optimal hemoglobin level in TBI patients is unknown but there is no benefit of a liberal transfusion strategy in moderate to severe TBI.
- Glucose-containing solutions should be avoided. Continuous or frequent glucose monitoring devices with algorithm-driven treatment protocols may reduce both extremes of hypoglycemia and hyperglycemia.
- Hyperthermia should be avoided.
- Decompressive craniectomy lowers ICP and length of stay in the ICU, but does not appear to affect mortality in severe TBI.

## Further reading

1. Clifton GL, Valadka A, Zygun D, et al. Very early hypothermia induction in patients with severe brain injury (the National Acute Brain Injury Study: Hypothermia II): a randomised trial. *Lancet Neurol* 2011;**10**:131–139.

2. Cooper DJ, Rosenfeld JV, Murray L, et al; DECRA Trial Investigators; Australian and New Zealand Intensive Care Society Clinical Trials Group. Decompressive craniectomy in diffuse traumatic brain injury. *N Engl J Med* 2011;**364**:1493–1502.

3. Faul M, Xu L, Wald MM, Coronado VG. *Traumatic Brain Injury in the United States: Emergency Department Visits, Hospitalizations, and Deaths.* Atlanta, GA: Centers for Disease Control and Prevention, National Center for Injury Prevention and Control; 2010.

4. Hutchinson PJ, Corteen E, Czosnyka M, et al. Decompressive craniectomy in traumatic brain injury: the randomized multicenter RESCUEicp study (www.RESCUEicp.com). *Acta Neurochir Suppl* 2006;**96**:17–20.

5. Myburgh J, Cooper DJ, Finfer S, et al. SAFE Study Investigators; Australian and New Zealand Intensive Care Society Clinical Trials Group; Australian Red Cross Blood Service; George Institute for International Health. Saline or albumin for fluid resuscitation in patients with traumatic brain injury. *N Engl J Med* 2007;**357**:874–884.

6.  Perel P, Roberts I, Shakur H, et al. Haemostatic drugs for traumatic brain injury. *Cochrane Database Syst Rev* 2010;(1): CD007877.

7.  The NICE-SUGAR Study Investigators. Intensive versus conventional glucose control in critically ill patients. *N Engl J Med* 2009;**360**:1283–1297.

# 14
# Anesthetic considerations for spinal cord injury

Armagan Dagal and Michael J. Souter

## Epidemiology

Approximately 12,000–20,000 new cases of non-fatal spinal cord injury (SCI) occur per year, according to the National Spinal Cord Injury Database, which populates data from an estimated 13% of these new SCI cases in the United States. Currently, some 250,000 Americans are living with the debilitating consequences of SCI.

Most SCIs are associated with an injury to the bony vertebral column as well as a coexisting traumatic injury to other regions. Between 20 and 60% of SCIs are associated with a concurrent traumatic brain injury (TBI). The median age at injury is 41 years and the United States population demographics are listed in Table 14.1.

Annual SCI costs are estimated to be $9.7 billion. In December 2009, estimates for average first year healthcare and living expenses ranged from $244,562 for incomplete motor function at any level to $829,843 for high tetraplegia (C1–C4). The subsequent recurring annual cost is reported to be well below first-year costs but is nonetheless a large economic burden on healthcare systems.

The life expectancy of individuals surviving at least one year following SCI varies with age and height of injury. For tetraplegics with C1–C4 level injury, life expectancy over one year post-injury is 37.4% at 20 years of age, 21.2% at 40, and 8.6% at 60. Pneumonia, septicemia, and pulmonary emboli are the leading causes of death among patients with SCI.

## Etiology

Etiology of SCI can be divided into traumatic or non-traumatic origin.

### Traumatic

- Motor vehicle collision 41.3%
- Falls 27.3%
- Violence 15%
- Sports-related injuries 7.9%
- Others/unknown 8.5%

### Non-traumatic

- Tumors
- Vascular disorders

---

*Essentials of Trauma Anesthesia*, ed. A. J. Varon and C. E. Smith. Published by Cambridge University Press.
© Cambridge University Press 2012.

**Table 14.1.** Spinal cord injury population demographics

| Feature | Incidence |
|---|---|
| Male | 81.0% |
| White | 66.2% |
| Employed | 57.5% |
| Married | 47.9% |
| College graduate | 26.5% |
| Veteran | 25.4% |
| Cervical injuries | 55.2% |
|     incomplete tetraplegia | 38.3% |
|     complete tetraplegia | 16.9% |

- Cysts
- Infections
- Arthropathy
- Iatrogenic (e.g., lumbar drain placement)

Advancing age is associated with a decreased frequency of acts of violence and sports injury, whereas falls increase in frequency, becoming the leading cause of SCI in those individuals over 50 years of age.

# Pathophysiology

SCI is divided into two separate but related categories – an initial or primary injury, and a subsequent secondary injury. Primary injury occurs at the time of the traumatic insult and includes shearing forces rupturing axons or blood vessels. Sources of mechanical force include:

- Bony fragments (e.g., vertebral body)
- Joint dislocation (e.g., facet joints, intervertebral joints)
- Arthropathy (e.g., spondylosis, spondylolisthesis)
- Ligamentous tears
- Intervertebral disc herniation

Secondary injury begins within minutes following the initial injury. Pathological mechanisms induce cord edema and, as a result of the rigid confines of the vertebral canal, increased pressure within that canal. This reaches its maximum between four and six days after the injury, with a consequent risk of ischemia. Central hemorrhagic necrosis may result from prolonged or severe ischemia.

The pathological consequences of injury include:

- Ischemia
- Hypoxia

- Inflammation
- Excitotoxicity
- Lipid peroxidation
- Neuron apoptosis

# Classification of spinal cord injury

## Complete spinal cord injury

- Loss of sensation and motor function in levels below the injury. In the acute stage, arreflexia, no response to plantar stimulation, and flaccidity exist. Male patients may have priapism. The bulbocavernosus reflex is usually absent. Urinary retention and bladder distension occur.

## Incomplete spinal cord injury

- Central cord syndrome. Disproportionate weakness in upper extremities below the level of the lesion compared with the lower extremities. More common in elderly patients with preexisting arthropathy.
- Anterior cord syndrome. Interrupted blood supply to the anterior portion of the spinal cord. Paraplegia/quadriplegia. Pain and temperature sensation loss (spinothalamic tract lesion), preserved two-point discrimination, position sense, deep pressure (posterior column).
- Brown-Sequard syndrome. Ipsilateral hemiplegia and contralateral pain and temperature sensation deficits due to injury to either side of the cord. More common with penetrating trauma.
- Posterior cord syndrome. Interrupted blood supply to the dorsal column of the spinal cord. Isolated ipsilateral loss of two-point discrimination, vibration, and conscious proprioception.
- Cauda equina syndrome. Compression of the nerves in the cauda equina, characterized by dull pain in the lower back and upper buttocks and lack of feeling (analgesia) in the buttocks, genitalia, and thigh, together with disturbances of bowel and bladder function.

# Initial assessment

The essential management principles of spine trauma include early detection and prevention of secondary injury through maintenance of adequate oxygenation, blood pressure support (volume replacement and cardiovascular support), and immobilization.

Spinal cord function is generally examined during the secondary trauma survey, after attending to airway, breathing, and circulation. Accurate assessment and documentation of the patient's neurological status helps to guide future management. The American Spinal Injury Association (ASIA) score is the grading scale employed for neurological assessment in patients with spinal injury (Figure 14.1). This comprises bilateral strength assessment of 10 muscle groups and pinprick discrimination assessment of 28 specific sensory locations. ASIA grade A refers to complete loss of motor and sensory function, whereas ASIA grade E describes intact function. Grades B, C, and D refer to progressively less severe involvement of motor and sensory pathways.

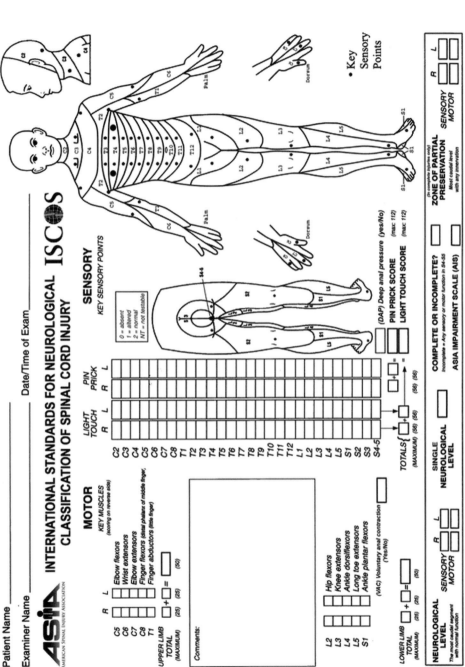

**Figure 14.1.** The American Spinal Injury Association (ASIA) score.

## Muscle Function Grading

**0** = total paralysis

**1** = palpable or visible contraction

**2** = active movement, full range of motion (ROM) with gravity eliminated

**3** = active movement, full ROM against gravity

**4** = active movement, full ROM against gravity and moderate resistance in a muscle specific position.

**5** = (normal) active movement, full ROM against gravity and full resistance in a muscle specific position expected from an otherwise unimpaired peson.

**5\*** = (normal) active movement, full ROM against gravity and sufficient resistance to be considered normal if identified inhibiting factors (i.e. pain, disuse) were not present.

**NT** = not testable (i.e. due to immobilization, severe pain such that the patient cannot be graded, amputation of limb, or contracture of >50% of the range of motion).

## ASIA Impairment (AIS) Scale

☐ **A = Complete.** No sensory or motor function is preserved in the sacral segments S4-S5.

☐ **B = Sensory Incomplete.** Sensory but not motor function is preserved below the neurological level and includes the sacral segments S4-S5 (light touch, pin prick at S4-S5: or deep anal pressure (DAP)). AND no motor function is preserved more than three levels below the motor level on either side of the body.

☐ **C = Motor Incomplete.** Motor function is preserved below the neurological level\*\*, and more than half of key muscle functions below the single neurological level of injury (NLI) have a muscle grade less than 3 (Grades 0-2).

☐ **D = Motor Incomplete.** Motor function is preserved below the neurological level\*\*, and at least half (half or more) of key muscle functions below the NLI have a muscle grade ≥ 3.

☐ **E = Normal.** If sensation and motor function as tested with the ISNCSCI are graded as normal in all segments, and the patient had prior deficits, then the AIS grade is E. Someone without an initial SCI does not receive an AIS grade.

\*\*For an individual to receive a grade of C or D, i.e. motor incomplete status, they must have either (1) voluntary anal sphincter contraction or (2) sacral sparing with sparing of motor function more than three levels below the motor level for that side of the body. The Standards at this time allows even non-key muscle function more than 3 levels below the motor level to be used in determining motor incomplete status (AIS B versus C).

NOTE: When assessing the extent of motor sparing below the level for distinguishing between AIS B and C, the *motor level* on each side is used; whereas to differentiate between AIS C and D (based on proportion of key muscle functions with strength grade 3 or greater) the *single neurological level* is used.

## Steps in Classification

The following order is recommended in determining the classification of individuals with SCI.

1. Determine sensory levels for right and left sides.

2. Determine motor levels for right and left sides.
   *Note: in regions where there is no myotome to test, the motor level is presumed to be the same as the sensory level. If testable motor function above that level is also normal.*

3. Determine the single neurological level.
   *This is the lowest segment where motor and sensory function is normal on both sides, and is the most cephalad of the sensory and motor levels determined in steps 1 and 2.*

4. Determine whether the injury is Complete or Incomplete. (i.e. absence or presence of sacral sparing)
   *If voluntary anal contraction = No AND all S4-5 sensory scores = 0 AND deep anal pressure = No, then injury is COMPLETE. Otherwise, injury is incomplete.*

5. Determine ASIA Impairment Scale (AIS) Grade:
   **Is injury Complete?** If YES, AIS=A and can record ZPP (lowest dermatome or myotome on each side with some preservation)

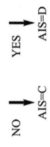

   If NO, AIS=B
   (Yes=voluntary anal contraction OR motor function more than three levels below the motor level on a given side, if the patient has sensory incomplete classification)

   **Are at least half of the key muscles below the single neurological level graded 3 or better?**

   NO → AIS=C    YES → AIS=D

   If sensation and motor function is normal in all segments, AIS=E
   *Note: AIS E is used in follow-up testing when an individual with a documented SCI has recovered normal function. If at initial testing no deficits are found, the individual is neurologically intact; the ASIA Impairment Scale does not apply.*

**Figure 14.1.** (cont.)

# Airway management

Airway interventions may be required during the hospital course of the patient with known or suspected traumatic SCI (see Chapter 3).

SCI occurs in up to 2–5% of all major trauma cases and at least 14% of these cases have the potential to have an unstable spine. Techniques to minimize cervical spine (C-spine) movement should be employed during airway management, while considerations should be given to other potential injuries. Cervical SCI occurs in up to 10% of head injured patients. As such, a high index of suspicion should be employed during airway management of traumatically injured patients, especially with head injury.

Although there is little evidence to support its practice, spinal immobilization is a logical course in all trauma victims. In the prehospital setting, neck immobilization with cervical collar, lateral supports, straps, and spinal hardboard should be used. Patients should be transferred off the hardboard as soon as it is practical and safe, to minimize pressure injury. Padded boards or inflatable beanbags help to reduce pressure on the occiput and sacrum. In the hospital, C-spine immobilization should continue by these methods and must be applied until appropriately trained clinicians clear the spine. Collar use in isolation is not ideal and could lead to C-spine misalignment.

In the normal spine, direct laryngoscopy leads to extension of the C-spine, predominantly at the atlanto-occipital junction, and to a lesser extent at the C1 to C2 joint. The sub-axial cervical segments (C4-C7) are minimally displaced but additional flexion occurs at the cervico-thoracic junction. Pressure exerted by the laryngoscope blade on airway soft tissue is generally transmitted to the spinal cord. Instability of the occiput–atlas–axis complex may lead to anterior movement of the atlas during direct laryngoscopy, thereby reducing the space available for the spinal cord.

The urgent nature of airway interventions usually requires direct or indirect laryngoscopy with manual in-line immobilization (MILI). The goal of MILI is to apply sufficient stabilizing force to the head and neck to limit spine movement during airway intervention. MILI provides better cervical stability but impairs the view of the vocal cords during conventional laryngoscopy. Use of increased laryngoscope blade force to overcome poor views does have the potential to increase cervical motion at an unstable fracture site when MILI is applied. Nevertheless, when MILI is utilized, the incidence of neurological impairment due to endotracheal intubation is extremely rare.

A minimum of jaw thrust and chin lift should be used and early employment of an oral or nasal airway helps to reduce the force required for airway maintenance.

Elective fixation of known spine or associated injuries requires careful planning for safe airway intervention. The patient may present in cervical traction or a halo, which impedes access to the airway.

Prevailing cervical spinal pathology including spondylosis, rheumatoid arthritis, Klippel–Feil syndrome, ankylosing spondylitis, tumor, cervical instrumentation, and upper (versus lower) cervical disease may increase the difficulty of airway interventions. Several methods of tracheal intubation exist, but no one technique has been proven superior to others (see Chapter 3). Awake fiberoptic intubation has not been shown to be superior to an asleep procedure. Awake fiberoptic intubation does enable a neurological exam to be performed after intubation and positioning. It requires cooperation, and may increase stress, discomfort, and disability in acutely injured patients. Patients without preexisting neurological impairment and acceptable radiological findings can be managed with MILI and direct laryngoscopy (with a tracheal tube introducer for grade III views) or Glidescope. If the airway is potentially difficult and the patient has an existing neurological deficit with C-spine instability, an alternative technique should be considered. A reinforced endotracheal tube may reduce the risk of kinking during patient positioning and also prevents tracheal compression during retraction employed in anterior cervical procedures.

Rigid indirect videolaryngoscopy has become an alternative to conventional direct laryngoscopy. There are a large number of small studies on normal subjects with significant population heterogeneity, but it is difficult to draw meaningful conclusions on their efficacy in SCI. The view of the vocal cords is usually superior with these devices compared with conventional laryngoscopy.

Supraglottic devices are part of the failed or difficult intubation algorithm. In the "can't intubate, can't ventilate" scenario, early consideration should be given to the surgical airway or cricothyroidotomy. These techniques may still produce movement of the C-spine, but this should not prevent their use in life-threatening circumstances.

The tracheal tube introducer, often referred to as the "gum elastic bougie," is a well-established adjunct to direct laryngoscopy, allowing successful intubation of the trachea in more limited views, and resulting in the application of less force during laryngoscopy.

The decision to extubate the trachea postoperatively is influenced by many factors. These include the ease of intubation, extent and duration of surgery, surgical complications (e.g., recurrent laryngeal nerve injury), prone positioning, blood loss, and subsequent fluid resuscitation. The presence of a cuff leak demonstrated on either inspiration or expiration in the spontaneously breathing patient has not consistently been shown to predict subsequent airway obstruction. Extubating the trachea with an airway exchange catheter in situ may facilitate emergent reintubation in the event of an obstruction from airway edema or hematoma. Good clinical judgment is paramount, and if there is concern, the trachea should be extubated at a later time.

As in most trauma situations, adequate neuromuscular blockade is required for successful intubation. Succinylcholine is the preferred agent for emergent intubation but should be avoided between two days and nine months following SCI due to the risk of induced hyperkalemia caused by denervation hypersensitivity. Rocuronium is an acceptable alternative.

## Cardiovascular management

Traumatic SCI is frequently complicated by systemic hypotension and reduced spinal cord perfusion pressure (SCPP). This in turn may contribute to secondary ischemic neurologic injury and should be avoided. SCPP is determined by the difference in mean arterial pressure (MAP) and cerebrospinal fluid pressure ($CSF_P$) ($SCPP = MAP - CSF_P$). Spinal cord perfusion is autoregulated over a wide range of systemic blood pressure (BP) in the same fashion as cerebral blood flow. Systemic vasodilation occurs in increasing severity with ascending levels of SCI above L2, leading to hypotension. Injuries above T6 are generally accompanied with bradycardia due to compromise of the sympathetic cardiac accelerator fibers.

Causes of systemic hypotension in SCI include:

**Direct**

- Neurogenic shock

### Indirect

- Hemorrhage (associated traumatic injuries)
- Tension pneumothorax
- Myocardial injury
- Pericardial tamponade
- Sepsis

Currently, there is little evidence regarding blood pressure elevation and the required duration to improve outcome in SCI. The American Association of Neurological Surgeons (AANS) published recommendations on the hemodynamic goals for management of the SCI patient. These include maintaining MAP to 85–90 mmHg and avoiding systolic BP less than 90 mmHg for over 5–7 days. Despite the lack of evidence, many consider that aggressive hemodynamic goal-directed management may provide a significant improvement in axonal function both in the motor and somatosensory tracts of the cord and may improve outcome.

Adequate fluid resuscitation is an important step in patients presenting with acute SCI. Conversely, excessive fluid administration in a prone patient is associated with significant edema (including airway edema), cardiac failure, electrolyte abnormalities, coagulopathy, and prolonged duration of postoperative intensive care unit stay. Hypotonic crystalloids such as D5W and 0.45% saline may exacerbate cord swelling and should be avoided. The use of albumin has become debatable, similar to the concerns of increased mortality in TBI (see Chapters 4 and 13). Goal-directed treatment using static and dynamic hemodynamic parameters such as pulse pressure variation, systolic pressure variation and cardiac output monitoring devices may improve intraoperative fluid administration and possibly reduce the morbidity associated with excessive fluid administration (see Chapter 9).

Injuries above T6 warrant an agent with cardioselective (inotropic, chronotropic) as well as vasoconstrictive properties. Agents such as dopamine, norepinephrine, or epinephrine fulfil these requirements with both $\alpha_1$- and $\beta_1$-agonist properties. Phenylephrine preferentially works as a $\alpha_1$-receptor agonist with minimal $\beta_1$ effects. It can be used to counteract the peripheral vasodilation observed in lower thoracic and lumbar cord injuries, but has the potential to induce reflex bradycardia. Vasopressin has a vasoconstrictive and catecholamine sparing effect that may be useful in hypotension. However, its antidiuretic effects may lead to increased water retention and hyponatremia, with potential exacerbation of intracellular edema after injury. Thus, its role in SCI is not well defined, and it should be used with some caution. Dobutamine is predominantly an inotropic agent but its use in SCI is limited because of its vasodilatory effects.

Persistent bradycardia may be seen in high cervical (C1–C5) lesions in the first two weeks after traumatic SCI and requires the use of anticholinergic agents or application of cardiac pacemakers.

$CSF_P$ may become elevated postoperatively, which may lead to a concomitant reduction in spinal cord perfusion. This suggests a possible role for intrathecal pressure monitoring, similar to TBI management. However, there is no direct evidence of improved outcome.

## Blood loss prevention

Maintenance of normovolemia in patients with SCI requiring operative intervention can be challenging.

Predictors for high-volume blood loss include:

- Multiple level thoracolumbar spine surgery
- Preoperative hemoglobin level less than 12 g/dl
- Age greater than 50 years
- Procedures requiring transpedicular osteotomy
- Procedures requiring instrumentation

Known risks of blood component transfusion are well established. While there is usually no benefit in correcting a hematocrit above 21% after surgery, optimal perioperative transfusion strategy remains uncertain in the context of active bleeding and loss of coagulation factors (see Chapter 6).

Several strategies have been used to minimize intraoperative blood loss. Use of the Jackson table, where the abdomen hangs free from compression, reduces the vena cava pressure. This in turn lessens epidural venous bleeding when compared to prone positioning on the Wilson frame. There are no existing studies in spine surgery that adequately compare the effectiveness of normovolemic hemodilution with hypotensive anesthesia, with regard to outcome or transfusion reduction. However, hypotensive anesthesia should be avoided in patients with SCI, as it may exacerbate secondary injury.

Antifibrinolytic agents have been shown to decrease intraoperative and total perioperative blood loss. A randomized study in patients undergoing antero-posterior spinal fusion comparing aminocaproic acid or aprotonin against controls showed an absolute decrease in both total perioperative blood loss and transfusion requirements, but effects in the aminocaproic acid group did not achieve significance. A randomized trial of tranexamic acid versus placebo in patients undergoing posterior thoracic or lumbar instrumented fusions showed significantly less perioperative blood loss compared to placebo; however, there was no difference in the amount of blood products transfused between the two groups. There was no increase in thromboembolic complications. In a recent Cochrane review of 252 randomized clinical trials involving over 25,000 patients, antifibrinolytic drugs used at the time of major surgery were associated with reductions in bleeding, the rate of further surgical procedures to control hemorrhage, and red cell transfusion. With the exception of aprotinin, these drugs appear reasonably safe.

Studies of the use of recombinant factor VIIa (rFVIIa) in multiple level posterior spinal fusion showed an absolute decrease in intraoperative blood loss but no significant decrease in transfusion requirements for the rFVIIa groups at any dose studied.

The effectiveness of using cell savers to reduce the need for homologous transfusion is variable. Studies conducted on cell savers are mostly retrospective with significant bias. There is little in the literature to support its cost-effective use in routine elective spine surgery.

During spine surgery, coagulopathy may occur subsequent to massive blood transfusion. It is a general rule that loss of red cells is accompanied by the loss of coagulation factors and this must be monitored with hemostasis assays and deficits actively replaced (see Chapter 6). Results obtained from standard coagulation testing are too slow to be used in actively bleeding surgical patients, and frequently empiric transfusion is required. In penetrating trauma, viscoelastic point-of-care coagulation assays have been reported as useful with rapid turnaround time and comprehensive assessment of the hemostatic system. The drawbacks of point-of-care testing include less accuracy, errors in predicting transfusion need, the lack of whole blood controls, operation by non-laboratory-trained staff, and cost.

The emergency hemorrhage panel is a recent development offering more accurate results with a short turnaround time. Prothrombin time, fibrinogen, platelet count, and hematocrit have been identified as pivotal factors in coagulation assessment, guiding decision-making on transfusion. This approach will appropriately shape transfusion strategies and prevent unnecessary donor product exposures.

# Electrophysiological monitoring

The ideal monitoring technique should provide:

- Early warning to permit injury to be reversed or minimized
- Continuous real-time assessment of neurologic condition
- Minimal false positives and false negatives
- Ease of interpretation
- Ready availability
- Cost effectiveness

Available intraoperative monitoring techniques include:

- Wake-up test
- Somatosensory evoked potentials (SSEP)
- Motor evoked potentials (MEP)
- Electromyography (EMG)

The Stagnara wake-up test, described in 1973, provides only a discontinuous assessment of neurological function. The intraoperative wake-up test involves a gradual lightening of anesthesia until the patient can voluntarily move the lower extremities. The test provides gross assessment of the motor function on the descending pathways. It does not measure any components of the sensory system. It has limited applicability in SCI, and the reduction in anesthesia is impractical in trauma victims due to their possible associated injuries including TBI.

## Somatosensory evoked potentials

SSEP are elicited by delivering a small electrical current to stimulate peripheral sensory nerves, with the response monitored by cutaneous electrodes positioned over the sensory pathway and somatosensory cortex. The median and posterior tibial nerves are used to monitor the integrity of upper extremity and lower extremity pathways respectively. Depending on the level of surgery, their comparison can offer insight in determining whether change is focal or generalized, suggesting surgical or anesthetic attribution respectively. The operator response time to meaningful change ranges from two to five minutes. Change is assessed by comparison to initial baseline values. These are best acquired immediately after incision, permitting the stabilization of anesthesia and temperature effects.

Amplitude changes of greater than 50% and latency increases of 10% are considered abnormal with amplitude changes being slightly more sensitive to onset of injury. SSEP changes are assumed as significant after alternative causes of change have been addressed (i.e., change in the level of anesthesia, technical faults, hypothermia, and hypotension).

Postoperative paraparesis with normal SSEP is commonly the result of anterior spinal artery syndrome. This syndrome selectively affects the anterolateral columns of the spinal cord with preservation of posterior column function.

# Motor evoked potentials

MEP monitor corticospinal track activity via stimulation at the level of the motor cortex or spinal cord and are selective for motor pathways, although they monitor only 4 to 5% of the motor neuron pool.

MEP are generated by stimulation of the cerebral cortex, and responses are measured from the epidural space or spinal cord (D-wave) or from the compound muscle action potential (CMAP). The CMAP is best monitored at the distal limb muscles, which are rich in corticospinal tract innervation. Common sites include abductor pollicis brevis, long forearm flexors and extensors in the upper extremity, or adductor hallucis brevis and tibialis anterior in the lower extremity. Amplitude changes of more than 50% from baseline are deemed significant while latency of response is less relevant.

Relative contraindications to MEP monitoring include epilepsy, cortical lesion, skull defect (e.g., fontanelle or prior craniectomy), proconvulsant medication, cardiac pacing, and implantable device.

Spontaneous EMG activity is recorded by an electrode placed in the muscle innervated by the nerve to be monitored. This is particularly useful in monitoring the mechanical irritation of nerve roots.

The proposed benefit of evoked potential monitoring is to identify the deterioration of spinal cord function, offering an opportunity to correct offending factors before permanent damage. Such factors include patient position (e.g., neck position, shoulder position), hypotension, hypothermia, and the surgical procedure itself. In elective spinal surgery without EP monitoring, iatrogenic neurological injuries have been estimated to be 0.46% for anterior cervical discectomy, 0.23–3.2% with scoliosis correction, and between 23.8 and 65.4% with intramedullary spinal cord tumor resection.

A recent systematic review indicated that while there is a high level of evidence that continuous real-time neuromonitoring is sensitive and specific in detecting intraoperative neurologic injury during spine surgery, there is a low level of evidence that the overall rate of new or worsening perioperative neurological deficits is reduced. There is little evidence that an intraoperative response to a neuromonitoring alert reduces the rate of perioperative neurologic deterioration.

The effects of anesthesia on synaptic signal transmission degrade monitoring quality in a dose-dependent fashion. This is most marked with nitrous oxide and volatile anesthetics, but also occurs with intravenous agents such as propofol and barbiturates. Volatile anesthetics may be used when SSEP are being monitored, provided their dosing does not exceed 1 MAC, and for spontaneous EMG recording, provided neuromuscular blocking agents are avoided. MEP are even more sensitive to these effects, and total intravenous anesthesia (TIVA) without paralysis is preferred. Nitrous oxide is best avoided. The relative utility of desflurane as compared to other volatile agents remains controversial, with some small studies suggesting preservation of MEP sensitivity.

Conversely, complete neuromuscular blockade should be applied for D-wave epidural recordings to reduce muscle reactivity. Opioids do not impact upon evoked potential monitoring. Ketamine and etomidate have been shown to enhance evoked potential monitoring. Dexmedetomidine has been used as a supplement to TIVA, allowing reduction of propofol dose, with no evidence of detriment to evoked potential monitoring. It needs to be stressed that stable anesthesia without significant changes in dose of any anesthetic agent, blood pressure, or temperature is required to detect those changes in evoked responses consequent upon the surgical procedure.

## Methylprednisolone

Methylprednisolone has been used as a treatment option in acute, non-penetrating SCI to theoretically decrease edema in injured areas of the spinal cord, increasing perfusion, improving impulse generation, and protecting the blood–spinal cord barrier. Proposed mechanisms include cell membrane stabilization as well as the anti-inflammatory properties of high doses (via reduction of interleukins, prostaglandins, and thromboxanes).

A bolus dose of 30 mg/kg over 1 hour, followed by an infusion of 5.4 mg/kg/hour continued for either 23 or 47 hours is used. When initiated between 3 and 8 hours following injury, methylprednisolone was shown to be associated with greater motor, but no functional recovery, when compared to other treatments.

The National Acute Spinal Cord Injury Studies (NASCIS) I, II, and III were multicenter, double-blind, randomized clinical trials conducted to investigate the use of methylprednisolone in acute SCI. After injury, as a result of transient swelling associated with injury, there is an expected nadir of function that subsequently improves. There was some variable timing of baseline assessments that may consequently have confused this expected change with a steroid treatment effect, and this remains an important methodological criticism of these studies, which were underpowered and lacking placebo arms to detect these effects with high-dose methylprednisolone. They also revealed an increased risk of serious side effects including pulmonary complications, wound infections, steroid myelopathy, and gastrointestinal hemorrhage.

Currently, the guidelines of the American Association of Neurological Surgeons/CNS Joint Section on Disorders of the Spine and Peripheral Nerves Guidelines Committee recommend the use of methylprednisolone only as a treatment option (while considering the risks and benefits associated with glucocorticoid use) and not as a standard of care.

## Recent advances in SCI management

Tirilizad mesylate, monosialotetrahexosylganglioside, thyrotropin releasing hormone, gacyclidine, naloxone, and nimodipine have all been investigated with largely negative results. Thyrotropin releasing hormone (Phase II trial) and monosialotetrahexosylganglioside (Phase II and III trials) showed some promise, but currently there are no future trials planned with these agents.

There are some emerging neuroprotective strategies currently under investigation.

### Riluzole

Riluzole is a sodium channel-blocking agent that is approved for use in persons with amyotrophic lateral sclerosis. It is reported to have neuroprotective properties via inhibition of excitotoxicity by blocking voltage-sensitive sodium channels and antagonism of the presynaptic calcium-dependent glutamate release. Based on the available preclinical evidence, riluzole has moved into Phase III clinical trials.

### Cethrin

Nogo-A is an inhibitory membrane protein, present in oligodendrocytes and central nervous system (CNS) myelin membranes. It has a crucial role in restricting axonal regeneration and compensatory fiber growth in the injured adult mammalian CNS. Nogo neutralizing antibodies, peptides blocking the Nogo receptor subunit NgR, and blockers of the postreceptor components Rho-A and ROCK have all been applied in animal models to induce long-distance axonal regeneration and compensatory sprouting, accompanied by an impressive enhancement of functional recovery. They are directly applied to the spinal cord after injury. The Rho antagonist Cethrin is currently undergoing a human clinical trial.

## Early surgical decompression

After SCI, damaged neural tissue may swell in the confined space of the spinal canal leading to further ischemia and excitotoxicity, and early surgical decompression ($< 24$ hours) should logically reduce these risks. Consequently, early surgical decompression has had an increasing role in the treatment of acute SCI. The potential benefit versus the risk inherent in the potentially unstable trauma patient demands careful appraisal. Clinical benefits of early surgery may include shorter length of both intensive care and overall hospital stay, with fewer medical complications (such as pneumonia and deep venous thrombosis). Preliminary results from the Surgical Treatment for Acute Spinal Cord Injury Study (STASCIS) suggest decompression of the spinal cord within 24 hours of injury is associated with improved neurologic recovery in persons with cervical injury.

## Hypothermia

Decompressive surgery within this early period of SCI can be logistically challenging. Transportation, stabilization, investigation (particularly radiological), and organization of surgery require delays of many hours. The ability to inhibit compressive injury to the spinal cord in the interim would be of great benefit in limiting neurological deterioration. There have been a wide range of reported biochemical, histological, and physiological effects attributed to the application of cooling. These include a reduction in polymorphonuclear leukocyte invasion, a lack of reduction in spinal cord blood flow in the injured spinal cord, a reduction in vasogenic edema at the injury site, and a reduction in glutamate levels in the CSF. Studies as long ago as 1966 utilized direct cooling of the spinal cord, but had small subject numbers and enjoyed variable success. Utilization of intravascular cooling catheters provides moderate systemic hypothermia more rapidly and precisely. Recent studies suggest that hypothermia may assist in limiting neuronal injury and apoptosis in the immediate neurotoxic environment induced by the secondary sequelae of spinal trauma. There are conflicting data on whether it affords any protection in circumstances of significant ongoing cord compression. Given the deleterious effects of hypothermia upon coagulation and immune function, well-designed human clinical outcome trials are needed before hypothermia can be recommended as a routine treatment strategy.

# Key points

- Many SCIs are associated with coexisting traumatic injury. It is uncommon for an SCI to present as an isolated injury.
- A high index of suspicion for C-spine instability should be maintained during airway management in blunt trauma patients. Standard precautions for spine protection should be employed at all times, including in-line immobilization. Tracheal intubation with conventional laryngoscopy can be complicated by poor visualization of the glottis. Alternatives to conventional laryngoscopy are often indicated.

- Traumatic SCI is frequently complicated by hypotension and reduced spinal cord perfusion pressure. Hemodynamic goals include MAP to 85–90 mmHg for up to five days. Aggressive hemodynamic goal-directed management may provide a significant improvement in axonal function and may improve outcome.

- Large volume blood loss may occur during spinal cord surgery. Strategies should be utilized to minimize intraoperative blood loss. Massive hemorrhage is usually accompanied by the loss of coagulation factors. Deficits should be replaced, ideally guided by the results of hemostatic assays.

- Intraoperative evoked potential monitoring offers an opportunity to correct offending factors like neck position, hypotension, and the surgical procedure itself before permanent damage occurs. Anesthetic technique requires modification, according to the monitoring modality, to prevent deterioration of the signal quality.

- Methylprednisolone is not recommended as a standard of care, but may be used as a treatment option.

- Decompression of the spinal cord within 24 hours of injury is associated with improved neurologic recovery. The potential benefits of early decompression must be carefully evaluated in the setting of hemodynamic instability in the multiple trauma patient.

- There are possible theoretical advantages of therapeutic hypothermia in SCI. Appropriately designed clinical trials are needed, however, before it can be recommended as a routine treatment strategy.

# Further reading

1. AANS/CNS. Blood pressure management after acute spinal cord injury. *Neurosurgery* 2002;**50**,S58–S62.

2. American College of Surgeons, Committee on Trauma. *Advance Trauma Life Support for Doctors: ATLS® Student Course Manual.* Chicago, IL: American College of Surgeons; 2008.

3. Casha S, Christie S. A systematic review of intensive cardiopulmonary management after spinal cord injury. *J Neurotrauma* 2011;**28**:1479–1495.

4. Crosby ET. Airway management in adults after cervical spine trauma. *Anesthesiology* 2006;**104**:1293–1318.

5. Dietrich WD, Levi AD, Wang M, Green BA. Hypothermic treatment for acute spinal cord injury. *Neurotherapeutics* 2011;**8**:229–239.

6. Fehlings MG, Brodke DS, Norvell DC, Dettori JR. The evidence for intraoperative neurophysiological monitoring in spine surgery: does it make a difference? *Spine (Phila Pa 1976)* 2010;**35**:S37–S46.

7. Furlan JC, Noonan V, Cadotte DW, Fehlings MG. Timing of decompressive surgery of spinal cord after traumatic spinal cord injury: an evidence-based examination of pre-clinical and clinical studies. *J Neurotrauma* 2010;**27**:1–29.

8. Miller SM. Methylprednisolone in acute spinal cord injury: a tarnished standard. *J Neurosurg Anesthesiol* 2008;**20**:140–142.

9. National Spinal Cord Injury Statistical Centre [database on the Internet]. https://www.nscisc.uab.edu/public_content/pdf/Facts%20and%20Figures%20at%20a%20Glance%202010.pdf. Accessed May 1, 2011.

10. Wilson JR, Fehlings MG. Emerging approaches to the surgical management of acute traumatic spinal cord injury. *Neurotherapeutics* 2011;**8**:187–194.

# Anesthetic considerations for ocular and maxillofacial trauma

Olga Kaslow and Suneeta Gollapudy

The multidisciplinary approach to managing ocular and maxillofacial trauma often requires involvement of the anesthesiologist, especially with regard to establishing and maintaining a patent airway in the emergency department, and provision of anesthesia for urgent or elective repair of injuries.

## Ocular trauma

Eye injuries are a common cause of serious morbidity, which could result in a devastating outcome – blindness. Surgery for ocular trauma presents a unique challenge for the anesthesiologist because of its specific physiologic and pharmacologic requirements.

## Mechanisms of ocular trauma

Loss of vision following trauma may occur due to direct injury to the eye globe from laceration, rupture, and contusion, injury to the optic nerve, hypoperfusion of eye structures, or loss of eyelid integrity.

Direct injuries to the eye are classified as open or closed globe. Open globe injury involves a full-thickness wound through the eye wall, comprised of cornea and sclera. Closed globe injury occurs if the ocular wall is preserved.

The type of eye injury determines the urgency of the surgery and the requirements for anesthetic management. Anesthetic goals essential for successful surgical repair of an injured eye include the following:

- Smooth induction and emergence
- Akinesia (eye muscle paralysis)
- Analgesia
- Attenuation of elevated intraocular pressure
- Ablating the oculo-cardiac reflex
- Minimizing bleeding

## Intraocular pressure

Understanding the physiology of intraocular pressure (IOP) and the mechanisms by which it may be altered is of paramount importance to the anesthesia provider. Normal IOP range is 10 to 20 mmHg. Elevation above 25 mmHg is abnormal and eventually leads to loss of

---

*Essentials of Trauma Anesthesia*, ed. A. J. Varon and C. E. Smith. Published by Cambridge University Press.
© Cambridge University Press 2012.

**Table 15.1.** Factors leading to increased intraocular pressure (IOP)

| | |
|---|---|
| ↑ Intraocular blood volume | Sustained systemic hypertension<br>↓ Intraocular vascular tone: choroidal arterial vasodilation due to hypercarbia and hypoxemia |
| ↓ Aqueous humor outflow | ↑ Venous pressure:<br>– Coughing<br>– Vomiting<br>– Valsalva maneuver<br>– Trendelenburg position<br>↓ Aqueous humor drainage:<br>– α-adrenergic stimulation → mydriasis → increase outflow resistance |
| External compression of the eye | – Forceful mask ventilation<br>– Surgical compression of the eye<br>– Contraction of the extraocular muscles (e.g., from succinylcholine) |

vision. The anesthetic technique may have a detrimental effect on IOP. Main determinants of IOP under control of the anesthesiologist are presented in Table 15.1.

# The oculocardiac reflex

The oculocardiac reflex (OCR) might be triggered by ocular trauma and is common in patients undergoing eye surgery. Repeated stimulation leads to fatigue of the OCR. Common causes of OCR include pressure on the eye globe, traction on the extraocular muscles, placement of a retrobulbar or intraorbital block, and orbital compression due to hematoma or edema.

OCR has a trigeminal vagal mechanism:

- Afferent limb: long and short ciliary nerves → ciliary ganglion → gasserian ganglion along the ophthalmic branch of the trigeminal nerve → main trigeminal sensory nucleus in the floor of the fourth ventricle.
- Efferent limb: along the vagus nerve.

OCR may result in negative inotropic and conduction effects such as sinus bradycardia, ectopic beats, heart block, ventricular bigeminy, multi-focal premature ventricular beats, ventricular tachycardia, and even asystole.

Treatment of OCR includes asking the surgeon to remove the pressure on the globe and intravenous (IV) atropine at doses of 0.01 to 0.4 mg/kg (e.g., 0.5–1.0 mg atropine in an adult). Recurrent episodes can be treated with local infiltration of lidocaine near the extrinsic eye muscles.

# Preoperative evaluation of the patient with eye injury

Ocular trauma often presents in combination with injuries to the orbit, face, head, and neck, as well as traumatic brain injury and cervical spine cord damage. The full extent of polytrauma needs to be addressed to establish surgical priorities. The ophthalmologist should perform a thorough eye exam as early as possible. Eye surgery may be delayed in an unstable patient with life-threatening injuries. Definitive surgical repair for an open globe injury requires primary closure within 24 hours of the injury together with antibiotics to prevent endophthalmitis.

Aspiration prophylaxis is a high priority in trauma patients. These drugs do not affect ocular physiology. By promoting gastric emptying or reducing acidity, they decrease the risk of aspiration and vomiting leading to elevated IOP. The following are commonly used agents:

- Serotonin antagonist (ondansetron, 0.15 mg/kg IV, maximum dose 16 mg) prevents emesis.
- Non-particulate antacid (sodium citrate, 30 mL) has a fast pH-lowering effect and a short duration – 30–60 minutes.
- Metoclopramide (0.15 mg/kg IV at the time of admission and then every 2–4 hours until surgery) accelerates gastric emptying.
- H2-histamine antagonist (famotidine, 20 mg IV) should be administered 1.5–2 hours before surgery. Although it inhibits gastric acid secretion, it does not lower the pH of gastric acid already present in a stomach.

## Anesthetic management

General anesthesia with tracheal intubation is necessary for the repair of penetrating eye injuries. General anesthesia is also used in uncooperative or intoxicated adults and in the pediatric patient population. Although regional anesthesia with a retrobulbar block can be administered in cooperative patients with limited trauma to the eyelid and cornea, it is generally contraindicated since it may increase IOP leading to extrusion of intraocular contents. Topical anesthesia is generally contraindicated since it does not allow ocular akinesia and intraocular manipulation.

Rapid sequence induction (RSI) and intubation in a patient with ocular trauma presents certain challenges to the anesthesiologist (see Chapters 3 and 7). A key goal is to achieve smooth, rapid, airway control with minimal sympathetic stimulation and hemodynamic changes to avoid increase in IOP.

- Preoxygenate with gentle application of the face mask minimizing external pressure to the injured eye and face.
- Carefully apply cricoid pressure to avoid interruption of the venous return from the head.
- Avoid bucking, coughing, or crying to prevent detrimental rise in IOP.
- Blunt sympathetic response to laryngoscopy and intubation by pretreatment with IV lidocaine (1.5 mg/kg) and opiates (e.g., remifentanil 0.5–1 mcg/kg).
- Place the patient in reverse Trendelenburg position to increase venous return from the head.

### Induction agents

Most of the induction agents have a protective effect on IOP, except ketamine. Both propofol and thiopental decrease IOP. Propofol also possesses antiemetic properties. Etomidate is the preferred agent for preserving hemodynamic stability, although it carries a risk of myoclonus that might potentially elevate IOP. Pretreatment with midazolam or remifentanil is advocated to attenuate this side effect. Ketamine is known for increasing IOP. It also triggers blepharospasm and nystagmus which makes this agent unsuitable for the patient with eye trauma.

## Neuromuscular blocking agents

Complete neuromuscular block is essential for penetrating eye surgery, since patient movement, especially coughing, can dramatically increase IOP. Succinylcholine is a preferred drug for RSI in trauma for its rapid onset, assuring optimal intubation conditions (see Chapters 3 and 7). Succinylcholine raises IOP by a few mmHg. As with intracranial pressure (ICP), inadequate anesthesia or paralysis is more likely to produce increased IOP and extrusion of vitreous humor than succinylcholine. In open globe eye injuries, non-depolarizing agents are preferred, but inadequate anesthesia and struggling to secure the airway are more detrimental than succinylcholine. There is no convincing evidence that succinylcholine has ever been associated with loss of an eye. Succinylcholine-induced elevation in IOP may be related to choroidal vascular dilatation or decrease in vitreous drainage. Defasciculating with non-depolarizing relaxants is not effective in blunting the increase in IOP. Pretreatment with IV lidocaine and opioids (fentanyl, sufentanil, remifentanil, and alfentanil) is advocated for blunting the rise in IOP. Non-depolarizing muscle relaxants lower IOP by relaxing the extraocular muscles. To achieve rapid onset of neuromuscular relaxation allowing intubation in 60 to 90 seconds, high doses of rocuronium (1.2 mg/kg), vecuronium (0.2 mg/kg), or cisatracurium (0.4 mg/kg) can be utilized.

## Maintenance of anesthesia (see also Chapter 7)

Inhalational anesthetics have been shown to lower IOP in proportion to the depth of anesthesia. Maintaining normocapnia with controlled ventilation is also an important contributing factor in controlling IOP. Total intravenous anesthesia (TIVA) with propofol and remifentanil (and/or dexmedetomidine) has been advocated for both IOP lowering effect and prevention of postoperative nausea and vomiting. Nitrous oxide should be avoided when intravitreal gas injection is used in the case of retinal detachment because of possible re-expansion of a gas bubble leading to IOP increase.

## Emergence of anesthesia

Achieving a smooth emergence and extubation of a patient with an eye injury might be challenging since any acute rise in intrathoracic and intra-abdominal pressure from bucking and coughing, frequently observed on awakening from anesthesia, might dramatically increase IOP. However, deep extubation of a trauma patient with a full stomach and unprotected airway is impractical due to a high aspiration risk. In addition, mask ventilation and placement of a nasal trumpet can aggravate damage to the eye and orbit. The ultimate goal is tracheal extubation without coughing and gagging with an awake patient. The following maneuvers may help achieve these conditions:

- Spraying the upper and lower airway with lidocaine or giving IV lidocaine (1.5 mg/kg) 5–10 minutes before awakening.
- Administration of short-acting opioids (e.g., remifentanil 0.5–0.7 mcg/kg) at the end of the case.
- Continuous infusion of dexmedetomidine, 0.2–0.7 mcg/kg/hr, during surgery until after the trachea is extubated.

# Maxillofacial trauma

Care of the patient with maxillofacial injuries represents a unique challenge for the anesthesia provider since trauma-related anatomic distortions directly involve the airway.

# Mechanisms of maxillofacial trauma

Common mechanisms of maxillofacial trauma are the following:

- Penetrating injury secondary to gunshot or motor vehicle accident.
- Blunt trauma secondary to motor vehicle accidents, falls, violent crimes.
- Chemical, electrical, or flame burns (see also Chapter 19).

Penetrating injuries result in loss of anatomical landmarks secondary to broken bones and teeth. Hemorrhage and tissue edema make airway assessment and face mask ventilation more difficult. Blunt trauma results in somewhat less obliteration of the facial structure than penetrating trauma, although midface trauma results in severe loss of airway definition and may be associated with cervical spine and head injuries (see also Chapters 13 and 14). Chemical, electrical or flame burns (see also Chapter 19) may cause severe obliteration of the airway secondary to tissue edema and soft tissue friability and may necessitate immediate airway management as the airway could become compromised with the passage of time secondary to ongoing tissue injury and edema.

# Classification of facial trauma

Facial skeleton fractures follow specific lines of weakness and can be characterized according to their anatomic location and displacement pattern.

Mandible fractures usually occur in two or more places due to its "U" shape; therefore, a second fracture should be suspected until proven otherwise. Bilateral (bucket handle) or comminuted fractures of the anterior mandible could lead to a loss of tongue support and its posterior displacement resulting in airway obstruction.

Zygomatic arch and condylar neck fractures may significantly limit jaw opening, leading to failed direct or video laryngoscopy.

Midface fractures may result in injuries to posterior structures and cause airway edema and compromise. They are also associated with head and C-spine injuries. Significant blood may be swallowed, resulting in a stomach full of blood and vomiting. In the early 20th century, Rene Le Fort classified midface fractures as follows (see Figure 15.1):

- Le Fort I: horizontal fracture that separates the tooth-bearing part of the maxilla from the rest of the maxilla; does not complicate intubation.
- Le Fort II: pyramid-shaped fracture separating the maxilla and the nose from the upper lateral midface and zygoma. This type of fracture should raise suspicion of a concomitant fracture of the skull base.
- Le Fort III: midface is separated and often displaced posteriorly. This type of fracture is often associated with fractures of the skull base. Blind attempts at nasotracheal intubation or nasogastric tube placement may result in intracranial penetration of the tube. Face mask ventilation is often difficult or impossible.

# Preoperative assessment

Anesthesia providers may be involved with the management of patients with facial trauma in the emergency department, as well as during urgent or elective repair of facial fractures in the operating room. Preoperative assessment in these patients should include the following:

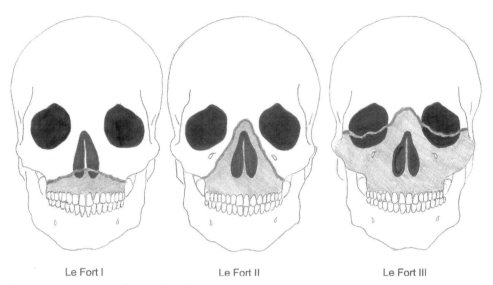

| Le Fort I | Le Fort II | Le Fort III |

**Figure 15.1.** Le Fort classification of midface fractures.

- History from the patient and prehospital personnel.
- Results of the primary and secondary surveys (see Chapter 2).
- Preliminary or final radiological results, including chest X-ray, spine evaluation, and head computed tomography.
- Neurological assessment, especially for the presence of altered level of consciousness, lateralizing neurologic symptoms, paralysis, pupillary size, and clinical signs of increased ICP such as hypertension, bradycardia, and irregular breathing pattern.
- The airway should be assessed since the rapid development of facial edema may obstruct the upper airway quickly. Assessment should include evaluation of facial deformity, swelling, neck motion, dental injury, nasal patency, mouth opening, and Mallampati score. Any evidence of impending respiratory compromise – cyanosis, dysphonia, agitation, dyspnea, or accessory muscle recruitment – usually indicates urgent or emergent need for a definitive airway.
- Close attention to the patient's request or attempts to sit up. This is an early sign of airway compromise. The sitting position and leaning forward allow passive drainage of oral and nasal secretions and blood; it relieves the airway obstruction from the tongue's displacement following a comminuted mandible fracture. Sitting should be allowed, with careful assistance to maintain cervical spine immobilization; if the sitting position is contraindicated due to spine, pelvic, or extensive extremity trauma, tracheal intubation should be performed expeditiously.
- An anesthesia provider must maintain a high index of suspicion for impending airway compromise and frequently reassess the patient. Airway obstruction in a patient with maxillofacial trauma results from multiple factors, as summarized in Table 15.2.

**Table 15.2.** Factors resulting in airway obstruction in a patient with maxillofacial trauma

| | |
|---|---|
| Displaced facial bone fragments | – Comminuted mandibular fractures resulting in loss of tongue support<br>– Posterior displacement of midface structures into the oropharynx |
| Soft tissue swelling | – Face, tongue, and neck tissue swelling develops within a few hours after injury |
| Retropharyngeal hematoma from C-spine fracture | – Contributes to airway collapse and complicates visualization of the larynx during intubation |
| Foreign bodies | – Blood and secretions may accumulate in the pharynx of a supine patient who is unable to swallow due to pain or loss of consciousness<br>– Teeth, dentures, food pieces<br>– Vomit due to full stomach, swallowed blood, alcohol intoxication |
| Impaired level of consciousness | – GCS score less than 9 due to brain injury, shock, or intoxication resulting in loss of protective airway reflexes |
| Inability to swallow and clear secretions | – Secondary to pain, swelling, and loss of consciousness |
| Associated C-spine injury | – Associated with midface and mandibular trauma<br>– Should be assumed until proven otherwise (see Chapter 14)<br>– Hard collar and manual in-line immobilization make airway evaluation difficult and limit glottic visualization during conventional laryngoscopy (see Chapters 3 and 14) |
| Associated neck trauma | – Hyoid bone fractures, trauma to cricoid or laryngeal cartilages and trachea lead to significant swelling and distortion of the airway<br>– Injury to the jugular vein or carotid artery results in hematoma |

Abbreviations: GCS = Glasgow Coma Scale; C-spine = cervical spine.

# Emergency airway management in maxillofacial trauma (see also Chapter 3)

The anesthesia provider must have a clear plan of action before attempting to intubate the trachea in a patient with facial trauma. Preparation to deal with the "difficult airway" and a backup plan, including the ability to rapidly perform a surgical airway, are of paramount importance.

- Assure immediate availability of adequate equipment and experienced assistance:
  - Oxygen, ventilation devices, and working suction.
  - Laryngoscopes, different types of blades, video-assisted intubating devices (e.g., Glidescope).
  - Oral airway, tracheal tube introducer (bougie), laryngeal mask airway (LMA), laryngeal tube airway.
  - Cricothyroidotomy kit should be readily available in case of failure to intubate.
- Considerations for selecting awake versus asleep intubation:
  - Ability to preserve airway patency after inducing unconsciousness.
  - Conscious patients are usually able to control their own airway, which is not the case of the uncooperative or unresponsive patient.

- Jaw thrust or traction to the mandible can relieve airway obstruction, but should be used with caution without displacing the fractures and providing a counter-support of the head to prevent any movement of the C-spine.
- If difficulty in laryngoscopy is anticipated, and the patient is cooperative, an awake intubation should be planned. The advantage would be proper oxygenation in a spontaneously breathing patient. The airway mucosa is prepared with local anesthetics and vasoconstrictors.
- Considerations for nasal versus oral route of intubation:
  - Blind nasotracheal intubation is contraindicated in patients with midface fractures or with suspected fractures of the base of the skull. Common symptoms and signs of basilar skull fracture include peri-orbital ecchymosis or "raccoon eyes", retro-auricular ecchymosis ("Battle's sign"), cerebrospinal fluid leak, and facial nerve palsy. Fiberoptic guided nasotracheal intubation may be performed in selected patients when the facial fracture does not cross midline.
  - In bilateral temporomandibular joint fractures, there could be restricted mouth opening due to pain or trismus. It should not be assumed that limited mouth opening will improve after induction and neuromuscular blockade.

## Preoxygenation and tracheal intubation

Adequate preoxygenation is difficult to achieve in the unconscious patient with significant facial injuries. Bag-mask ventilation can be attempted, but may also prove to be difficult or impossible because adequate mask seal is difficult to attain, may further displace the facial bone fragments and worsen airway obstruction, or may force air into the subdural space.

RSI and intubation with cricoid pressure is usually the technique of choice in patients with adequate mouth opening. Alternative techniques like the LMA, lighted stylet, fiber-optic bronchoscope, retrograde intubation, and others could be used depending on availability of equipment and expertise of the anesthesiologist (see Chapter 3):

- The fiberoptic bronchoscope is a useful instrument in experienced hands for awake intubation in cooperative, spontaneously breathing patients. Disadvantages include poor visualization secondary to copious blood, secretions, and significant airway swelling or deformity.
- The LMA can provide sufficient oxygenation and ventilation to the patient with a difficult airway. The LMA can also be used as a conduit for tracheal intubation with a fiberoptic bronchoscope. The LMA Fastrach™ (intubating LMA) is a helpful adjunct for tracheal intubation, especially in the emergency setting. Both types of LMA are not definitive airways and do not provide protection from aspiration of gastric contents. They may, however, provide protection from aspiration of upper airway material.
- Intubating lighted stylet (light wand) is another useful device in the hands of skilled providers, even in patients with limited mouth opening. A distinct disadvantage is that room lights must be dimmed during the procedure, which may not be feasible in the trauma setting.
- Retrograde wire technique utilizes a blind approach to secure the airway when direct visualization is not possible.

A surgical airway may be the first choice for definitive airway management, or may be needed when intubation and ventilation by other means prove difficult or impossible.

- Both cricothyroidotomy and tracheotomy require experienced surgical skills and may pose problems in patients with severe edema and anatomic distortions.
- An awake tracheostomy with local anesthesia may be indicated in an otherwise cooperative patient who is not in respiratory distress.
- An emergency cricothyroidotomy should be converted to a definitive tracheotomy once the patient is stabilized.
- Transtracheal jet ventilation – tracheal cannulation through the cricothyroid membrane followed by jet ventilation – may be life-saving during difficult airway situations. However, extreme care is needed to avoid barotrauma.

## Bleeding from maxillofacial injuries

Maxillofacial injuries alone are unlikely to be the cause of hemorrhagic shock. Most injuries result in minor slow venous bleeding from the nose or mouth and can be controlled. The bleeding may not be apparent if a patient is unable to clear their oral secretions due to pain or an altered sensorium. Blood and saliva accumulated in the oropharynx may cause airway obstruction and obscure visualization of the glottis when intubation is attempted, or be aspirated in an unconscious patient. Blood is often swallowed in a supine position, predisposing to vomiting and subsequent aspiration.

Control of bleeding from facial fractures improves airway patency and may be achieved with "damage control" maneuvers such as rapid manual reduction and stabilization of displaced bone fragments, nasal and oral gauze packing, and occlusion with nasal balloons or Foley catheters.

Profuse bleeding from panfacial fractures is often difficult to control due to the complex vascularization of the oromaxillofacial region. When packing and fracture reduction is ineffective in controlling hemorrhage, angiographic embolization in the intervention radiology suite may be necessary.

## Anesthetic management in elective maxillofacial repair

### Surgical considerations

The timing of surgical repair of facial trauma depends on the extent and severity of associated injuries. In the multiply injured patient, life, sight, or limb-threatening injuries are addressed first. Definitive repair may be deferred until the patient's overall condition is stable, pertinent clinical evaluations and imaging studies are completed, and the facial edema is resolved, allowing easier manipulation of bone fragments and soft tissue.

Mandibular fractures are usually repaired within 24 to 48 hours; other facial fractures within 7 to 10 days. After 10 to 14 days, the fractures are more difficult to reduce correctly.

Re-establishing proper dental occlusion is usually achieved first, followed by reduction of the other bony fractures. The ultimate goal of surgical repair is to restore nasal function, mastication, orbital integrity, and ocular position and mobility.

### Airway considerations

Since the airway is shared between the surgeon and anesthesiologist, the decision on appropriate placement of an endotracheal tube should be made and agreed upon by both physicians.

Facial fractures with malocclusion are managed with maxillomandibular fixation that usually precludes oral intubation (with exception of the patients with missing teeth in the molar region). Nasotracheal intubation is usually required for mandibular and midface fractures. Nasotracheal intubation with fiberoptic bronchoscopy is acceptable in patients with Le Fort II/III fractures provided that the fracture does not cross the midline or that the cribiform plate is intact on imaging studies. Blind nasotracheal intubation is discouraged because of the potential to intubate the cranial vault in the presence of Le Fort II/III fractures. Risks of nasotracheal intubation also include epistaxis and sinusitis.

Repair of complex panfacial fractures requires access to both the nose and the mouth. When neither oral nor nasal route of intubation is appropriate for the surgical repair, formal tracheostomy or submental intubation is performed. The submental route for intubation consists of pulling the free end of a tracheal tube (universal connector removed) through a submental incision, after a conventional orotracheal intubation has been performed.

- Submental intubation is performed by surgeons for intra- and postoperative maxillomandibular fixation in order to avoid a tracheostomy.
- After intubation, the proximal end of the tube is passed through a surgical incision in the floor of the mouth.
- This technique is advocated for patients who do not require prolonged ventilation.
- Submental intubation is technically easier, cosmetically better, and causes less complications than a tracheostomy, resulting in less hemorrhage, tracheal damage, and infection.

### Anesthetic considerations

The anesthetic plan should be based on the extent and time of facial reconstructions, airway issues, possibility of blood loss, hemodynamic status, and requirement for postoperative mechanical ventilation.

Induction and intubation should be smooth; wide variations in blood pressure could either cause excessive bleeding or impair perfusion to vital organs, especially if there is closed head injury with increased ICP. Other injuries should also be considered when selecting the drugs.

Maintenance can be provided by either inhalational anesthetic or TIVA with propofol and remifentanil (and/or dexmedetomidine). Advantages of TIVA include smooth awakening with minimal coughing and without postoperative nausea and vomiting.

Arterial line monitoring and a urinary catheter are often indicated for these surgeries (see Chapters 5 and 9). Controlled hypotension during surgery may improve operative conditions and reduce bleeding. Some surgeries require intraoperative assessment of nerve integrity and therefore maintaining an adequate level of anesthesia without neuromuscular relaxants. Fluid management should be targeted to assure adequate blood and fluid replacements and maintaining hemodynamic normality, especially in long reconstructive flaps.

Emergence and extubation should be carefully planned. If there are no contraindications to extubation such as edema, bleeding, compromised airway, or altered level of consciousness from other injuries, tracheal extubation can proceed.

The airway should be suctioned and the degree of airway edema assessed. Full recovery of airway reflexes and consciousness should also be assured before proceeding with extubation. If a nasal pack was used, its position must be checked to avoid migration and further airway obstruction.

Patients with maxillomandibular fixation should have wire cutters at their bedside in case of vomiting or airway compromise. Patients at risk for further swelling or hemorrhage (all Le Fort II and III fractures) require postoperative observation in an intensive care setting for 12–24 hours.

# Key points

- The goal of anesthesia for a patient with ocular trauma is to avoid increases in IOP. The anesthesiologist should be familiar with the main determinants of IOP and the mechanisms by which it may be altered.
- Complete neuromuscular block is essential for penetrating eye surgery, since patient movement, especially coughing, can dramatically increase IOP.
- In open globe eye injuries, non-depolarizing agents are preferred, but inadequate anesthesia and struggling to secure the airway are more detrimental than succinylcholine. There is no convincing evidence that succinylcholine has ever been associated with loss of an eye.
- Patients with maxillofacial trauma should be assessed early, and a plan to secure their airway in a safe manner should be outlined.
- Bag-mask ventilation may be difficult or impossible in patients with significant facial injuries.
- The anesthesiologist must have a clear plan of action before attempting to intubate a patient with facial trauma. Preparation to deal with the "difficult airway" and a backup plan are of paramount importance.
- Nasotracheal intubation with fiberoptic bronchoscopy is acceptable in patients with Le Fort II/III fractures provided that the fracture does not cross the midline or that the cribiform plate is intact on imaging studies.
- Coexisting injuries and potential for significant blood loss should be kept in mind when designing the anesthesia plan for patients with maxillofacial trauma.

## Further reading

1. Bramhall J. Anesthesia for maxillofacial trauma. *Lecture* (2004). http://faculty. washington.edu/bramhall/lectures/ trauma/max.html. Accessed January 10, 2011.

2. Chesshire NJ, Knight D. The anesthetic management of facial trauma and fractures. *British Journal of Anaesth* 2001;**1**:108–112.

3. Curran JE. Anaesthesia for facial trauma. *Anaesth Intens Care Med* 2008;**9**:338–343.

4. Dauber M, Roth S. Eye trauma and anesthesia. In: Smith CE, ed. *Trauma Anesthesia*. New York, NY: Cambridge University Press; 2008.

5. Donati F. Pharmacology of neuromuscular blocking agents and their reversal in trauma patients. In: Smith CE, ed. *Trauma Anesthesia*. New York, NY: Cambridge University Press; 2008.

6. Kohli R, Ramsingh H, Makkad B. The anesthetic management of ocular trauma. *Int Anesthesiol Clin* 2007;**45**:83–98.

7. Parekh KP, Ash CS. Oral and maxillofacial trauma. In: Smith CE, ed. *Trauma Anesthesia*. New York, NY: Cambridge University Press; 2008.

8. Perry M, Dancey A, Mireskandari K, et al. Emergency care in facial trauma – a maxillofacial and ophthalmic perspective. *Injury, Int J Care Injured* 2005;**36**:875–896.

9. Sinha AC, Baumann B. Anesthesia for ocular trauma. *Curr Anaesth Crit Care* 2010;**21**:184–188.

10. Vachon CA, Warner DO, Bacon DR. Succinylcholine and the open globe. Tracing the teaching. *Anesthesiology* 2003;**99**:220–223.

11. Wilson WC. Trauma airway management. In: Smith CE, ed. *Trauma Anesthesia*. New York, NY: Cambridge University Press; 2008.

# 16 Anesthetic considerations for chest trauma

Brendan Astley and Charles E. Smith

## Introduction

Chest trauma is the second most common cause of mortality after head trauma.

- Immediate deaths are usually due to massive injury of the heart, great vessels, or lungs.
- Early deaths occurring within 30 minutes to 3 hours are secondary to airway obstruction, hypoxemia, hemorrhage, cardiac tamponade, hemo-pneumothorax, and aspiration.
- Associated abdominal injuries are common.
- Multi-system injuries such as head, face, spine, and extremities frequently coexist in patients sustaining blunt chest trauma.

Overall, most chest injuries only need conservative management such as control of the airway and tube thoracostomy. Those injuries that do need surgical intervention, however, will likely need aggressive management (Table 16.1). As a consultant anesthesiologist, one needs to be aware of the clinical presentations, differential diagnoses, investigations, and treatment options when it comes to life-threatening chest trauma. Initial assessment includes mechanism of injury, history and physical exam, and resuscitation of vital functions according to Advanced Trauma Life Support (ATLS) principles. In the operating room (OR), priorities include definitive airway management, monitoring of hemodynamics, support of vital signs and organ perfusion, a high suspicion for associated injuries, measurement of pertinent lab values, provision of general anesthesia (see Chapter 7), and treatment of injuries. Hemorrhagic shock is treated with warmed fluid resuscitation using rapid infusion devices and large-bore intravenous (IV) access (see Chapter 4). If the patient does not respond to fluid and blood resuscitation, blood pressure support should be considered with vasopressors and inotropes. Other diagnoses should be entertained including tension pneumothorax and cardiac tamponade. This chapter will focus on the perioperative care of patients with chest trauma. The role of ultrasound in chest trauma, including echocardiography, is discussed in Chapter 10.

## Mechanism of injury

Chest trauma can be classified as penetrating or blunt.

- Penetrating wounds of the chest such as gunshot and stab wounds can directly injure any or all structures in the trajectory of the missile or weapon, causing rib fractures, pneumothorax, hemothorax, pulmonary injury, cardiac injury, and great vessel injury.

*Essentials of Trauma Anesthesia*, ed. A. J. Varon and C. E. Smith. Published by Cambridge University Press. © Cambridge University Press 2012.

**Table 16.1.** Indications for operative intervention after chest trauma

| Emergent | Sub-acute |
|---|---|
| • Cardiac tamponade | • Traumatic diaphragmatic hernia |
| • Acute deterioration or cardiac arrest in the trauma center | • Cardiac septal or valvular lesion |
| • Penetrating truncal trauma | • Non-evacuated clotted hemothorax |
| • Vascular injury at the thoracic outlet | • Chronic thoracic aortic pseudoaneurysm |
| • Loss of chest wall substance | • Post-traumatic empyema |
| • Massive air leak from chest tube | • Lung abscess |
| • Tracheobronchial tear | • Tracheoesophageal fistula |
| • Great vessel laceration | • Missed tracheal or bronchial tear |
| • Mediastinal traverse of a penetrating object | • Innominate artery/tracheal fistula |
| • Missile embolism to the heart or pulmonary artery | • Traumatic arterial venous fistula |
| • Placement of inferior vena caval shunt for hepatic vascular injury | |

Modified from Wall MJ, Storey JH, Mattox KL. Indications for thoracotomy. In: Mattox KL, Feliciano DV, Moore EE, eds. *Trauma*, 4th edition. New York, NY: McGraw-Hill; 2000.

- Gunshot and shrapnel wounds cause both direct injury to structures encountered by the weapon and secondary injury due to the blunt trauma-like shock wave created by the missile. The extent of internal injuries cannot be judged by the appearance of a skin wound alone. Furthermore, the extent of tissue injury, even on initial direct examination in the OR, is imprecise. These wounds occasionally require a staged approach with planned re-exploration.
- Blunt forces applied to the chest wall cause injury by rapid deceleration, direct impact, and compression. Rapid deceleration is the usual force involved in high-speed motor vehicle collisions and falls from a height. Suspicion of pulmonary, cardiac, and great vessel trauma should be heightened in patients who have sustained high-energy decelerating trauma.

With severe blunt trauma, the heart and great vessels are most often disrupted at one of four "anchor points": the aortic root, the posterior left atrium, the cavo-atrial junction in the right atrium, and the proximal descending thoracic aorta (Figure 16.1). Direct impact by a blunt object can cause localized fractures of the bony chest wall with underlying lung parenchymal injury, blunt cardiac injury, pneumothorax, and/or hemothorax. Compression of the chest by a very heavy object impedes ventilation and may result in traumatic asphyxia because of marked increases in pressure within veins of the upper thorax. Compression often causes severe bony chest wall fractures.

## Pathophysiology

- Chest trauma may result in respiratory insufficiency with resultant hypoxia, hypercarbia, and acidosis.

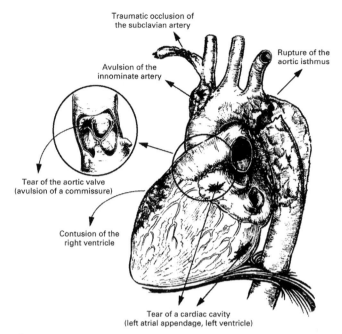

Traumatic occlusion of
the subclavian artery

Rupture of the
aortic isthmus

Avulsion of the
innominate artery

Tear of the aortic valve
(avulsion of a commissure)

Contusion of the
right ventricle

Tear of a cardiac cavity
(left atrial appendage, left ventricle)

**Figure 16.1.** Commonly encountered injuries to the heart and great vessels in patients with blunt cardiac trauma. Reproduced with permission from Pretre RM, Chilcott M. Blunt trauma to the heart and great vessels. *N Engl J Med* 1997;**336**:626–632.

- Respiratory insufficiency occurs as a result of chest wall injury (especially multiple rib fractures with flail chest), pneumothorax, pulmonary contusion, aspiration, tracheal injury, or hemothorax.
- Chest trauma can also result in circulatory collapse due to hemorrhagic shock (e.g., massive hemothorax), cardiogenic shock, tamponade, or tension pneumothorax.
- Tracheal intubation, mechanical ventilation, tube thoracostomy, and shock resuscitation are key features of anesthetic management.

## Pulmonary contusion

Pulmonary contusions are defined as injuries to the lung parenchyma. If the injury is significant, hypoxia may result. Pulmonary contusion may affect 25–75% of severe chest trauma patients. The mortality rate can be as high as 40%, depending on the severity of the contusion and underlying injuries. Most pulmonary contusions resolve in five days without any further insults. About 50% of patients with pulmonary contusion develop acute respiratory distress syndrome (ARDS). If more than 20% of the lung is involved, the percentage increases to 80% developing ARDS.

This diagnosis is usually made on chest X-ray (CXR) if there is a large area affected, especially in the presence of multiple rib fractures and flail chest (discussed below). Pulmonary contusion may occur without rib fractures in pediatric patients who don't have completely ossified ribs. Contusions will be found on the lung periphery as a white, opaque area and extend deeper into the lung depending on the severity of the lesion. Sometimes the CXR may just appear hazy and look as if there was aspiration pneumonia. The diagnosis

**Table 16.2.** Indications for tracheal intubation and mechanical ventilation after flail chest and pulmonary contusion

| Pulmonary function criteria | Indication |
| --- | --- |
| Arterial oxygen | < 70 mmHg with rebreathing mask |
| Arterial carbon dioxide | > 50 mmHg |
| Respiratory rate | > 35/min or < 8/min |
| Vital capacity | < 15 mL/kg |
| Negative inspiratory force | < 20 cm $H_2O$ |
| $PaO_2/FiO_2$ ratio | ≤ 200 |
| Dead space to tidal volume ratio | > 0.6 |
| $FEV_1$ | ≤ 10 mL/kg |
| Shunt fraction (Qs/Qt) | > 0.2 |

Modified from Cogbill TH, Landercasper J. Injury to the chest wall. In: Mattox KL, Feliciano DV, Moore EE, eds. *Trauma*, 4th edition. New York, NY: McGraw-Hill; 2000.
Abbreviations: $PaO_2/FiO_2$ ratio = ratio of arterial oxygen tension to fraction of inspired oxygen; $FEV_1$ = forced expiratory volume in 1 second

may be made on computed tomography (CT) scan if a smaller area is affected. However, the diagnosis may not have clinical significance if it is very small. Physical exam may reveal overlying soft tissue injury, multiple rib fractures, flail chest, and/or crackles heard over the affected lung field. Crackles, however, are fairly non-specific and often do not present until the lung injury blossoms over the ensuing 48 hours. Pulmonary contusions may not lead to hypoxia and ventilation issues until the injury evolves. When the pulmonary contusions are significant, they can lead to pneumonia, ARDS, atelectasis, and respiratory failure.

Management goals include supportive care. This may include supplemental oxygen, tracheal intubation, and mechanical ventilation as the situation dictates (Table 16.2). Secretions should be managed aggressively. When pulmonary contusions initially present, they may be small and not cause severe changes in gas exchange. However, these injuries become much more difficult to manage over the ensuing two to three days, as the lung becomes less compliant. During this time period, if the patient presents to the OR, one should have a low threshold for managing the airway with tracheal intubation and maintaining that secure airway until the contusion resolves.

- Limiting peak and plateau pressures and tidal volume, and avoiding overdistension during mechanical ventilation, are important management strategies in patients with lung injury.
- Pressure-controlled ventilation minimizes peak and plateau airway pressures and may help prevent barotrauma.
- The goal of fluid management should be to keep the patient euvolemic.
- Hypovolemia or fluid restriction can lead to a stress response and hypoperfusion state. It can further lead to acute lung injury (ALI), ARDS, and multiple organ failure.
- Hypervolemia, on the other hand, can lead to pulmonary edema that would further complicate the patient's clinical course.

**Table 16.3.** Incidence of injuries in patients with blunt thoracic trauma presenting to the operating room for emergency surgery

| Type of injury | Incidence, % |
|---|---|
| Rib fractures | 67 |
| Pulmonary contusion | 65 |
| Pneumothorax | 30 |
| Hemothorax | 26 |
| Flail chest | 23 |
| Diaphragmatic injury | 9 |
| Myocardial contusion | 5.7 |
| Aortic tear | 4.8 |
| Tracheobronchial injury | 0.8 |
| Laryngeal injury | 0.3 |

Modified from Devitt JH, McLean RF, Koch JP. Anaesthetic management of acute blunt thoracic trauma. *Can J Anaesth* 1991;**38**,506–510.

- Fluid status can be monitored in multiple ways. In the intraoperative environment with invasive monitors, the authors have found systolic pressure variation (from the arterial line tracing) and central venous pressure (CVP) trends to be reliable indications of volume status (see also Chapter 9).

# Rib fractures/flail chest

Rib fractures are the most commonly identified injuries of the chest (Table 16.3). Flail chest occurs when two or more ribs are fractured in two or more places. This disrupts the bony continuity of the chest wall with the remainder of the thoracic cage. The injury may or may not be apparent on CXR. In the lower thoracic region, rib fractures and flail chest may be associated with diaphragm rupture and liver and spleen lacerations. In the upper thoracic region one should consider injury to the heart, lungs, and great vessels. Pneumothorax and hemothorax are possibilities that also need to be addressed emergently and closely watched in this situation.

Respiratory insufficiency is mainly due to the contusion that occurred at the instance of trauma. As the bruised lung attempts to heal from the injury, the lung parenchyma becomes less compliant and has increased elastic recoil. This is associated with increased work of breathing and hypoxemia (Figure 16.2). Pain control is very important in this situation. If neuraxial analgesia is not contraindicated, it would be prudent to provide epidural analgesia to decrease pain and improve pulmonary dynamics (see Chapter 8).

- Although thoracic epidural placement may not be practical in the setting of the initial trauma, it should strongly be considered for pain control after life-threatening injuries and coagulopathy issues have been addressed.

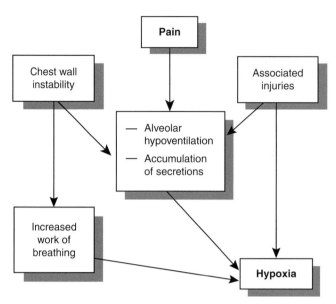

**Figure 16.2.** Pain after chest trauma limits the ability to cough and breathe deeply. Elderly patients and those with poor respiratory reserve are particularly vulnerable to hypoxia and respiratory failure after rib fractures and flail chest. Reproduced with permission from Orliaguet G, Carli P. Thoracic blocks. In: Rosenberg AD, Grande CM, Bernstein RL, eds. *Pain Management and Regional Anesthesia in Trauma*. London: Saunders; 2000.

- Early epidural placement may not prevent a patient's trachea from being intubated; however, most experts believe it may decrease duration of mechanical ventilation and intensive care unit (ICU) stay.

Pneumothorax and hemothorax (see below) may also be caused by rib fractures. Depending on the size, these injuries require chest tube placement for drainage of air and fluid.

Ventilator support decisions should be based on physical exam findings, serial CXRs, chest CT, and arterial blood gas (ABG) monitoring. If the gas exchange deteriorates, treatment options include increasing oxygen concentration ($FiO_2$), fluid management toward euvolemia, and consideration for non-invasive or invasive ventilatory support depending on the situation. In an emergent chest trauma situation requiring surgical intervention in the OR, it is very likely that the patient's trachea will be intubated and will stay intubated until respiration and hemodynamics improve, and underlying issues and injuries are identified and managed. Of particular note, if the first rib is fractured, attention should be paid to the underlying structures including the aorta because it takes a large amount of energy to fracture this specific rib; scapular fractures also suggest heart and lung injury.

Surgical repair of rib fractures is occasionally required. Ribs may be resected or removed if they are displaced into the lung or externally through the skin.

## Tracheobronchial injury

Tracheobronchial injuries are usually due to penetrating trauma; however, high-energy blunt trauma can also cause these injuries, usually within 1 inch of the carina.

Symptoms and physical exam findings may include:

- Subcutaneous crepitus
- Hemoptysis
- Dyspnea
- Air leaks and failure of the lung to expand after chest tube placement

If the injury occurred secondary to blunt chest trauma, this was likely a high-energy accident and other vital organs have likely been injured as well. CXR may show subcutaneous air. There may be a persistent air leak through the chest tube. CT scan may show the actual tear. Fiberoptic bronchoscopy is the gold standard for making this diagnosis (see also Chapter 3).

Definitive treatment is often surgical and may include airway reconstruction, lobectomy, or pneumonectomy. However, initial treatment management options include placing the tracheal tube distal to the air leak or if the leak is too far distal then lung isolation with a double-lumen tube (DLT) or bronchial blocker (see section on One-lung ventilation). After this has been achieved, a more permanent surgical repair, if warranted, should be attempted. Invasive monitors will likely be required, including arterial and central venous pressure and adequate peripheral IV access. Of note, if tracheal repair is completed surgically, positive pressure ventilation should ideally occur distal to the lesion (or not at all) as this may further disrupt the tissue that was injured and repaired.

# Pneumothorax

A pneumothorax is defined as air present outside the pleural cavity and inside the chest wall. This is likely the second most common chest injury after trauma. A primary pneumothorax occurs in the absence of known lung disease such as in trauma. A secondary pneumothorax occurs because of known lung disease. The size of the pneumothorax can affect pulmonary function and cardiac function if enough pressure is present to compress essential structures such as the heart or great vessels.

Pneumothoraces can be due to blunt or penetrating trauma. These are usually diagnosed with physical exam findings and CXR. Symptoms and physical exam findings may include:

- Decreased breath sounds over one lung field
- Deviated trachea
- Dyspnea
- Tachycardia
- Distended neck veins
- Cyanosis

CXR classically will show decreased lung markings over the affected lung field. Lung markings should be viewed from the hilum to the periphery of each lung field. If there is an area that is devoid of lung markings, there may be a small pneumothorax present. A larger pneumothorax may further show deviation of the trachea, such as in a tension pneumothorax. CT scan will show even the smallest pneumothorax and these can be followed for resolution over the ensuing days. A small pneumothorax can progress to a larger one especially if a decision is made to start positive pressure ventilation. In the trauma situation, some authors would recommend placement of a chest tube for even the smallest pneumothoraces, especially if the patient will undergo general anesthesia or receive positive pressure ventilation.

Common practice is to place a chest tube in patients who have hemodynamic changes, pulmonary changes, and for larger pneumothoraces. When hemodynamic changes start to occur, it is quite possible that the patient has a tension pneumothorax.

Tension pneumothorax may shows signs of a simple pneumothorax but also include the more severe signs such as:

- Decreased blood pressure
- Hypoxia
- Mental status changes

In the event a chest tube is not immediately available or personnel are not available that can place a chest tube successfully, needle decompression of the affected side should be performed. This is achieved by inserting a long 14-gauge needle into the second intercostal space on the affected side in the mid-clavicular line. Needle decompression is only a temporary procedure that functions as a bridge until a chest tube is placed. However, it can rapidly improve hemodynamics and airway mechanics.

## Hemothorax

Hemothorax is defined as blood that is present outside the pleural cavity and inside the chest wall. Usually the bleeding is caused by intercostal blood vessels that have been lacerated by fractured ribs. Other vascular structures may be affected including lung parenchyma and great vessels.

- This diagnosis can be suggested by a "white out" on the CXR.
- Other findings on CXR may include displacement of the chest contents away from the side of the chest that has the "white out" appearance.
- Physical exam findings include decreased breath sounds over the affected lung field and dyspnea.
- If a large amount of blood has been lost, hemodynamic and pulmonary compromise are possible and the vital signs will reflect this problem.

Definitive treatment may be chest tube placement if blood loss through the chest remains low (< 200 mL/hr). If immediately after the chest tube is placed, one liter or more of blood is drained, then a decision should be made to continue to thoracotomy for surgical repair. Ongoing blood loss > 200 mL/hr is usually an indication for surgical repair. One-lung ventilation (OLV) facilitates surgery, especially for video-assisted thoracic procedures (VATS).

## Vascular air embolism after chest trauma

Systemic air embolism is a rare and often unrecognized complication of chest trauma with a high mortality rate. It is thought to be due to communication between pulmonary blood vessels and the airway (traumatic alveolar to pulmonary venous fistula). Cardiovascular collapse may occur soon after intubation and positive pressure ventilation. Delayed presentation may occur following lung recruitment strategies. Treatment strategies consist of minimizing the pressure gradient between the airways and the pulmonary venous circulation (e.g., reduced tidal volume, avoidance of positive pressure ventilation, lung isolation, high frequency oscillatory ventilation). Emergency thoracotomy with hilar clamping can be done. Hyperbaric oxygen therapy may minimize secondary damage to affected organs.

# One-lung ventilation

The majority of the time, OLV is indicated to facilitate surgical procedures such as thoracotomy and thoracoscopy. OLV can also prevent contralateral soiling from blood or infection and controls the distribution of ventilation (e.g., bronchopleural fistula, vascular air embolism). Options for OLV and lung isolation include DLT, Univent, and bronchial blocker (Table 16.4). Leftsided DLTs are preferred by the authors because they provide excellent lung isolation, are quickest to place successfully, permit bronchoscopy and suction to the isolated lung, and allow addition of continuous positive airway pressure (CPAP). The main disadvantage is non-optimal postoperative two-lung ventilation. Bronchial blockers are mainly used for patients with known difficult airway anatomy whose tracheas are already intubated. Tube exchange from single lumen to DLT is also an option.

Fiberoptic bronchoscopy is vital for positioning DLTs. The Glidescope and Wuscope can facilitate DLT placement in patients with cervical spine precautions. With the Glidescope, the DLT is placed into the mouth with the same curvature as the Glidescope. With the Wuscope, the tube is placed inside the channel created by the Wuscope blades (only suitable for sizes 35 and 37 Fr). Once the tube is past the vocal cords, fiberoptic bronchoscopy is used to position the tube into the mainstem bronchus.

If the patient requires postoperative mechanical ventilation, the previously placed DLT may be withdrawn so that the bronchial cuff is in the mid-tracheal position. The bronchial tube is then used as a single lumen tube and the tracheal tube is clamped. This may be necessary when the risk of reintubation with a single-lumen tube is judged to be unacceptably high. Otherwise, tube exchange is generally done using an airway exchange catheter. A step-by-step approach to airway tube exchange is shown in Table 16.5. Complete neuromuscular blockade significantly increases the chance of successful tube exchange. There is always a risk of losing the airway during a tube exchange. Therefore, a back-up plan (including a surgical airway) is prudent.

# Cardiac injuries

Penetrating cardiac injuries involving the pericardium, cardiac wall, interventricular septum, valves, chordae tendineae, papillary muscles, and coronary vessels can occur. Blunt cardiac trauma presents clinically as a spectrum of injuries of varying severity. Within this spectrum, injuries can manifest as:

- Free septal rupture
- Free wall rupture
- Coronary artery thrombosis
- Heart failure
- Rupture of chordae tendineae or papillary muscles
- Severe valvular regurgitation
- Wall motion abnormalities
- Arrhythmias

Most patients with myocardial contusion and wall motion abnormalities have external signs of thoracic trauma such as abrasions, rib or sternum fractures, pneumothorax, or hemothorax (Table 16.6). Myocardial cell damage produces electrical instability, which may result in supraventricular or ventricular arrhythmias (Table 16.7). The right ventricle

**Table 16.4.** Options for lung isolation in patients with chest trauma

| Options | Advantages | Disadvantages |
|---|---|---|
| **Double-lumen tube** 1. Direct laryngoscopy 2. Via tube exchanger 3. Glidescope, Wuscope, flexible fiberscope | – Quickest to place successfully<br>– Repositioning rarely required<br>– Bronchoscopy to isolated lung<br>– Suction to isolated lung<br>– CPAP easily added<br>– Can alternate OLV to either lung<br>– Placement possible if bronchoscopy not available | – Size selection more difficult<br>– Harder to place in patients with difficult airways or abnormal tracheas<br>– non-optimal postoperative two lung ventilation<br>– Laryngeal trauma<br>– Bronchial trauma |
| **Bronchial blockers** 1. Arndt 2. Cohen 3. Fuji 4. Fogarty catheter | – Size selection rarely an issue<br>– Easily added to regular TT<br>– Allows ventilation during placement<br>– Easier placement in patients with difficult airways and in children<br>– Postoperative two-lung ventilation easily accomplished by withdrawing blocker<br>– Selective lobar lung isolation possible<br>– CPAP to isolated lung possible | – More time needed for positioning<br>– Repositioning needed more often<br>– Bronchoscope essential for positioning<br>– Non-optimal right lung isolation due to RUL anatomy<br>– Bronchoscopy to isolated lung impossible<br>– Minimal suction to isolated lung<br>– Difficult to alternate OLV to either lung |
| **Univent** | – Same as bronchial blockers<br>– Less repositioning compared to bronchial blockers | – Same as bronchial blockers<br>– TT portion has higher air flow resistance than regular TT<br>– TT portion has larger outside diameter than regular TT |
| **TT advanced into mainstem bronchus** | – Easiest placement in patients with difficult airways or emergency situation | – Does not allow for bronchoscopy, suctioning, or CPAP to isolated lung<br>– Cuff not designed for lung isolation<br>– Poor conditions for right lung OLV due to RUL obstruction |

Modified from Kanellakos GW, Slinger P. Intraoperative one-lung ventilation for trauma anesthesia. In: Smith CE, ed. *Trauma Anesthesia*. New York, NY: Cambridge University Press; 2008.

Abbreviations: OLV = one-lung ventilation; CPAP = continuous positive airway pressure; RUL = right upper lobe; TT = tracheal tube.

**Table 16.5.** Stepwise approach to airway tube exchange

| Steps | Comments |
|---|---|
| A. Is tube exchange indicated? | – There is always a risk of losing the airway. Indications for tube exchange should always be reviewed |
| B. Assemble equipment | – Laryngoscope, fiberoptic bronchoscope<br>– TTs (at least two sizes)<br>– Airway exchange catheter<br>– Lubricant<br>– Dry gauze or sponge (to provide traction when rotating tube in Step I below)<br>– Oxygen insufflation source<br>– Suction<br>– Assistance for handling equipment |
| C. Test equipment | – Add lubricant liberally to catheter, internal lumen of TT, and bronchoscope<br>– Test exchanger and bronchoscope in DLT and TT to confirm easy passage<br>– Remove TT and exchange catheter connectors for easier passage<br>– Ensure suction is working<br>– Confirm bronchoscope is connected |
| D. Ventilate with 100% oxygen | – All airway maneuvers should begin with preoxygenation |
| E. Ensure complete neuromuscular block | – A patient that begins coughing during airway manipulation significantly reduces tube exchange success |
| F. Insert laryngoscope and maintain optimal view throughout the tube exchange | – This displaces the tongue and provides a more direct path for the tube exchange<br>– Establish a view of the larynx<br>– Apply suction, if necessary |
| G. Insert exchange catheter into patient's DLT (or TT) | – This requires an assistant<br>– Take into consideration depth of insertion by observing markings on exchange catheter (premeasure with an external tube, if necessary)<br>– An exchange catheter advanced too deep can cause severe injuries, especially since they are very stiff. Consider using the newest models equipped with a soft, flexible tip<br>– An exchange catheter not advanced deep enough risks losing the airway during the exchange |
| H. Remove patient tube | – Care must be taken to keep exchange catheter from moving out with tube |
| I. Insert new tube over exchange catheter and advance into airway Maintain optimal view throughout the tube exchange (*most difficult step) | – Again, it is important to keep exchange catheter depth constant in order to avoid injury |

**Table 16.5.** (cont.)

| Steps | Comments |
|---|---|
| (*most difficult step) | – Care must be taken not to damage the cuff along the patient's teeth |
| | – When the tube touches the larynx, resistance will be felt. Excessive pressure here only makes advancement more difficult and causes injury. Moderate to low pressure should be applied while slowly rotating the tube. This allows the bevel of the TT to "unhook" itself from the obstruction and then it will advance. If the advancing pressure is too strong, then the distal tip of the TT will not rotate well. Instead, the tube itself might twist. Use gauze to help grip tube, if necessary |
| | – The obstruction is usually visible with laryngoscopy, helping to direct tube rotation |
| | – Often, complete 360° rotation is necessary to overcome obstruction |
| J. Remove tube exchanger | – Immediately check correct tube placement with bronchoscope, ETCO$_2$, and auscultation |

Modified from Kanellakos GW, Slinger P. Intraoperative one-lung ventilation for trauma anesthesia. In: Smith CE, ed. *Trauma Anesthesia*. New York, NY: Cambridge University Press; 2008.
Abbreviations: TT = tracheal tube; DLT = double lumen tube; ETCO$_2$ = end tidal carbon dioxide

**Table 16.6.** Clinical manifestations of myocardial contusion

| |
|---|
| Arrhythmias |
| Impaired cardiac function |
| Elevated troponin |
| Right heart failure |

Modified from Gerhardt MA, Gravlee GP. Anesthesia considerations for cardiothoracic trauma. In: Smith CE, ed. *Trauma Anesthesia*. New York, NY: Cambridge University Press; 2008.

(RV) is more frequently injured than the left ventricle (LV) due to its anterior anatomic location. Cardiac enzymes, especially troponin-I, may be elevated but do not have the same prognostic value as that after acute coronary syndrome. Echocardiography is critical for accurate diagnosis (see Chapter 10).

RV contusion can result in RV contractile dysfunction, which in turn leads to systemic hypotension from decreased LV filling. RV contusion is frequently associated with pulmonary contusion, which can synergistically contribute to right heart failure. Pulmonary contusion results in increased interstitial pulmonary edema and hemorrhage, diffusion abnormalities, and hypoxia, which all contribute to increased pulmonary artery resistance and can cause acute pulmonary hypertension, diminished RV function, and right heart failure.

**Table 16.7.** Arrhythmias associated with myocardial contusion

| |
|---|
| Sinus tachycardia |
| Sinus bradycardia |
| First-degree atrioventricular block |
| Right bundle branch block |
| Complete heart block |
| Atrial fibrillation |
| Premature ventricular contractions |
| Ventricular tachycardia |
| Ventricular fibrillation |

Modified from Aydin NB, Moon MC, Gill I. Cardiac and great vessel trauma. In: Smith CE, ed. *Trauma Anesthesia*. New York, NY: Cambridge University Press; 2008.

# Tamponade

Cardiac tamponade in the trauma environment is usually due to a rapidly expanded pericardial effusion after blunt or penetrating trauma. Rapid accumulation of fluid in the pericardial space, particularly following penetrating cardiac trauma or aortic injury, can result in cardiac tamponade and hypotension. Tamponade physiology results when sufficient pressure is exerted on the myocardium that interferes with diastolic filling and systolic output. There is a compensatory rise in catecholamines leading to tachycardia and increased right heart pressure with septal shift to the left, further compromising LV stroke volume (Figure 16.3). This is a potentially life-threatening and reversible condition in a trauma situation. As little as 60 to 100 mL of blood in the pericardial sac can produce tamponade physiology. Diagnosis can be made by echocardiography (transthoracic or transesophageal, TEE), and suspected based on electrocardiographic (ECG) findings that include low voltage across all leads. The combination of shock and jugular venous distension in a patient with cardiac trauma is suggestive of tamponade, although the differential diagnosis includes tension pneumothorax, right ventricular failure, and tricuspid valve rupture. Neck veins may not be distended if tamponade is accompanied by hemorrhagic shock.

Clots form quickly in the setting of trauma and is therefore not usually amenable to needle drainage. If hemodynamic compromise is occurring, then a decision should be made to proceed to the OR for a pericardial window to relieve the tamponade followed by careful inspection of the heart for a source of continued bleeding. If hemodynamic collapse is imminent, then immediate pericardiocentesis can be done to relieve the pressure. Definitive repair will be required in the OR. Prompt recognition and operative management can be life-saving. Pericardial window can also be performed under local anesthesia to stabilize the patient while preparations are made for transport. Depending on severity, wounds of the heart may be reparable without the use of cardiopulmonary bypass (CPB). If temporary asystole is required for surgical control of bleeding, the authors have found that rapid bolus of adenosine, 6–12 mg IV, is useful, especially when dealing with lateral wall bleeding. Asystole lasts for approximately 15–20 seconds.

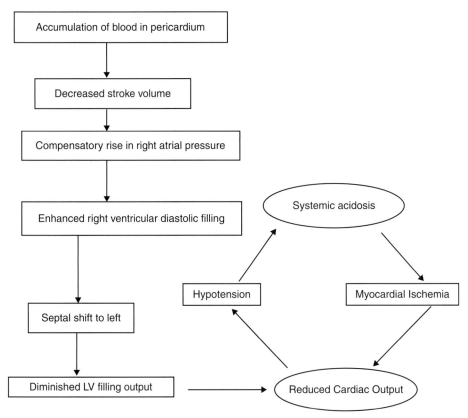

**Figure 16.3.** Tamponade physiology results when sufficient pressure is exerted on the myocardium that interferes with diastolic filling and cardiac output. Echocardiographic findings include pericardial effusion, right atrial systolic collapse, right ventricular diastolic collapse, respiratory variation in right and left ventricular diastolic filling, and inferior vena cava plethora.
Reproduced from Barach P. Perioperative anesthetic management of patients with cardiac trauma. *Anesth Clin North Am* 1999;**17**:197–209.

If CPB is required for more complex repair (e.g., valves and supporting structures, atrial or ventricular septal defects, coronary vessels), preparations for systemic heparinization and a full cardiac team including perfusionist will be necessary. TEE is essential for diagnosis and monitoring of traumatic cardiac injuries and should always be interpreted by a credentialed provider.

Gunshot wounds (GSWs) of the heart have several unique considerations with respect to anesthetic management. The potential exists for transmediastinal injury including the great vessels and the esophagus. Traumatic esophageal perforation may be worsened with TEE. Placement of a TEE probe may therefore be contraindicated. Missile embolus can occur with GSW of the heart. This occurs when the bullet or shrapnel fragment penetrates a vascular structure and then is carried by blood flow until it lodges in the arterial tree at a remote site where it can produce end-organ ischemia. The trauma care team can be distracted by the penetrating cardiac trauma and neglect to search for missile embolus preoperatively. Appropriate evaluation for missile embolus should occur prior to leaving the OR to avoid prompt return for embolectomy.

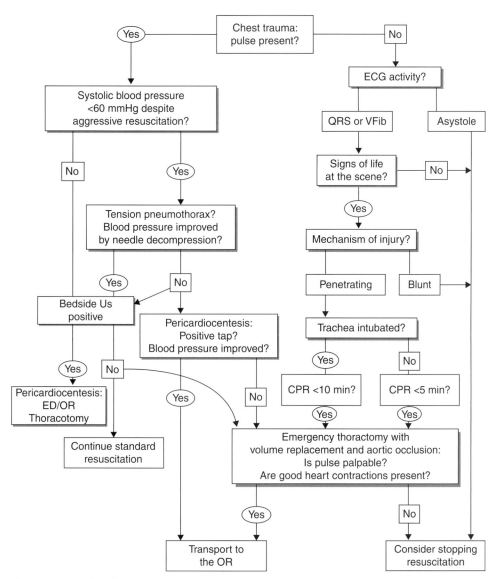

**Figure 16.4.** An algorithmic approach to chest trauma. Bedside echocardiography should be performed as quickly as possible to establish the diagnosis of pericardial effusion with tamponade physiology, which then mandates urgent surgical repair. Patients with penetrating cardiac injury invariably require surgical repair. The location (operating room versus emergency department) and timing (immediate versus urgent) depends on the patient's clinical status. QRS = organized electrical activity; VFib = ventricular fibrillation; positive tap = pericardial tap yielding blood; US = ultrasonography; CPR = cardiopulmonary resuscitation; ED = emergency department; OR = operating room. Reproduced from Boczar ME, Rivers E. Resuscitative thoracotomy. In: Roberts JR, Hedges JR. *Clinical Procedures in Emergency Medicine*, 4th edition. Philadelphia, PA: Saunders; 2004.

# Emergency department thoracotomy

Emergency department (ED) thoracotomy is a drastic, dramatic, and potentially life-saving procedure. With thoracotomy, the goal is to relieve cardiac tamponade, support cardiac function with direct cardiac compression and/or cross-clamping of the aorta to improve coronary perfusion, and perform internal defibrillation when indicated (Figure 16.4). The decision should be based on a realistic judgment that the patient has a chance of survival but will not tolerate any delay in operative intervention. It is also important to consider not performing thoracotomy for cases in which there is virtually no chance of salvaging a neurologically intact patient (e.g., prehospital cardiac arrest after blunt trauma). Pertinent information in formulating a decision to perform ED thoracotomy includes time of injury, transport time, and time that vital signs or cardiac electrical activity ceased. Patients with penetrating trauma with signs of life in the field, even if only electrical activity on cardiac monitor or agonal respirations, are candidates for thoracotomy if transport times are less than 10 minutes.

## Traumatic aortic injury

Traumatic aortic injury can occur following blunt or penetrating trauma. Injuries to the aorta can include a tear or outright rupture. Aortic disruptions typically occur at the attachment site of the ligamentum arteriosum in the proximal descending aorta (junction between the aortic arch and the descending aorta or aortic isthmus). These often cause immediate exsanguination and mortality is high. If the tear is incomplete, the adventitia or parietal pleura contains the rupture with development of a pseudoaneurysm or intramural hematoma.

One must have a high index of suspicion for aortic injury. Clinical suspicion should be raised by mechanisms such as high-speed crashes and rapid deceleration. Associated injuries are common. CXR may show widened mediastinum, first rib fractures, clavicular fractures, and pulmonary contusions. The diagnosis is by chest CT, although aortography, TEE, and magnetic resonance imaging all play a role depending on availability, expertise, and other factors.

In the past, these injuries were cared for in the OR on an emergency basis using open repair via thoracotomy with substantial morbidity and mortality. More recently, a push has been made to delay surgical repair until other management issues have been addressed. Beta-blockers are used to decrease the heart rate and LV contractile force, which in turn will attenuate the shear stress of blood flow at the site of rupture/transection. The goal in this scenario would be to take the patient to the OR for endovascular repair when they are as optimized for this surgery as possible. Anesthesia goals include:

- Accurate control of blood pressure and heart rate to alleviate shearing forces on the aortic wall.
- Smooth induction with blunted sympathetic response when securing the airway.
- Adequate beta-blockade and blood pressure with short-acting agents such as esmolol and nitroglycerin.
- Maintaining a target heart rate of 60–80 beats/min and systolic blood pressure in a range of 90–120 mmHg to minimize aortic disruption, while at the same time preserving an adequate perfusion pressure in other organs like the brain and spinal cord.

Benefits of an endovascular approach to blunt thoracic aortic disruption include:
- Avoids thoracotomy
- Avoids OLV
- Avoids aortic cross-clamping
- Avoids requirement for partial cardiopulmonary bypass

Avoidance of thoracotomy minimizes postoperative pain and associated respiratory compromise. Endovascular repair reduces blood pressure shifts, surgical blood loss, and ischemic time of the visceral organs and spinal cord. The requirement for anticoagulation is minimal, which is desirable in patients with other injuries like head, spine, abdomen, and musculoskeletal. Disadvantages of endovascular repair include the potential complication of an endoleak following exclusion of the aortic disruption and a lack of long-term outcome data.

Maintaining spinal cord perfusion (the difference between mean arterial pressure and cerebrospinal fluid pressure, CSFp) is vital with open or endovascular techniques to prevent paraplegia. Insertion of an intraspinal catheter to measure CSFp is sometimes required depending on anatomical factors and surgeon preference. With the spinal catheter, CSF can be drained in an effort to decrease CSFp and improve spinal cord perfusion.

Invasive pressure monitoring is routine (see also Chapters 5 and 9). Right radial or brachial arterial cannulation is preferred for proximal endovascular or open descending thoracic injuries because the injury may involve the left subclavian artery; a left radial (or brachial) arterial line is done for ascending aortic or proximal arch tears to avoid problems with innominate artery cross-clamping. Aortic arch repair may necessitate deep hypothermic circulatory arrest. A cardiac anesthesia team should be available for this type of surgery, and a pulmonary artery catheter is typically indicated. TEE monitoring is done for complex cardiac and great vessel surgery (see Chapter 10).

# Key points

- Blunt chest trauma is frequently associated with multi-system injuries including head, face, spine, abdomen, and extremities.
- Chest trauma can result in respiratory insufficiency due to pulmonary contusion, multiple rib fractures, pneumothorax, aspiration, tracheal injury, or hemothorax.
- Chest trauma can result in circulatory collapse due to hemorrhagic shock, cardiogenic shock, cardiac tamponade, or tension pneumothorax.
- Tracheal intubation, mechanical ventilation, tube thoracostomy, and shock resuscitation are key features of anesthetic management for chest trauma.
- Limiting peak and plateau pressures and tidal volume and avoiding overdistension during mechanical ventilation are important management strategies in patients with lung injury.
- Although thoracic epidural placement may not be practical in the setting of the initial trauma, it should be strongly considered for pain control in patients with multiple rib fractures once other issues have been addressed.
- Lung isolation techniques may require tube exchange. There is always a risk of losing the airway during a tube exchange.
- Blunt trauma can cause myocardial contusion, more often to the anteriorly located right ventricle, which can present as heart failure or arrhythmias. Patients who display any arrhythmia during a procedure or have hypotensive episodes attributed to blunt cardiac injury should have increased postoperative observation and monitoring.
- Penetrating wounds to the heart may present as cardiac tamponade. Pericardial window is life-saving.
- Surgical and anesthetic management of descending thoracic aortic traumatic disruptions has evolved and endovascular repair is preferred to avoid thoracotomy and aortic cross-clamping.

# Further reading

1. Aydin NB, Moon MC, Gill I. Cardiac and great vessel trauma. In: Smith CE, ed. *Trauma Anesthesia*. New York, NY: Cambridge University Press; 2008.

2. Barach P. Perioperative anesthetic management of patients with cardiac trauma. *Anesth Clin North Am* 1999;**17**:197–209.

3. Barash PG, Cullen BF, Stoelting RK, Cahalan M, Stock MC, eds. *Clinical Anesthesia*, 6th edition. Philadelphia, PA: Lippincott Williams & Wilkins; 2009.

4. Boczar ME, Rivers E. Resuscitative thoracotomy. In: Roberts JR, Hedges JR. *Clinical Procedures in Emergency Medicine*, 4th edition. Philadelphia, PA: Saunders; 2004.

5. Brederlau J, Muellenbach RM, et al. Delayed systemic air embolism in a child with severe blunt chest trauma treated with high-frequency oscillatory ventilation. *Can J Anesth* 2011;**58**:555–559.

6. Cogbill TH, Landercasper J. Injury to the chest wall. In: Mattox KL, Feliciano DV, Moore EE, eds. *Trauma*, 4th edition. New York, NY: McGraw-Hill; 2000.

7. Devitt JH, McLean RF, Koch JP. Anaesthetic management of acute blunt thoracic trauma. *Can J Anaesth* 1991;**38**,506–510.

8. Duan Y, Smith CE, Como JJ. Anesthesia for major cardiothoracic trauma. In: Wilson WC, Grande CM, Hoyt DB, eds. *Trauma: Resuscitation, Anesthesia, and Critical Care*. New York, NY: Informa Healthcare; 2007.

9. Gerhardt MA, Gravlee GP. Anesthesia considerations for cardiothoracic trauma. In: Smith CE, ed. *Trauma Anesthesia*. New York, NY: Cambridge University Press; 2008.

10. Kanellakos GW, Slinger P. Intraoperative one-lung ventilation for trauma anesthesia. In: Smith CE, ed. *Trauma Anesthesia*. New York, NY: Cambridge University Press; 2008.

11. Morgan GE, Mikhail MS, Murray MJ. *Clinical Anesthesiology*, 4th edition. New York, NY: McGraw Hill; 2006.

12. Orliaguet G, Carli P. Thoracic blocks. In: Rosenberg AD, Grande CM, Bernstein RL, eds. *Pain Management and Regional Anesthesia in Trauma*. London: Saunders; 2000.

13. Pretre RM, Chilcott M. Blunt trauma to the heart and great vessels. *N Engl J Med* 1997;**336**:626–632.

14. Smith CE, Marciniak D. Comprehensive management of patients with traumatic aortic injury. In: Subramaniam K, Park KW, Subramaniam B, eds. *Anesthesia and Perioperative Care for Aortic Surgery*. New York: Springer; 2011.

15. Wall MJ, Storey JH, Mattox KL. Indications for thoracotomy. In: Mattox KL, Feliciano DV, Moore EE, eds. *Trauma*, 4th edition. New York, NY: McGraw-Hill; 2000.

Chapter

# 17

# Anesthetic considerations for abdominal trauma

Olga Kaslow and Robert Kettler

The surgical management of abdominal trauma is a dynamic situation. The patient's response to the initial injury and subsequent therapeutic interventions can present a rapidly evolving challenge to the anesthesiologist. This chapter will cover abdominal trauma by reviewing the relevant anatomy, preoperative evaluation, and general perioperative considerations, as well as the anesthetic considerations to specific procedures.

## Anatomic considerations

Surface landmarks to delineate the extent of the abdomen are:

- Superior: diaphragm.
- Inferior: inguinal ligaments and symphysis pubis.
- Lateral: anterior axillary lines.

The flank is the area between the anterior and posterior axillary lines down from the sixth intercostal space to the iliac crest. The abdominal compartments and their contents are listed in Table 17.1.

During exhalation the diaphragm may ascend to the level of the fourth intercostal space, so abdominal viscera can be injured by trauma to the thorax. During inhalation the descending diaphragm moves the spleen and liver down to the abdominal cavity, making them susceptible to abdominal trauma.

## Mechanisms of injury

Knowledge of the trauma mechanism allows prediction of the pattern of injury to abdominal organs and vascular structures, and facilitates decision-making about the diagnostic method to be used.

With blunt trauma, the most common forces are:

- Compression of the solid abdominal organs (liver, spleen) against a fixed or moving object (e.g., steering wheel, baseball bat) causing crushing and bleeding.
- Compression of the hollow organs, which creates a rapid increase in an intraluminal pressure, resulting in their rupture and subsequent peritoneal contamination.
- Deceleration, which generates shearing of the organ tissues between fixed and mobile structures, causing liver and spleen lacerations at the site of their fixed ligaments, and damage to the mesentery and large vessels.

*Essentials of Trauma Anesthesia*, ed. A. J. Varon and C. E. Smith. Published by Cambridge University Press.
© Cambridge University Press 2012.

**Table 17.1.** Anatomic considerations: Four abdominal compartments and their contents

| Thoracoabdominal compartment | Diaphragm<br>Liver<br>Spleen<br>Stomach<br>Transverse colon |
|---|---|
| Peritoneal cavity | Small bowel<br>Parts of the ascending and descending colon<br>Sigmoid colon<br>Omentum<br>Gravid uterus<br>Dome of distended bladder |
| Retroperitoneal space | Abdominal aorta<br>Inferior vena cava<br>Two thirds of duodenum<br>Pancreas<br>Kidneys and ureters |
| Pelvic space | Bladder and urethra<br>Rectum<br>Uterus and ovaries<br>Iliac vessels |

With penetrating trauma, the common mechanisms of injury are:

- Stab wounds, low velocity
  - Create direct damage by lacerations. The most frequently injured organs are the liver, diaphragm, and small and large bowel.
- Gunshot wounds, high velocity
  - Cause damage by a combination of direct laceration by the missile and its fragments, cavitation effect within the organs along the missile track, and crushing from the blast injury.
  - Solid organs like the liver, spleen, and kidneys are frequently injured by the cavitation effect.
  - Hollow organs (stomach, bowel, and bladder) are not affected by cavitation if they are empty, but they may suffer considerable damage if they contain fluid.

# Preoperative evaluation and management (see also Chapter 2)

## Early involvement

An anesthesiologist should evaluate the patient as early as possible on arrival to the hospital. The anesthesiologist's roles in a trauma bay include acting as a member of a multi-disciplinary trauma team conducting the initial assessment and resuscitation according to Advanced Trauma Life Support (ATLS) principles, an airway management expert, and a consultant demonstrating broad knowledge of trauma care, leading to an in-depth preoperative assessment. The anesthetic plan is formulated and adapted according to the urgency of surgical intervention.

# History

Findings at the scene from prehospital personnel reports are helpful and include vital signs, Glasgow Coma Scale (GCS) score (see Chapter 2, Table 2.3), and interventions at the scene and en route: airway and ventilation, intravenous (IV) access, administered fluid and medications, resuscitating maneuvers such as chest compressions, defibrillation, tourniquets, cervical collar, and pelvic binder.

# Physical exam of the abdomen

The physical exam of the abdomen is performed as part of the secondary survey and includes a systematic evaluation of the abdomen including inspection, palpation, percussion, and auscultation. The following abnormalities can be detected by physical exam:

- External signs of injury (abrasions, ecchymoses) and contusion patterns (lap belt and steering wheel marks) indicate a possibility of intra-abdominal injury.
- Abdominal distension is suspicious for intraperitoneal hemorrhage.
- Signs of peritonitis (rigidity, rebound tenderness) suggest gastric or intestinal perforation and leakage.
- Cullen's sign (periumbilical ecchymosis) and Grey-Turner's sign (flank bruising) are red flags for retroperitoneal hemorrhage.
- Assessment of pelvic stability may reveal pelvic fractures that are commonly associated with disruption of arteries and veins causing major hemorrhage. Manipulation of the fractured pelvis must be done with extreme caution to avoid aggravation of any vascular injury by bone fragments.
- Rectal, perineal, and vaginal exams are performed to rule out potential injury and bleeding; the loss of rectal sphincter tone is suggestive of spinal cord trauma; blood at the urethral meatus and a high riding prostate indicate urethral tear and disruption.

# Diagnostic studies

Laboratory studies are limited to a complete blood count, basic chemistry, and coagulation. If the patient is hemodynamically abnormal, an arterial blood gas (ABG) is drawn to assess tissue perfusion and a type and screen or type and cross is performed for 4–6 units of packed red blood cells (PRBCs). Chest X-ray findings associated with abdominal injuries include:

- Free air under the diaphragm secondary to a hollow viscous rupture.
- Rib fractures may predispose to hepatic or splenic injury.
- Displaced nasogastric (NG) tube, bowel, or stomach in the chest are diagnostic of a ruptured diaphragm and traumatic diaphragmatic hernia.

Pelvic X-ray assists with diagnosis of both retroperitoneal hemorrhage and genitourinary injuries. Focused assessment with sonography for trauma (FAST) is a rapid, portable, and non-invasive examination of pericardial, perihepatic, perisplenic, and pelvic anatomic spaces for free fluid indicative of hemopericardium or hemoperitoneum (see Chapter 10). However, the exam provides limited visualization in obese patients and does not identify the specific source of bleeding. Diagnostic peritoneal lavage is used for detection of intra-abdominal hemorrhage and injury of hollow organs. Despite being highly sensitive, it is invasive, painful, time consuming, and interferes with further abdominal exams. Computed tomography (CT) provides diagnosis of hemoperitoneum and specific abdominal, retroperitoneal, and pelvic organ injuries. Besides being highly sensitive, it allows grading and evaluation of concomitant injuries. Its disadvantages include the high cost and exposure to IV contrast and radiation. CT scan should not be performed on hemodynamically unstable patients and those requiring emergent surgical intervention.

## Hemodynamic instability in the preoperative period

In a patient with abdominal trauma who becomes hemodynamically unstable, additional studies should be deferred to expedite the transfer to definitive care. Hypotension and tachycardia in a patient with a normal chest X-ray, absence of a large scalp laceration or major extremity trauma, and that does not improve or only transiently improves after resuscitation with boluses of IV fluid (up to 2.0 L) should be attributed to active abdominal or retroperitoneal bleeding. Immediate intervention is required to control hemorrhage. Blood transfusion should be initiated with cross-matched or O Rh-negative (women of childbearing age) or O Rh-positive (men) PRBCs. In the absence of traumatic brain injury, a strategy of permissive hypotension may be utilized until hemostasis is achieved. Transfer to the operating room (OR) or interventional radiology suite for control of bleeding may be required urgently or emergently.

## Intraoperative management

### Airway

Rapid sequence induction (RSI) and intubation is highly recommended due to the high risk of aspiration (see also Chapters 3 and 7). This is because most trauma patients have not fasted and gastric emptying is delayed due to high catecholamine levels from the stress of trauma. Patients may also have high abdominal pressure from hemoperitoneum.

### Breathing

In a hemodynamically normal patient, stethoscope, capnography, and pulse oximetry may be sufficient for monitoring ventilation and oxygenation (see also Chapter 9). Arterial blood gas measurements are routine for unstable patients.

### Circulation

Significant bleeding requiring large volume resuscitation is common in abdominal trauma. Adequate IV access is imperative (see also Chapter 5). At least two large-bore peripheral IVs should be placed. Preferred sites for placement of IV lines are the veins that drain into the superior vena cava; the inferior vena cava (IVC) could be disrupted by injury or clamped during surgical resuscitation. Insertion of a large gauge introducer in the internal jugular or subclavian veins is helpful for volume resuscitation; however, central venous access should not delay emergent surgery. Optimal positioning and sterile condition for central venous access during ongoing laparotomy are difficult to achieve, predisposing to complications such as pneumothorax, neck hematoma, and infection. Placement of intraosseous lines (15 G) or ultrasound guided cannulation are useful in patients with difficult IV access. Large-bore IV tubing with a minimal number of stop-cocks/luer locks helps minimize resistance to flow during volume resuscitation. Pressure bags, fluid warmers, and rapid infuser and autologous blood salvage devices are useful. Availability of blood products should be confirmed and a prospectively established massive transfusion protocol should be activated if needed.

## Monitoring (see Chapter 9)

In addition to the American Society of Anesthesiologists' standard monitors, invasive monitors are needed for cases with significant hemorrhage and major fluid shifts requiring large volume resuscitation. Commonly used monitoring devices include an arterial line, pulse contour analysis, and transesophageal echocardiography (see Chapter 10).

## Drugs

### Induction agents

A moribund patient needs no induction agent, only neuromuscular blockade to facilitate intubation. Scopolamine, 0.4 mg IV, can be administered for amnesia. Small doses of midazolam may be given if there is restoration of blood pressure. An awake patient should be induced with an agent that better preserves cardiovascular stability (see Chapter 7). Induction agents and opioids may precipitate severe hypotension in a patient with hemorrhagic shock for the following reasons:

- The anesthetic is diluted in a smaller total blood volume resulting in higher serum levels.
- A much higher proportion of cardiac output is diverted to the brain and heart, increasing their anesthetic content.
- Direct myocardial depressant and vasodilator effects of the drug.
- Inhibition of endogenous catecholamines by the drug.

Etomidate (0.1–0.2 mg/kg) and ketamine (0.25–1 mg/kg) are preferred for the patient in severe shock. Propofol and thiopental may also be used, but in reduced and fractionated doses.

### Neuromuscular relaxants

Succinylcholine (1.0–1.5 mg/kg) has the fastest onset for RSI (30–60 seconds). Contraindications include malignant hyperthermia and demyelinating neurologic diseases (see Chapters 3 and 7). The patient with concomitant spinal cord injury or burn is at risk for life-threatening hyperkalemia 24–48 hours after the insult. Rocuronium (1.0–1.2 mg/kg) is a non-depolarizing agent used for RSI with only a slight delay in onset time (1–1.5 minutes), but longer duration (45–60 min).

### Maintenance of anesthesia

Providing adequate sedation, amnesia, and analgesia to a hemodynamically unstable patient with abdominal trauma is a challenging task. Administration of just a neuromuscular blocking agent alone might result in recall. Anesthetic techniques include the use of IV agents, volatile anesthetics, and regional anesthesia.

- Volatile anesthetics:
  - Although all volatile agents produce dose-dependent myocardial depression, there is no absolute contraindication to these anesthetic agents for abdominal trauma; however, their end-tidal concentration should be titrated to the patient's blood pressure. Most patients who are maintained in a range of minimum alveolar concentration (MAC)-awake (0.3–0.5 MAC) do not recall intraoperative events.

- In a bleeding patient, MAC is reduced by hypothermia, hypoxemia, severe anemia, and hypotension.
- Nitrous oxide ($N_2O$) is generally avoided in surgery for abdominal trauma because it may produce bowel distention; it can also enlarge a pneumothorax or pneumocephalus that may be present in patients with multiple injuries. $N_2O$ is also known to support combustion if a fire occurs.
- IV agents:
  - Incremental doses of narcotics and/or ketamine are the most commonly used.
  - Scopolamine or benzodiazepines may be added to assure amnesia.
  - Total IV anesthesia with propofol can also be used.
- Neuraxial and regional anesthesia:
  - Both spinal and epidural anesthesia are ill advised in abdominal trauma because of difficult positioning, time required, and most importantly sympathectomy, which may cause severe hypotension and cardiac arrest in hypovolemic patients.

# Exploratory laparotomy

## Surgical approach

A midline abdominal incision from xyphoid to pubis is employed with self-retaining retractors to facilitate exposure. Goals of surgery include:

- Control of hemorrhage, evacuation of the free blood, rapid packing of all four quadrants, identification and clamping of bleeding vessels
- Contamination control by suturing the bowel perforations
- Systematic exploration of entire abdomen
- Injury repair of specific organs
- Abdominal closure

## Anesthetic considerations

The anesthetic plan is based on knowledge of the patient's injuries, age, known preexisting conditions, response to initial resuscitation, and surgical interventions. Communication with the surgeon is the key with regard to how the surgery is progressing. The surgeon needs to be kept informed of anesthetic concerns and actions. Anesthesia goals include:

- Maintaining normothermia (see Chapter 7).
  - Monitor the patient's core temperature and keep the OR warm. Cover the patient with warm blankets and utilize forced air warming (convective warming). Use warmed IV fluids and blood products.
- Maximizing surgical exposure by maintaining adequate paralysis, stomach decompression with NG or gastric tube, and avoiding abdominal distension with $N_2O$.
- Ensuring adequate hemodynamics and blood volume tailored to the patient's needs:
  - Appropriately titrate anesthetic for extremes of blood pressure and heart rate. Treat hypotension with judicious administration of warmed IV fluid.
  - Use dynamic hemodynamic parameters (e.g., pulse pressure variation, systolic pressure variation, stroke volume variation), base deficit, and lactate levels to guide volume resuscitation (see Chapter 9). Excessive use of vasopressors should be avoided.

- Be aware of sudden hemodynamic changes associated with surgical occlusion of major vessels.
- Replace blood loss (see Chapters 4 and 6).
- Estimating blood loss is difficult in abdominal trauma due to mixture of shed blood with other body fluids (urine and bowel contents), irrigation solutions, and blood absorption in drapes and packing materials.
- Notify the surgeons about gross blood suctioned from stomach or detected in urine.
- Measurement of hematocrit, ionized calcium, and coagulation parameters is essential for guiding transfusion of blood products (PRBC, plasma, cryoprecipitate), fibrinogen, and/or prothrombin complex concentrate (PCC).
- Ongoing oozing in the operative field after achieving surgical hemostasis necessitates aggressive treatment of coagulopathy.

Use autologous blood salvage devices (cell saver). Non-contaminated intra-abdominal blood from injured liver, spleen, or retroperitoneum is being salvaged in many trauma centers. Cell saver wash cycle does remove many bacteria but not anaerobes. The source and degree of contamination (small intestine versus colon), and the addition of povidone-iodine or antibiotics in irrigation solution, should be considered when deciding on autotransfusion if life-threatening hemorrhage occurs.

## Damage control laparotomy

Damage control surgery is instituted on an unstable patient who would not be able to tolerate a long definitive repair (see also Chapter 7).

## Surgical considerations

Damage control laparotomy should be considered if the estimated surgical time is more than 90 minutes, the patient needs multiple surgeries to reassess and repair abdominal organs, and if there are associated injuries outside of the abdomen requiring surgical repair. Damage control should also be considered if there is hemodynamic instability with poor response to resuscitation, coagulopathy is identified as a major cause of bleeding, and in the setting of hypothermia with severe acidosis.

Initial control of bleeding is achieved by packing, vessel clamping, and ligation. Abdominal exploration without a definitive organ repair, splenectomy, nephrectomy, and ureter ligation are preferred over reconstruction. For contamination control, gastric and bowel contents are drained, bowel ends are stapled, and end-to-end anastomosis and stoma maturation are postponed. The abdominal cavity is packed and temporary abdominal closure is utilized.

## Anesthetic considerations

Consideration should be given to inducing anesthesia with RSI *after* the operative field is prepped and draped and the surgeons are gowned, gloved, and ready to cut. The role of the anesthesiologist consists of the following:

- Maintaining a high index of suspicion for the need of damage control based on both injury pattern and the patient's hemodynamics.
- Facilitating decision-making in initiating damage control surgery or converting a definitive abdominal surgery to damage control laparotomy.

- Tailoring resuscitation to sequential surgical repair.
- Discussing utilization of the cell saver.

The anesthesiologist needs to be aware of surgical maneuvers. Two-way communication is imperative. Aortic cross-clamping, vessel occlusion, and pressure held with temporary packing allow brief periods of anesthetic "catch ups" to restore the patient's intravascular volume. The Pringle maneuver may be required (temporary occlusion of portal triad) to gain operative exposure and vascular control of the liver. Decreased venous return may precipitate severe hypotension and cardiac arrest in the hypovolemic patient. Be prepared to treat.

Resuscitation principles and goals for damage control surgery (see also Chapters 4, 6, and 7) include the following:

- Hypotensive resuscitation:
  - Warm IV fluid is given in small boluses, with close attention to the rate of surgical bleeding.
  - Maintaining systolic blood pressure approximately 90 mmHg and heart rate < 120 beats/min (systolic blood pressure of at least 100 mmHg in patients with head trauma).
- Maintenance of blood composition and chemical equilibrium:
  - Initiating massive transfusion protocol with PRBCs, plasma, and platelets.
  - Reducing the volume of crystalloids.
  - Maintaining hematocrit > 25%, INR < 1.6, platelets > $50 \times 10^9$ per liter.
  - Consider Factor VIIa, fibrinogen, PCC, or tranexamic acid if coagulopathy is difficult to control.
- Preservation of homeostasis:
  - Restoration of end-organ perfusion: pH > 7.25, arterial carbon dioxide < 50 mmHg and decreasing lactate level.
  - Maintaining normothermia by increasing room temperature, warming IV fluids and irrigation solutions, and using convective warming blankets, radiant heat and gel pad warming.
- Analgesia and sedation should be continued in spite of hemodynamic instability:
  - Deep and stable level of anesthesia can be achieved with incremental doses of fentanyl.
  - Small boluses of ketamine and midazolam are also advocated.
  - Tracheal extubation is not expected at the end of surgery.

## Re-exploration ("Relook on demand surgery")

This is an emergent surgical procedure required for postoperative bleeding or abdominal compartment syndrome.

## Release of abdominal compartment syndrome

Abdominal compartment syndrome is the result of increased intra-abdominal pressure after massive fluid resuscitation (with bowel edema) or ongoing bleeding.

Normal abdominal pressure ranges from 0 to 5 mmHg; pressures exceeding 20–25 mmHg result in impaired circulation and tissue perfusion, and organ dysfunction. Respiratory dysfunction manifests as high peak airway pressures, decreased tidal volume, worsening atelectasis, and hypercarbia. Cardiovascular abnormalities include decreased thoracic venous return and low cardiac output. Renal hypoperfusion results in decreased kidney function and oliguria.

### Anesthetic considerations

Laparotomy and release of intra-abdominal pressure elicit rapid reperfusion syndrome and lactate washout prompting hypotension and even asystole.

IV fluid loading should begin before abdominal decompression. Vasopressors such as phenylephrine, norepinephrine, or vasopressin may be necessary to support blood pressure. Acidosis is treated by increasing minute ventilation; sodium bicarbonate should be considered as well. Calcium chloride is advocated to reduce the effects of hyperkalemia resulting from reperfused ischemic tissues.

# Definitive repair and repeat exploration

Definitive surgery is usually performed when the endpoints of resuscitation are met, commonly in 24–72 hours, and consists of removal of packing, definitive repair of bowel injuries and survey of other injuries, copious irrigation, and subsequent staged closure of the abdomen after bowel edema is resolved.

Late complications of exploratory laparotomy after abdominal trauma require urgent surgery. The most common indications are missed injuries presenting with delayed hemorrhage from colon, diaphragm, and chest wall vessels; peritonitis from breakdown of anastomosis; abscess or fistula formation; bowel obstruction or ischemia; and wound dehiscence and infection. Patients often present with serious illnesses such as pneumonia, acute respiratory distress syndrome (ARDS), and sepsis.

# Surgical and anesthetic considerations for specific abdominal injuries

## Intraperitoneal injuries

Hemodynamically normal patients with isolated blunt liver trauma are managed non-operatively with a high success rate. Severe hemorrhage from a liver injury is difficult to control. The Pringle maneuver may be performed by the surgeon to interrupt blood flow through the portal vein and hepatic artery; occlusion of thoracic or proximal abdominal aorta may also be necessary. Massive transfusion is frequently required. The surgeon may place a shunt from the infrahepatic IVC to the heart, and the anesthesiologist could attach an extension to the shunt for transfusion purposes.

Solitary injuries of the spleen in hemodynamically stable patients are managed non-operatively. When splenectomy is required, antipneumococcal vaccine must be given post-operatively to avoid pneumococcal infection and post-splenectomy sepsis due to depression of immune response.

Stomach, small bowel, and colon injuries are complicated by peritoneal contamination from release of gastric and intestinal contents into the abdominal cavity, resulting in bacterial peritonitis. Hemorrhage may be encountered as well.

The diaphragm may be injured in both blunt and penetrating trauma. Right hemi-diaphragm rupture occurs less often than the left, because of mechanical support of the liver on the right side. Holes in the diaphragm might create an air passage from abdomen to the chest causing pneumothorax. Herniation of abdominal organs through the diaphragmatic tear results in their strangulation, respiratory compromise, and increased risk of aspiration. Mechanical ventilation may mask diaphragmatic injury on chest X-ray by displacing herniating abdominal organs to near-normal position.

## Retroperitoneal injuries

Blunt injuries of the pancreas are difficult to diagnose. Repeat surgeries are often required for complications of pancreatic trauma such as fistulas, abscesses, pseudocysts, and secondary hemorrhage. Pancreatic duct damage prompts release of pancreatic enzymes in surrounding tissues causing severe pancreatitis.

Severe injuries of the duodenum and the head of the pancreas may require a Whipple procedure (pancreaticoduodenectomy), which is complex, time consuming, and unsuitable when a damage control laparotomy is required.

Kidney trauma may result in renal contusion, laceration, subscapular hematoma, shattered kidney, renal artery occlusion, and renal vein thrombosis. It may cause extensive retroperitoneal bleeding as well as urine leakage.

Great vessel injuries cause profound hemorrhagic shock.

- Arterial injury is associated with very rapid blood loss; at the same time venous injury causes low-pressure and high-volume bleeding, often very difficult to control.
- Activation of a massive transfusion protocol and initiating a rapid volume infusion is necessary.
- Adequate IV access is of paramount importance. The IV lines should be in the upper extremities, subclavian vein, or internal jugular vein. Saphenous or femoral venous lines cannot be used if surgery requires IVC occlusion.
- Temporary clamping of the abdominal aorta may be required to maintain perfusion of the heart and the brain.
- Occlusion of the IVC results in profound decrease of venous return and precipitation of cardiovascular collapse.

## Anesthetic considerations for non-operative management of abdominal trauma

Non-operative surgical management of abdominal trauma has become routine in most trauma centers. Utilization of various modern and highly accurate non-invasive radiographic methods allows for achieving hemostasis and salvaging organs without the need for surgery. Around-the-clock availability of a multi-disciplinary team of experts, such as trauma surgeons, emergency physicians, radiologists, and anesthesiologists, is necessary to successfully provide such complex and sophisticated management.

Traditionally, non-operative management of abdominal trauma has been reserved for hemodynamically stable patients and those who respond to fluid resuscitation, while unstable patients were treated by emergency laparotomy. Currently, angiographic embolization of arterial hemorrhage in a hemodynamically unstable patient may be used both as a first-line treatment modality and also as an adjunct to surgery that fails to achieve hemostasis.

A variety of injuries from both blunt and penetrating abdominal trauma may be amenable to angioembolization.

- Splenic embolization can be used as an alternative to splenectomy. Spleen preservation is important to retain immunological and hematological functions and to reduce the risk of post-splenectomy sepsis.
- There has been increasing success with early embolization of hepatic vascular injuries in hemodynamically unstable patients that previously were managed surgically.
- Embolization and endovascular stent placement have been employed in primary management of renal vascular injuries with high success.
- Angiography with selective embolization can successfully control a life-threatening pelvic arterial hemorrhage, reducing transfusion requirements (see Chapter 18).
- Open exploration of retroperitoneal hematomas may lead to a disaster, and surgery should be reserved only for repair of associated visceral injuries. (Severe pelvic fractures from blunt injury should undergo external fixation that itself significantly contributes to hemostasis.)

## Advantages of angiographic embolization

Avoiding open exploration of the abdomen and retroperitoneal space preserves tamponade effect of the hematoma and prevents hemodynamic collapse. Angiography provides early diagnosis of bleeding sites, and embolization treats bleeding in several locations simultaneously, accessing the areas that are difficult to approach surgically. It allows non-operative management of solid organ hemorrhage.

## Interventional radiology techniques

Embolization with coils, microcoils, or gelfoam slurry is the most common technique for solid organ hemorrhage. Stents or stent grafts are employed in direct arterial trauma, allowing control of hemorrhage with simultaneous preservation of blood supply. Occlusion balloons are placed selectively or temporarily within main visceral vessels, internal iliac arteries, or even within the aorta for temporary cessation of bleeding.

## Possible complications

Allergic reaction to contrast and contrast-induced nephropathy may occur, especially in patients with acute or chronic renal failure. Other complications include coil migration, parenchymal infarct, and abscess formation.

## Key points

- Surgery for abdominal trauma is a dynamic situation requiring early involvement and constant vigilance on the part of the anesthesiologist.
- The care of the patient with abdominal trauma has evolved to the point that one anesthesiologist may have to provide care to one patient receiving multiple interventions from multiple specialties at multiple locations.
- Clear communication among all parties involved is paramount. While this is important in the perioperative period, it is equally important (if not more so) in the non-operative, pre-trauma stage.

- CT provides accurate diagnosis of hemoperitoneum, and specific abdominal, retroperitoneal, and pelvic organ injuries. However, it should not be performed on hemodynamically unstable patients and those requiring emergent surgical intervention.
- Rapid sequence induction (RSI) and intubation is highly recommended for abdominal trauma patients due to the high risk of aspiration.
- Anesthesia goals for abdominal trauma include maintaining normothermia, maximizing surgical exposure, ensuring adequate hemodynamics tailored to the patient's needs, and refraining from excessive use of vasopressors.
- Adequate IV access is of paramount importance. IV lines should be placed in the upper extremities, subclavian vein, or internal jugular vein. Saphenous or femoral venous lines cannot be used if surgery requires IVC occlusion.
- Both spinal and epidural anesthesia are ill-advised in acute abdominal trauma.
- Exploratory laparotomy for abdominal compartment syndrome can elicit rapid reperfusion syndrome and lactate washout, and lead to hypotension and asystole. Adequate preparation is essential.
- Practice parameters can be established by team consensus so that care during an emergency can be provided effectively and efficiently. Planning and flexibility are keys to success in these circumstances.

## Further reading

1. American College of Surgeons, Committee on Trauma. *Advance Trauma Life Support for Doctors: ATLS® Student Course Manual.* Chicago, IL: American College of Surgeons; 2008.

2. Dutton R. Damage control anesthesia. *TraumaCare* 2005;**15**:197–201.

3. Dutton R. Trauma anesthesia. *ASA Refresher Courses in Anesthesiology* 2008;**36**:33–43.

4. Knight RG, Bellamy RF. Abdominal injuries. In: Zajtchuk R, Bellamy RF, Grande CM, eds. *Anesthesia and Perioperative Care of the Combat Casualty.* *Textbook of Military Medicine.* Part IV – surgical combat casualty care. Tacoma, WA: TMM Publications; 1995.

5. Moeng MS, Loveland JA, Boffars KD. Damage control: beyond the limits of the abdominal cavity. A review. *TraumaCare* 2005;**15**:189–196.

6. Wallis A, Kelly MD, Jones L. Angiography and embolization for solid abdominal organ injury in adults – a current perspective. *World J Emerg Surg* 2010;**5**:18.

7. Wilson CW. Anesthesia consideration for abdominal trauma. In: Smith CE, ed. *Trauma Anesthesia.* New York, NY: Cambridge University Press; 2008.

Chapter

# 18

# Anesthetic considerations for musculoskeletal trauma

Jessica A. Lovich-Sapola and Charles E. Smith

## Introduction

According to Miller, "musculoskeletal injuries are the most frequent indications for surgical operative management in most trauma centers" (see Further reading). It is important to achieve early stabilization and alignment of fractures after multiple trauma.

- Reduction and fixation of fractures will generally lead to reduced pain, improved resuscitation, restoration of function, and enhanced mobility.
- Failure to stabilize musculoskeletal injuries leads to increased morbidity and length of hospital stay, and worsens pulmonary complications.
- Timing of fracture repair in a multiple-trauma patient is complicated, requiring a team approach with ongoing communication.
- Early fracture reduction and fixation represents an important shift in the care of trauma patients to reduce morbidity, acute respiratory distress syndrome (ARDS), and sepsis (Table 18.1).
- Life-threatening and limb-threatening musculoskeletal injuries need to be addressed emergently (Table 18.2).

## Choice of anesthetic technique

### Regional anesthesia for musculoskeletal trauma (see also Chapter 8)

Advantages of regional anesthesia include:

- Ability to assess the patient's mental status.
- Increased vascular flow to the extremity.
- Decreased blood loss.
- Decreased incidence of deep venous thrombosis.
- Avoidance of airway intervention.
- Improved postoperative pain control and earlier mobilization.

Disadvantages of regional anesthesia include:

- Requirement for sedation.
- Hemodynamic instability.
- Unsuitability for multiple body regions.

---

*Essentials of Trauma Anesthesia*, ed. A. J. Varon and C. E. Smith. Published by Cambridge University Press.
© Cambridge University Press 2012.

**Table 18.1.** Musculoskeletal injury requiring urgent surgical treatment

| Surgery recommended within 6–8 hours | Surgery recommended within 24 hours |
|---|---|
| Open fracture | Unstable pelvis/acetabulum fracture |
| Traumatic arthrotomy | Unstable femur fracture |
| Dislocated joint | Proximal fracture in the elderly |
| Displaced femoral neck fracture in young adult | |

**Table 18.2.** Life-threatening and limb-threatening injuries

| Life-threatening injuries | Limb-threatening injuries |
|---|---|
| Pelvic ring injuries with hemorrhage | Traumatic amputation |
| Long-bone fractures with hemorrhage | Vascular injury |
| | Compartment syndrome |

- A potentially longer time to achieve anesthetic levels.
- Time lasting beyond what is necessary.
- Potential difficulty in evaluating peripheral nerve function.

## General anesthesia for musculoskeletal trauma (see also Chapter 7)

The advantages of a general anesthetic technique include:

- Speed of onset.
- Ability to better regulate duration.
- Allows for multiple procedures.
- Improved patient acceptance.

Disadvantages of general anesthesia include:

- Inability to do serial mental status examinations.
- Requirement of airway manipulation.
- More complex hemodynamic management.
- Increased risk for barotrauma.

## Perioperative preparation for orthopedic trauma surgery

It is imperative that a history and physical examination be performed prior to the patient going to the operating room. How extensive this evaluation is depends on the nature and urgency of the surgery. At a minimum, the anesthesiologist should review the primary and secondary Advanced Trauma Life Support (ATLS) surveys, interventions required, and tests performed including laboratory analyses and radiographs of the chest, pelvis, spine, head, and abdomen. Anesthesia considerations for orthopedic trauma are shown in Table 18.3. It is worthwhile to recall that certain fractures and dislocations are associated with specific neurologic and vascular injuries (Table 18.4).

**Table 18.3.** Anesthesia considerations for musculoskeletal trauma

| |
|---|
| Degree of urgency and inadequate time for evaluation of comorbidities and optimization of medical conditions |
| Full stomach and risk of aspiration |
| Uncleared cervical spine, inability to optimally position the head and neck for tracheal intubation leading to difficult airway management |
| Drug intoxication and substance abuse: alcohol, cocaine, amphetamines, cannabinoids, opioids, and other agents |
| Positioning injuries |
| Hypothermia |
| Major blood loss and coagulopathy |
| Long tourniquet times leading to injury of nerves, muscles, and blood vessels |
| Fat embolism syndrome with delayed emergence and ARDS |
| Deep venous thrombosis |
| Compartment syndrome |
| Postoperative pain |

**Table 18.4.** Fractures and dislocations associated with neurological or vascular injury

| Fracture or dislocation | Structure injured |
|---|---|
| Clavicle or first rib fracture | Subclavian artery |
| Shoulder dislocation | Axillary nerve or artery |
| Humeral shaft fracture | Radial nerve |
| Supracondylar humerus fracture | Brachial artery |
| Hip dislocation | Sciatic nerve |
| Femoral shaft fracture | Superficial femoral artery |
| Supracondylar femur fracture | Popliteal artery |
| Knee dislocation | Common peroneal nerve, popliteal artery |
| Proximal tibia or fibula fracture | Common peroneal nerve |

Reproduced with permission from: Vallier HA, Jenkins MD. Musculoskeletal trauma. In: Smith CE, ed. *Trauma Anesthesia*. New York, NY: Cambridge University Press; 2008.

Recommended preoperative testing:

- Complete blood count.
- Type and screen.
- Coagulation panel.
- Basic metabolic panel as needed per the patient's history.
- Electrocardiogram as needed per the patient's history.
- Further testing should be mandated by the specific patient and surgery planned.

Monitoring for an orthopedic trauma case should include standard American Society of Anesthesiologists monitors (see also Chapter 9). Specific monitors should be determined based on the patient's overall medical condition and status, but should always include measures of oxygenation, ventilation, circulation, and temperature.

- Oxygenation: pulse oximetry, patient color observation, inhaled and exhaled gas analysis, blood gas analysis.
- Ventilation: end-tidal carbon dioxide measurement, auscultation of breath sounds, monitoring the ventilator arterial blood gas.
- Circulation: ECG, blood pressure (non-invasive or invasive with an intra-arterial catheter), echocardiography, pulmonary artery catheter measurements, urine output.
- Temperature: esophageal, nasal, bladder, or rectal.

Fluid management should be determined on a case-by-case basis (see also Chapter 4). Options for fluid management include:

- Crystalloids:
  - Lactated Ringer's (LR) (standard for trauma patients).
  - LR is contraindicated for the co-infusion or dilution of packed red blood cells (RBCs) secondary to the 3 mEq/L of calcium.
  - 0.9% saline (used for the dilution of RBCs).
  - Glucose-containing solutions are generally avoided due to the risk of hyperglycemia
- Colloid:
  - More effective plasma expanders than crystalloid.
- Blood products:
  - RBCs.
  - Fresh frozen plasma.
  - Platelets.
  - Cryoprecipitate.

## Pain management

The acute management of pain in a patient with an orthopedic injury is often challenging, especially if there are multiple sites of injury (see also Chapter 8). Pain management should begin with small, frequent doses of rapidly acting intravenous agents until the patient begins to develop some pain relief. Once the patient is comfortable, the dose required to achieve this effect can be used to estimate the patient's basal requirements before starting long-acting medications or patient-controlled analgesia. The development of hypotension in response to the analgesic is usually a sign of hypovolemia and should be treated accordingly. Patient recovery will often require significant physical therapy; an appropriate increase in medication will be required during this therapy.

Pain relief can also be supplemented with comprehensive emotional support and counseling, since the mechanism of the trauma itself often has significant negative psychological associations. Referral to a psychiatrist for post-traumatic stress disorder treatment may be appropriate.

Orthopedic pain is often associated with neuropathic pain. This pain presents as burning and "electrical shocks," rarely responds well to narcotics alone, and should be treated with gabapentin and possibly selective regional anesthesia to "break the pain cycle."

Regional analgesia using an epidural or peripheral nerve block should be considered for any orthopedic trauma (see Chapter 8). Coagulation parameters and history of bleeding diathesis should be verified prior to performing any regional technique. Regional analgesic techniques are often associated with a high level of patient satisfaction, improved pulmonary function, and can facilitate earlier mobilization of the affected limb.

# Femur fracture management

Life-threatening hemorrhage can occur due to bilateral femur fractures or multiple long-bone fractures. Mortality rates can be as high as 25%. It is estimated that the average blood loss from a femoral shaft fracture is 1,500 cc. Placement of two large-bore intravenous lines or central venous access is required (see Chapter 5).

Early definite stabilization (within 24 hours of the injury) has been shown to be safe in most patients, including patients with multiple injuries such as severe abdominal, chest, or head injuries as long as adequate resuscitation and medical optimization has been achieved prior to surgery. A protocol for early appropriate definitive surgery of unstable axial fractures has been developed at MetroHealth Medical Center (Table 18.5). Optimization includes fluid resuscitation with crystalloid, colloid, and blood products as needed. Serial arterial blood gas samples to follow lactate, pH, and base deficit will help guide adequacy of resuscitation. Early consultation of other services is often required to address other injuries or comorbidities.

The benefits of early definite stabilization of a femur fracture include:

- Fewer pulmonary complications.
- Fewer ventilator days.
- Fewer deep venous thromboses.
- Shorter hospital stay.
- Lower healthcare costs.

# Pelvic fracture management

The mortality after a pelvic ring fracture ranges from 5 to 18%. The bleeding from a pelvic fracture is often into a closed space and therefore not immediately obvious to an examiner. Pelvic fractures can be associated with massive retroperitoneal hemorrhage. Urgent resuscitation and early stabilization of the fracture can minimize morbidity and mortality.

The benefits of early (within 24 hours of injury) stabilization or reduction and definitive fixation of an unstable pelvic fracture include:

- Control of bleeding and assists with resuscitation.
- Pain relief.
- Ability to mobilize the patient.
- Ease of reduction.
- Improved reduction quality.
- Elimination of traction and recumbency.
- Reduced risk of pulmonary, septic, and thromboembolic complications.
- Less organ failure.
- Reduced morbidity and mortality.
- Decreased length of stay in the intensive care unit.
- Shorter hospital stay.

**Table 18.5.** Early appropriate care. A protocol for treatment of unstable axial fractures at MetroHealth Medical Center

| | |
|---|---|
| Inclusion criteria | Mechanically unstable fracture of the proximal or diaphyseal femur, pelvic ring, acetabulum, and/or thoracolumbar spine requiring surgical stabilization<br>AND at least one of the following:<br>• Associated major injury to one or more other body systems<br>• Hemodynamic instability on presentation as defined by hypotension, tachycardia, and/or transfusion requirements<br>• One or more of the fractures of interest (listed above)<br>• Presenting Injury Severity Score $\geq 16$ |
| Exclusion criteria | • Severe head injury (Abbreviated Injury Score 4 or 5)<br>• Fracture associated with vascular injury requiring repair<br>• Patients undergoing digit or limb replantation<br>• Pregnant women<br>• Advanced age ($> 80$ years old)<br>• Severe baseline dementia<br>• Low energy fractures, such as a fall from standing height<br>• Skeletally immature patients<br>• Fractures secondary to neoplasm<br>• Known malignancy at other site<br>• History of chemotherapy, steroid use (prednisone $> 10$ mg/day or equivalent within past year)<br>• Expected survival less than one year due to baseline condition |
| Protocol | • On admission check ABG, lactate, CBC, platelets, INR, BMP<br>• Repeat labs every 8 hours until normal<br>• Recommend definitive stabilization within 36 hours of injury if:<br>  • pH $\geq 7.25$<br>  • Base deficit $\geq -5.5$<br>  • Lactate $< 4.0$<br>  AND<br>  • Patient is responding to resuscitation without vasopressor support (this may require serial lab measurements if there is persistent bleeding or hypotension)<br>• If these criteria are not met within 8 hours of presentation, proceed with a damage control strategy; i.e. external fixation of those femur and pelvis fractures amenable to this tactic. Then continue to reassess until the patient meets stabilization criteria before proceeding with definitive management<br>• If these criteria are not met within 8 hours and the patient is worsening, consider definitive fixation if it is projected to control active bleeding at surgeon discretion<br>• Postoperative management<br>  • Will include CBC, platelets, ABG, lactate, and INR every 8 hours until normal<br>  • Antibiotics will be standardized<br>  • DVT prophylaxis per trauma protocol |

Courtesy of Heather A. Vallier, MD, Department of Orthopaedic Surgery, MetroHealth Medical Center, Cleveland, OH.

Abbreviations: CBC = complete blood count; ABG = arterial blood gas; DVT = deep venous thrombosis; INR = international normalized ratio.

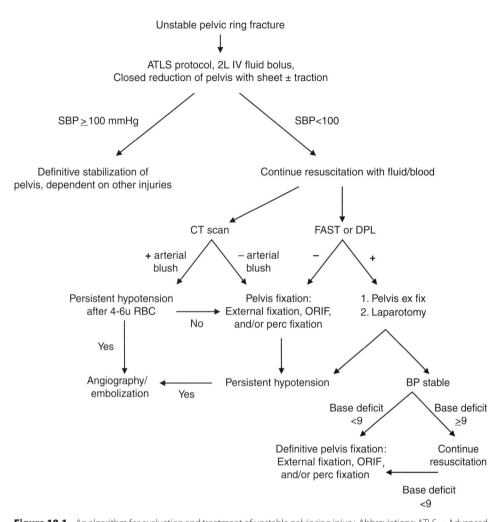

**Figure 18.1.** An algorithm for evaluation and treatment of unstable pelvic ring injury. Abbreviations: ATLS = Advanced Trauma Life Support; IV = intravenous; SBP = systolic blood pressure; CT = computed tomography; FAST = focused assessment with sonography for trauma; DPL = diagnostic peritoneal lavage; RBC = packed red blood cells; ex fix = external fixation; perc = percutaneous; ORIF = open reduction internal fixation.
Reproduced with permission from Vallier HA, Jenkins MD. Musculoskeletal trauma. In: Smith CE, ed. *Trauma Anesthesia*. New York, NY: Cambridge University Press; 2008.

Bleeding is a significant problem associated with a pelvic fracture. Bleeding can be from the bone itself, the iliac vessels, venous and arterial structures in close proximity to the sacroiliac joint, or the sacral venous plexus. Bleeding from the sacral venous plexus can result in significant blood loss. Four liters of blood can be retained in the retroperitoneal space before a tamponade would occur. If the patient remains hemodynamically unstable after aggressive fluid replacement, pelvic reduction and emergent angiography should be performed. Angiography may show the site of the bleed and allow therapeutic embolization (Figure 18.1).

Treating an unstable pelvic arterial bleed in the angiography suite is not without risks. Safe patient transfer to the angiography suite requires a coordinated approach between surgery, radiology, anesthesia, and intensive care unit staff. Following transcatheter embolization, the patient may then require further surgery and transfer to the operating room or intensive care unit to optimize perfusion and ventilation, correct acidosis and blood volume, and reverse coagulopathy. Anesthesia equipment and monitors used during interventional radiology should meet the same standards used in the operating room. The anesthesiologist must have a reliable way to communicate for help if needed.

## Two or more mechanically unstable fractures

For patients with multiple injuries, sequencing of fixation together with repair of other injuries is done in consultation with the surgical teams. This is frequently coordinated by trauma surgery and requires excellent communication and frequent reassessments to determine the safety of continuing surgery. Lab studies should be repeated at intervals to aid in decision-making. Consideration must be given to projected surgical time, anticipated blood loss, and patient positioning.

## Hip dislocation

Hip dislocation often results from high-impact trauma. Hip dislocations may be associated with neurologic and vascular injuries. Patients often have an associated acetabulum fracture. The treatment of the fracture may be delayed, but the treatment of the dislocation is a medical emergency. If the hip dislocation is not recognized and treated, the patient is at a high risk for developing avascular necrosis of the femoral head. Hip reduction often requires a deep level of sedation. If the patient requires further surgery, tracheal intubation and neuromuscular blockade are often recommended to facilitate the hip reduction and allow for future surgeries. It is important to remember that the trauma patient is always at risk for aspiration.

## Open fractures

Open fractures are surgical emergencies. The infection rate increases after a delay of 6–8 hours. Debridement and irrigation in the operating room plus provisional or definite fixation of the fracture should happen as soon as it is safely possible.

Early treatment with antibiotics (e.g., 2 g IV loading dose of cefazolin or 1.5 g IV of cefuroxime for an adult), followed by repeat doses at appropriate intervals is recommended to help prevent infection. Clindamycin 900 mg IV for an adult is appropriate if the patient has a cephalosporin or penicillin allergy. In a case where the open wound has obvious gross contamination, gram-negative coverage with 4–5 mg/kg of gentamicin IV every 24 hours is effective. Patients with soil contamination of the open fracture should receive 4 million units of IV penicillin every 4 hours to treat anaerobes.

The Centers for Disease Control and Prevention recommend tetanus vaccination every 10 years, but in a trauma situation, the vaccine is often given secondary to the fact that most patients are unaware of the date of their most recent booster. The tetanus vaccination should be given immediately after the injury but can be given days or weeks after the injury (see Chapter 11). Following the tetanus vaccination, it may take up to two weeks for antibodies to form, so a tetanus reaction from this wound may still occur if the patient has not had a recent vaccination. If a patient with a traumatic wound has not been previously fully immunized, then a dose of tetanus immune globulin (TIG) should be given. A single injection of TIG provides protective levels of passive antibodies for at least four weeks. The TIG and tetanus toxoid may be given at the same time, but should be placed at separate sites.

## Traumatic amputation

Treatment of a traumatic amputation requires immediate pressure to control the bleeding, early intravenous antibiotics, and tetanus prophylaxis. Emergent surgery is often necessary to control the bleeding and perform surgical debridement.

## Vascular injury

Injury to the arterial vascular supply of a limb is a surgical emergency. This is most commonly seen with penetrating trauma, but can also occur with blunt trauma. Traumatic knee dislocations are the most common etiology of vascular injury in blunt trauma. A major arterial injury should be suspected when a patient presents with pallor, coolness, and decreased pulses in the extremity. The patient may also present with an expanding hematoma or massive bleeding; blood and fluid replacement by the anesthesia team is critical to the patient's survival.

## Fat embolism

It has been shown by intraoperative transesophageal echocardiography that most patients undergoing a long-bone repair experience some microembolization of fat and marrow. While most patients show no significant clinical impact, some can develop a significant acute inflammatory response. Clinically significant fat embolism syndrome occurs in 3 to 10% of patients having a long-bone repair, with a higher incidence if the patient has multiple long-bone fractures. The onset of symptoms can be gradual (over 12 to 72 hours) or very sudden, presenting with acute respiratory failure and cardiac arrest (Table 18.6). The treatment for fat embolism syndrome is supportive. Treatment requires early recognition, appropriate ventilatory management with supplemental oxygen and increased positive end-expiratory pressure (PEEP), and judicious fluid management.

**Table 18.6.** Clinical manifestations of fat embolism syndrome

| |
|---|
| Hypoxia |
| Tachycardia |
| Mental status change: drowsiness, confusion, obtundation, coma* |
| Petechial rash of the upper body: conjunctiva, oral mucosa, skin folds of the neck and axilla |
| Elevated pulmonary artery pressure |
| Decreased cardiac output |
| Lab results: fat microglobulinemia, anemia, thrombocytopenia, high erythrocyte sedimentation rate, fat globules in the urine |
| Chest radiograph: bilateral alveolar infiltrates |

* Fat embolism syndrome may be responsible for delayed emergence after anesthesia.

## Compartment syndrome

Acute compartment syndrome occurs when increased pressure within a limited space compromises the circulation and function of the tissues within that space. The most susceptible regions to develop compartment syndrome are the distal leg and volar forearm.

Medical conditions that can result in compartment syndrome include the following:

- Fractures
  - Tibial shaft.
  - Radius.
  - Ulna.
- Gunshot wounds.
- Contusions.
- Bleeding disorders.
- Burns.
- Post-ischemic swelling.
- Reperfusion injury.
- Drug overdose resulting in a prolonged immobile state.
- Prolonged limb compression.
- Iatrogenic (e.g., extravasation of a pressurized infusion).

The diagnosis of compartment syndrome is mainly clinical. The initial symptoms are pain out of proportion to the injury, pain on passive motion, and tense swelling of the affected area. Decreased distal sensation and loss of proprioception are seen next, followed by complete anesthesia and muscle weakness. The late-onset symptoms of pulselessness, pallor, paralysis, and paresthesias often do not present themselves until irreversible loss of function has occurred.

Diagnosis frequently includes compartment pressure measurements. The normal compartment pressures are 0–15 mmHg. Compartment pressures greater than 30 to 50 mmHg can produce significant muscle ischemia. The ischemic threshold for normal muscle is reached when the compartment pressure is elevated to 20 mmHg below the diastolic pressure or 30 mmHg below the mean arterial pressure.

Certain anesthetic techniques have been reported to contribute to delay in the diagnosis of compartment syndrome. These techniques include regional and neuraxial anesthesia (see Chapter 8). In situations where a patient has an altered state of consciousness or is receiving deep sedation, anesthesia, or large doses of pain medication, a high index of suspicion is required along with serial physical exams so that compartment syndrome is not missed.

Treatment for compartment syndrome includes a fasciotomy of all involved compartments. To be effective, fasciotomy must be performed as early as possible to prevent irreversible ischemic damage (Table 18.7).

## Crush injuries

Common mechanisms of crush injury (i.e., skeletal muscle compression) that result in rhabdomyolysis include the following:

**Table 18.7.** Skeletal muscle damage as a function of warm ischemia time

| Duration of ischemia (hours) | Result |
| --- | --- |
| < 2 | No permanent histologic damage |
| 2–4 | Irreversible anatomic and functional changes |
| 6 | Muscle necrosis |
| 24 | Maximal reperfusion injury |

Reproduced from Malinoski DJ, Slater MS, Mullins RJ. Crush injury and rhabdomyolysis. *Crit Care Clin*, 2004;**20**:171–192. With permission from Elsevier.

- Alcohol intoxication with a subsequent fall, immobility, and coma.
- Improper intraoperative positioning
  - Extended lithotomy.
  - Lateral decubitus.
- Blunt trauma.
- Electrical injuries.
- Sudden automobile deceleration.
- Earthquakes, landslides, building collapses.
- Vascular compromise: arterial thrombosis, embolus, traumatic interruption, or external compression.
- Soft tissue infections.
- Prolonged use of a tourniquet.

Clinical manifestations after crush injury include the following:
- Shock.
- Swollen extremities.
- Rhabdomyolysis.
- Dark urine secondary to myoglobin.
- Acute renal failure.
- Electrolyte abnormalities.

Crush syndrome is defined as rhabdomyolysis secondary to the associated hypovolemia and toxin exposure from crush injury. Cellular components of the affected muscle are released into the circulation after muscle compression is relieved or vascular interruption is corrected. In addition, large volumes of intravascular fluid can be sequestered in the involved extremity due to increased capillary permeability.

Rhabdomyolysis occurs when the components of damaged skeletal muscle enter the patient's circulation. The compression of the muscle leads to ischemia followed by reperfusion of that muscle. Serum creatinine kinase correlates with the degree of muscle injury. Acute renal failure from rhabdomyolysis occurs in 4 to 33% of cases, and is associated with a mortality rate of 3 to 50%.

Mechanisms by which rhabdomyolysis can lead to renal failure include:
- Decreased renal perfusion
  - Hypovolemia.
  - Stimulation of the sympathetic nervous system.

- Renin-angiotensin-aldosterone axis.
- Renal vasoconstriction secondary to vasoconstrictors released in the presence of myoglobin in the plasma.
- Myoglobin cast formation with tubular obstruction.
- Direct toxic effects of myoglobin on the renal tubules.

Rhabdomyolysis leads to electrolyte and laboratory abnormalities including:

- Hypocalcemia.
- Hyperkalemia.
- Acidemia.
- Hypophosphatemia.
- Increased tissue thromboplastin levels leading to disseminated intravascular coagulation.
- Decreased platelet levels.
- Increased myoglobin levels.

Treatment and prevention of renal failure after a crush injury include:

- Early and vigorous volume replacement to treat hypovolemic shock and hyperkalemia
  - Crystalloid (total body deficit may be up to 15 L).
- Confirm urine flow prior to forced mannitol-alkaline diuresis
  - Mannitol.
  - Alkalinization of the urine with sodium bicarbonate.
- Closely monitor urine output and electrolytes.
- Experimental therapy:
  - Free-radical scavengers: glutathione and vitamin E.
  - Desferrioxamine, an iron chelator.
  - Platelet activating factor receptor blockers.
  - Endothelin receptor antagonists.
- Daily hemodialysis or continuous hemodialysis/hemofiltration.

## Key points

- Early stabilization and definitive fixation of a fractured femur or pelvis results in improved morbidity and mortality rates in trauma patients.
- Advantages of general anesthesia for orthopedic trauma include speed of onset, ability to better regulate duration, allows for multiple procedures, and improved patient acceptance.
- Advantages of regional anesthesia for musculoskeletal trauma include ability to perform serial mental status examinations, no requirement for airway manipulation, less complex hemodynamic management, decreased risk for barotrauma, increased vascular flow to the extremity, decreased blood loss, decreased incidence of deep venous thrombosis, improved postoperative pain control, and earlier mobilization.
- Pelvis and femur fractures are associated with major blood loss mandating reliable venous access and vigilant monitoring.
- Fat embolism syndrome may result in delayed emergence, cardiovascular complications and ARDS. Treatment is supportive. It requires early recognition,

appropriate ventilatory management with increased oxygen and PEEP, and judicious fluid management.

- Compartment syndrome is a condition in which increased pressure within a limited space compromises the circulation and function of the tissues within that space. The most susceptible regions to developing compartment syndrome are the distal leg and volar forearm. Regional and neuraxial anesthesia can contribute to delayed diagnosis of compartment syndrome. Consultation with the surgical team prior to block performance is prudent.

- Clinical manifestations after crush injury include shock, swollen extremities, rhabdomyolysis, dark urine secondary to myoglobin, acute renal failure, and electrolyte abnormalities.

# Further reading

1. Malinoski DJ, Slater MS, Mullins RJ. Crush injury and rhabdomyolysis. *Crit Care Clin* 2004;**20**:171–192.

2. Marx J, Hockberger R, Walls R. *Rosen's Emergency Medicine*, 7th edition. Philadelphia, PA: Mosby Elsevier; 2009.

3. Miller RD, Eriksson LI, Fleisher LA, et al. *Miller's Anesthesia*, 7th edition. New York, NY: Churchill Livingstone; 2009.

4. Nahm NJ, Como JJ, Wilber JH, Vallier HA. Early appropriate care: definite stabilization of femoral fractures within 24 hours of injury is safe in most patients with multiple injuries. *J Trauma* 2011;**71**:175–185.

5. Olsen SA, Glascow RR. Acute compartment syndrome in lower extremity musculoskeletal trauma. *J Acad Orthop Surg* 2005;**13**:436–444.

6. Smith CE, ed. *Trauma Anesthesia*. New York, NY: Cambridge University Press; 2008.

7. Vallier HA, Cureton BA, Ekstein C, Oldenburg FP, Wilber JH. Early definitive stabilization of unstable pelvis and acetabulum fractures reduces morbidity. *J Trauma* 2010;**69**:677–684.

8. Vallier HA, Jenkins MD. Musculoskeletal trauma. In: Smith CE, ed. *Trauma Anesthesia*. New York, NY: Cambridge University Press; 2008.

Chapter

# 19

# Anesthetic management of the burn patient

Edgar J. Pierre and Albert J. Varon

## Introduction

The management of thermally injured patients is challenging. Effective treatment is mandatory at the scene of the accident, in the resuscitation bay, the operating room (OR), and the intensive care unit (ICU). Anesthesiologists trained in resuscitation, intraoperative management, and postoperative support are essential members of the burn patient management care team. As our surgical colleagues concentrate on surgical diagnosis and therapy, the anesthesiologist must also provide anesthesia and preserve vital organ functions.

Severe burn injuries, defined as burns exceeding 40% of total body surface area (TBSA), occur in approximately 35,000 patients annually. In 15 to 30% of fire victims, smoke inhalation and carbon monoxide intoxication complicate the burn injury. Risk factors associated with mortality include:

- Age greater than 60 years
- More than 40% of body surface area (BSA) burned
- Presence of inhalation injury

Mortality can be predicted as 0.3%, 3%, 33%, or approximately 90%, depending on whether zero, one, two, or three of these risk factors are present, respectively.

## Pathophysiology

A thorough knowledge of the pathophysiologic changes that accompany burn injuries facilitates anesthetic management during the three phases of burn injury:

1. Early resuscitation
2. Debridement and grafting
3. Reconstructive phases

The pathophysiology of thermal injury is related to the initial distribution of heat within the skin. Most burns involve only the epidermis (first-degree burns) or portions of the dermis (second-degree burns), but, with prolonged exposure, burns may involve the entire dermis (third-degree burns) or extend beneath into fat, muscle, and bone. Burn injuries induce a systemic hypermetabolic response, resulting in inflammation, immune system compromise, catabolism, and endocrine dysfunction. Early excision and grafting have been demonstrated to reduce inflammation and decrease the risks of infection, wound sepsis, and multi-organ failure.

*Essentials of Trauma Anesthesia*, ed. A. J. Varon and C. E. Smith. Published by Cambridge University Press.
© Cambridge University Press 2012.

# Hypovolemia

Hypovolemia is often evidenced in severely burned patients as hemoconcentration and hypotension. Hypovolemia may occur unexpectedly in the conscious, extensively burned patient who is hemodynamically stable in the emergency department, only to become hypotensive as fluid sequestration progresses. Peripheral edema in burn patients results from loss of plasma into the interstitium and usually takes several hours to develop. Patients with burns and inhalation injury require more fluids for resuscitation than patients who only have burns. Large amounts of resuscitation fluids are necessary to maintain intravascular volume and cardiac output. Pain, fear, decreased cardiac output, hypotension, and reflex responses to hypovolemia induce catecholamine release.

The rate of fluid administration is dependent on the rate of fluid loss, the latter being assessed by monitoring of organ perfusion. An initial rate for the first 24 hours can be estimated using the size of the burn (combined second and third degree) relative to BSA and body weight:

- Adult formula (Parkland): fluid first 24 hours = 4 mL/kg/% BSA burn (one half is administered in first 8 hours).
- Children's formula (Cincinnati-Shriner): fluid first 24 hours = 4 mL/kg/% BSA burn + 1500 mL/m$^2$ BSA (for children, especially those under 6 years of age, replacement includes normal daily requirements not considered in the adult formula).

Estimation of TBSA burned is based on the "rule of nines" as follows:

For adults:

- Head and neck = 9%
- Anterior torso = 18%
- Posterior torso = 18%
- Single arm = 9%
- Single leg = 18%
- Genitalia/perineum = 1%

For children:

- Head and neck = 18%
- Anterior torso = 18%
- Posterior torso = 18%
- Single arm = 9%
- Single leg = 14%
- Genitalia/perineum = 1%

The palmar surface of an adult or pediatric patient's hand represents approximately 1% TBSA and can be used for estimating patchy areas.

In general, fluids that contain salt, in at least plasma isotonic quantities, are appropriate for use in resuscitation if given in sufficient volume. Restoration of the sodium loss is essential. Fluids should be free of glucose (except in children < 20 kg), since glucose intolerance is characteristically present due to high circulating levels of stress hormones. The oral route can be used for small burns. The most appropriate fluid is lactated Ringer's solution because its composition is the closest to that of extracellular fluid. In addition, lactate is a source of base for conversion to bicarbonate by the liver. Hypoproteinemia and edema formation complicate the use of isotonic crystalloids for resuscitation. Hypertonic saline has a theoretical advantage of improved hemodynamic response and diminished overall fluid needs as intracellular water is shifted into extracellular space by the hyper-osmolar solution. However, a clear role for hypertonic saline has not yet been defined. Some clinicians add colloid (protein formulations or dextran) to the resuscitation fluid regimen after capillary leak has subsided.

One of the best indicators of fluid resuscitation in burn patients is urine output. A urine output of 0.5–1.0 mL/kg/hr in adults and 1.0–1.5 mL/kg/hr in children is considered an indicator of adequate organ perfusion. Smaller hourly urinary outputs in the first 48 hours post-burn almost always indicate inadequate resuscitation. Patients with electrical or crush injuries, presenting with myoglobin in the urine, have an increased risk of renal failure. Fluids should be increased and urine output maintained at 1–2 mL/kg/hour as long as the pigments are in the urine. The administration of bicarbonate may facilitate clearance of myoglobin by preventing its entry into the tubular cells.

With adequate fluid resuscitation, cardiac output increases dramatically. This is in contrast to a decrease in cardiac output in the first 18 hours post-burn injury during which time there is continued capillary leak.

## Inhalation injury

Inhalation injury refers to injury due to inhalation or exposure to hot gaseous products of combustion; it can cause serious respiratory complications. It is estimated that 50 to 80% of fire deaths are the result of inhalation injuries that include burns to the respiratory system. Hot smoke injures or kills by a combination of thermal damage and pulmonary irritation and swelling, caused by carbon monoxide, cyanide, and other combustion products. Changes in the airway microcirculation appear immediately after smoke inhalation. Fiber-optic bronchoscopy, performed by the anesthesiologist while the patient is undergoing surgery, may demonstrate evidence of soot particles, hyperemia, and edema – which are accepted criteria for diagnosing inhalation injury.

An important judgment decision must be made during the initial assessment as to whether the injured airway can be maintained safely without an endotracheal tube. When in doubt of whether progressive edema is likely, it is safest to intubate the trachea.

The following is a list of the major patient categories at risk for airway compromise:

- Heat and smoke injury, no facial burn. If there is no evidence of severe upper-airway edema, this group can be carefully observed. The lack of facial and mouth distortion makes it feasible to intubate the trachea later.
- Oral burns but no smoke injury. These patients have difficulty controlling secretions as edema evolves. Early intubation is a safe approach because anatomical distortion of the mouth makes intubation at a later time very difficult.
- Heat and smoke injury plus extensive face and neck burns. This group invariably requires tracheal intubation. If intubation is performed, the endotracheal tube must be well secured because, as the process of edema evolves, it may be extremely difficult to replace if dislodged. Anticipate a two to three week period of upper-airway symptomatology, since this is the time frame for mucosal re-epithelialization to occur.

Edema forms much faster than it resolves, thus, early preventive measures are important. In both the non-intubated and intubated patients, it is beneficial to maintain a semi-erect or 45-degree position if hemodynamically stable, to minimize the airway and facial edema process.

Associated inhalation injury can increase mortality rates 30–40%. Although, over the last three decades, mortality levels appear to be decreasing, burns associated with inhalation injury still pose significant challenges in trauma management. Three distinct injuries – carbon monoxide (CO) intoxication, upper airway injury, and pulmonary inhalation injury – may occur individually or concurrently. CO intoxication often occurs in patients involved in structural fires. Anoxia is the most likely cause of early mortality in these patients.

- CO has over 200 times the affinity of oxygen for hemoglobin binding sites.
- CO shifts the oxyhemoglobin dissociation curve to the left, inhibiting the release of oxygen to tissues.
- Carboxyhemoglobin saturations greater than 15% are toxic; those greater than 50% are typically lethal.
- Symptoms include throbbing headache, nausea, and vomiting when CO levels measure 20–30%.
- Altered consciousness, ranging from minor changes in mental status to coma, and convulsions and cardiac arrest are seen with CO levels >60%.

Because CO-intoxicated patients may have a normal $PaO_2$, and show no cyanosis, it is essential to measure arterial concentrations of oxy- and carboxyhemoglobin by co-oximetry.

Treatment includes displacement of CO from hemoglobin by delivering 100% oxygen. The elimination half-life of CO can be reduced from 4 hours to 40 minutes by breathing 100% oxygen rather than room air. Administering 100% oxygen at 2.5 atmospheres in a hyperbaric chamber decreases the half-life to 24 minutes.

## Electrical burns

An electrical burn is a unique form of trauma. The clinical picture following cellular damage due to electrical current represents more of a syndrome than a specific injury. The electrical insult results in progressive tissue necrosis in excess of the original trauma, and resembles the injury of crush trauma. Clinically, three types of skin damage may result from electrical injury:

1. Contact burn at points of current entry and exit from the body
2. Arc burns caused by current exiting and re-entering adjacent parts or body parts in close proximity
3. Thermal injury from ignition of clothing

In severe electrical injuries, death of large volumes of muscle may occur resulting in large fluid volume shifts, as well as rhabdomyolysis. Significant blood loss may occur as a consequence of vascular injury or from associated fractures. The possibility of associated hemorrhage or perforation of an intra-abdominal organ should always be considered. Both myoglobin and hemoglobin may be present in the urine; these pigments will precipitate and can cause renal failure. Creatinine and creatinine phosphokinase levels may be elevated. Damage of cardiac muscle will be reflected by a rise in cardiac enzyme levels, such as troponin.

A 12-lead electrocardiogram (ECG) should be obtained. If ECG findings are abnormal, continuous cardiac monitoring is necessary along with pharmacologic treatment for any dysrhythmia. Prolonged respiratory support may be required. Maintenance of adequate fluid to support the intravascular volume is difficult in patients with major electrical burns. Fluid requirement exceeds the predicted Parkland formula due to underlying deep muscle damage. Because of the possibility of renal failure from precipitation of myoglobin and hemoglobin, a brisk urine flow must be encouraged; urine output over 1 mL/kg is preferred. An osmotic diuretic, such as mannitol, may be useful to achieve this goal. As in crush injury, succinylcholine should be avoided due to the risk of hyperkalemia.

## Chemical injuries

A patient's airway can be affected by chemical injury in various ways. Ingestion will cause contact burns of the upper airway as well as inhalation injury. If the injury is to the face and lips only, with no intraoral exposure, airway compromise is unlikely. If there is any injury from the lips to the larynx, the trachea should be intubated before resuscitation begins as edema may progress rapidly and cause airway obstruction. Airway patency should be assessed regularly, and the trachea should be extubated only when it is safe to do so. A "cuff-leak" test, which involves demonstrating a leak around the tracheal tube with the cuff deflated, has been advocated to determine the safety of extubation in patients with upper airway edema. Although the presence of cuff leak indicates that extubation is likely to be successful, a failed cuff-leak test does not preclude uneventful extubation.

Lavage of the affected areas should be done with copious quantities of fluid. Large quantities are necessary since certain strong acids and caustics can contaminate large quantities of water. Some institutions have advocated the use of neutralizing solutions. The solutions used should be of the buffered variety, with a pH near 6. This has been shown to be useful if applied after 10 minutes of intensive water irrigation.

The absorption of an offending agent may result in direct myocardial depression, decreased systemic vascular resistance, and hypotension leading to inadequate tissue perfusion. Proper intravenous (IV) access and fluid resuscitation are necessary to maintain perfusion and adequate urine output. Inotropic support should be considered and instituted if necessary.

## Pharmacology

The pathophysiologic effects of burn injury alter drug pharmacokinetics. These changes depend on the severity of injury and the timing between injury and drug administration.

Protein binding is altered in both the resuscitation and recovery phases of burn injury. Albumin concentration is decreased, but alpha-1-acid glycoprotein (acute phase reactant) is increased. Binding of albumin-bound drugs (e.g., benzodiazepines) is decreased, resulting in increased free fraction and a larger volume of distribution for the drug. However, since most anesthetic drugs are not highly protein-bound, the effect of protein binding on the pharmacologic effects of anesthetics is minimal. On the other hand, fluid loss to the burn wound and surrounding tissue edema can decrease plasma concentrations of many drugs below those expected in the unburned patient.

After the initial resuscitation phase, a hypermetabolic state develops and the concomitant increase in cardiac output increases blood flow to the kidneys and liver, favoring drug clearance. However, because of a wide patient-to-patient variability in renal and hepatic function following burns, drug therapy should be individually tailored.

Finally, pharmacodynamic changes are common after burns and appear to account for many of the clinically relevant alterations in anesthetic drug pharmacology.

## Anxiolytic agents and analgesia

Burn patients appear to require higher doses of sedation and analgesia than non-burned patients. However, the pharmacokinetics of these drugs do not explain the increased requirements. Lorazepam is eliminated by conjugation, which is little affected by age, disease, or concurrent administration of drugs. In contrast, the cytochrome P450 system, which plays a part in the elimination of diazepam, is sensitive to these factors. The pharmacokinetics of morphine are not altered in burned patients. Although fear of addiction to narcotics has led to underdosing in burn patients, iatrogenic addiction in this setting is rare. Morphine, hydromorphone, or fentanyl administered via patient-controlled analgesia (PCA) are suitable options.

## Neuromuscular blocking drugs (NMBDs)

Burn injuries profoundly influence responses to both succinylcholine and non-depolarizing NMBDs. A hyperkalemic response after succinylcholine exposure is related to dose, severity of burn, and time elapsed since the injury. Cardiac arrest in burned patients after succinylcholine was first reported in 1958. It was not until 1967 that an exaggerated hyperkalemic effect was identified as the cause of this phenomenon. Hyperkalemia can occur after succinylcholine administration in these patients as early as 24–48 hours after injury and as late as two years post-burn. This may be due to a denervation-like phenomenon with increased extrajunctional acetylcholine receptors throughout the muscle membrane. Denervation and immobilization increase the number of extrajunctional acetylcholine receptors and enlarge the area sensitive to acetylcholine. As a result of receptor proliferation, the entire membrane becomes sensitive to cholinergic agonists and depolarization can cause release of potassium from a large portion of muscle cell surface rather than just the motor endplate. The resulting large-scale shift of intracellular potassium can generate life-threatening hyperkalemia. In the event of hyperkalemic cardiac arrest, calcium chloride, bicarbonate, glucose, and insulin are indicated, in addition to chest compressions and basic and advanced life support.

The response to non-depolarizing muscle relaxants can also be altered by burn injury. Burn patients have decreased sensitivity to non-depolarizing agents and may require two to three times the normal dose for similar effect. Resistance is apparent by 7 days after injury and peaks by approximately 70 days. The mechanism of the altered response appears to involve pharmacodynamic rather than pharmacokinetic changes; an increased number of acetylcholine receptors at the neuromuscular junction and along muscle fibers seems to be the pharmacodynamic mechanism. Increases in acute phase reactant proteins can also decrease free drug available for action.

## Other drugs

The anesthesia provider must also consider the possibility of impaired hepatic and renal clearance in burn patients with organ failure. Antibiotics such as aminoglycosides, clindamycin, and piperacillin/tazobactam can potentiate neuromuscular blockade in these patients.

# Airway management

The anesthesia provider caring for a burn patient must always consider potential airway management complications. Edema from resuscitation with large amounts of fluid can be significant enough to compromise the airway, causing partial or complete obstruction. Tracheal intubation is essential in patients with TBSA burn greater than 40% and patients with frank stridor or airway obstruction. Preferably, intubation should be facilitated using the largest tube the larynx can accommodate, as thick secretions may obstruct a smaller tube. Reintubation may be very difficult in these patients because of anatomical distortion by edema. In such instances, fiberoptic bronchoscopy is a useful approach. Patients at risk for airway edema must be monitored continuously and assessed at frequent intervals if a tracheal tube has not been placed.

# Transport to and from the OR

Transport of a critically ill burn patient from the emergency room or ICU to the OR may require movement through isolated areas of the hospital such as hallways and elevators. Careful planning and preparation can minimize the risks of transport. The patient's hemodynamic status should be optimized prior to transport. It is wise to secure the airway before transporting patients who are unconscious or sedated and present with posterior pharyngeal swelling or circumferential facial burns. Special consideration should be given to determining the degree of respiratory dysfunction and the amount of ventilatory support necessary for transport. At times, a portable ventilator is essential for this purpose. During transport, there should be no interruption in the monitoring or maintenance of a patient's vital functions. In addition, the accompanying personnel and equipment should be selected to provide for any ongoing or anticipated acute care patient needs. The American College of Critical Care Medicine has published detailed guidelines for the intrahospital transport of critically ill patients (see reference 11 in Further reading).

# Anesthetic management
## Pre-anesthestic evaluation

Initial management of the burn patient involves the ABCs of trauma care. Determining the percentage of the BSA and the depth of the burn are essential for planning fluid therapy. Volume resuscitation should start immediately and a urinary catheter should be inserted to monitor urine output. History of preexisting disease, allergies, and current management should be obtained as soon as possible. Cardiovascular status should be evaluated and evidence of respiratory distress and smoke inhalation assessed.

## Intraoperative management

American Society of Anesthesiologists (ASA) standard monitors may be difficult to place due to skin loss. A non-invasive blood pressure cuff may be applied over burned skin, however, insertion of an arterial line is usually necessary for patients with major burns. ECG lead placement may also be difficult, resulting in non-standard lead monitoring. Needle electrodes or stapling of electrodes to the skin may be necessary. Capnography represents the single best method to rule out esophageal intubation and provides fast and reliable insight into ventilation, circulation, and metabolism. This is especially important in burn patients, where energy expenditure and carbon dioxide production may greatly exceed normal.

Urine output is an indicator of not only kidney function, but also of overall organ perfusion, as renal blood flow decreases early in circulatory dysfunction. The urinary catheter not only allows monitoring of urinary output, it can also be used to measure bladder temperature. In addition, urine appearance may reveal additional trauma, which may manifest as hematuria or myoglobinuria.

Arterial catheters provide on-line measurement of blood pressure and access for frequent sampling of arterial blood. Blood gas analysis and determination of hematocrit and electrolytes help guide ventilatory and fluid management during excision of extensive burns.

In general, large-lumen IV catheters are necessary for volume replacement. Although recommended sites for central venous catheter insertion include the femoral, jugular, and subclavian veins, the incidence of infection is lowest when the subclavian approach is selected (see also Chapter 5). Central venous catheters should be removed as soon as no longer needed. If a burn patient develops septic shock or high output cardiac failure, insertion of a pulmonary artery catheter may permit estimation of the determinants of heart function (preload, afterload, contractility) and allow calculation of oxygen delivery and consumption. However, the use of oxygen delivery targets has not yet found a place in the management of burn shock. Transesophageal echocardiography (TEE) is a less invasive technique that allows evaluation of volume status and cardiac function, and may guide fluid and pharmacological support in the perioperative setting (see Chapter 10).

IV access: at least two peripheral catheters, or one central multi-lumen catheter, for fluid resuscitation and drug infusion. Transfusion requirements, including fresh frozen plasma and platelets, may be significant since for each 1% TBSA excised and grafted, about 2% blood volume is lost. Some estimates are as high as 3–6% blood volume lost.

Temperature: warm everything! Warm the operating room, fluids, gases, and irrigation fluids. Because most burn surgeries are not emergency procedures, if the patient's temperature decreases 1°C from baseline, consider discontinuing surgery to avoid the complications of hypothermia.

## Selection of anesthetic agents

Many different techniques for induction and maintenance of anesthesia have been described. Ketamine at a dose of 0.5–2.0 mg/kg IV has been used for induction. Ketamine offers many advantages, including preservation of hypoxic and hypercapnic ventilatory stimulation and reduction of airway resistance. Heart rate, blood pressure, and cardiac index increase in response to ketamine. Circulatory stimulation is attributed to ketamine's sympathetic activity. A side effect of ketamine is the occurrence of unpleasant hallucinations during the postoperative period. The incidence of emergence delirium can be reduced by the use of benzodiazepines (e.g., midazolam, 0.02–0.1 mg/kg IV). Anesthetic induction can also be achieved by combining an IV opioid such as fentanyl (2.0 to 6.0 µg/kg) with a sedative hypnotic and an NMBD relaxant. Sufentanil or remifentanil are alternative opioids. Propofol can be used for induction (1.5 to 2 mg/kg) and maintenance (75–200 mcg/kg/min) as long as the patient is hemodynamically stable. Hypotension and cardiovascular collapse may occur after rapid bolus dosing of propofol in burn patients with absolute or relative hypovolemia. Etomidate (0.2–0.3 mg/kg) is considered a better choice for induction in the hypovolemic critically ill patient due to its more favorable hemodynamic profile. Although a single IV induction dose of etomidate can result in temporary adreno-cortical suppression, the clinical significance of this phenomenon remains unclear.

Anesthesia maintenance can be achieved with low concentrations of potent inhaled anesthetics such as isoflurane or sevoflurane, with or without nitrous oxide, and additional fentanyl (intermittent boluses or infusion). Volatile anesthetics produce dose-dependent cardiac depression and vasodilation. These agents also tend to abolish hypoxic pulmonary vasoconstriction and therefore may affect ventilation/perfusion matching.

## Postoperative pain management

Although frequent assessments of pain severity are needed, evaluations recorded by professionals generally correlate poorly with the patient's own assessment. A distinction needs to be made between background, breakthrough, and procedural pain since each will require a different control strategy. Background pain is best addressed through the use of long-acting analgesic agents. Breakthrough and procedural pain are managed with short-acting agents via an appropriate route.

The mainstay regimen of early postoperative pain management in burn patients is usually opioid-based. Opioids can be administered orally or IV with a combination of background infusion and boluses. Intramuscular opioid administration is undesirable due to injection site discomfort and unpredictable absorption.

There is a proclivity for the use of patient-controlled analgesia (PCA), which has been found to be effective in burns. However, PCA is not a panacea, because it requires a cooperative patient able to use the device (not possible with burned hands) and the serum opioid concentration may decrease during sleep. Although a background infusion will reduce the likelihood of the latter, opioids have a propensity to accumulate, leading to undesirable side effects such as respiratory depression. A high level of vigilance must be maintained and protocols need to be in place to prevent or address these events. Similar requirements apply to the use of opioids by continuous infusion, which is an effective strategy in the early postoperative period. Use of non-steroidal anti-inflammatory drugs (NSAIDs) can reduce the inflammatory component of pain and opioid consumption, unless the risk of hematoma outweighs these benefits. Antidepressant therapy may be beneficial in burn patients with disturbed sleep patterns or chronic pain.

The concept of balanced analgesia promotes the additional use of regional blocks and NSAIDs, depending on the extent of injury and site of graft harvest. Large raw areas produced during surgery, in particular donor sites, are amenable to analgesia by a number of methods.

Regional blocks are used less often than might be expected because of practical difficulties such as infection close to the insertion site, generalized sepsis, and coagulation abnormalities. For the lower limbs and abdomen, the use of a continuous epidural infusion is feasible. Opioids may be added to the regimen to reduce the risk of local anesthetic toxicity and side effects. Postoperative pain from split skin donor sites is often more intense than pain at the grafted site. The fascia iliaca compartment block is a simple and efficient peripheral nerve block for diminishing pain at the thigh donor site.

Providing anesthesia care to burned patients is challenging, but it can be successfully managed when the anesthesiologist is experienced and vigilant in taking a severely ill patient through a devastating, deforming, painful, and stressful process. Training and experience in providing anesthesia care for patients with burns should be complemented by a provider's familiarity with advances in the field. The competent and informed anesthesiologist is a valuable member of the burn team, and is encouraged to participate fully in the care of these patients.

# Key points

- Burn injuries induce a systemic hypermetabolic response, resulting in inflammation, immune compromise, catabolism, and endocrine dysfunction.
- Thermal injury to the upper airway causes edema and potential airway obstruction. The combination of facial burns and a history of entrapment in a closed space should prompt active airway management.
- Edema from resuscitation with large amounts of fluid in a patient with extensive burns can also compromise the airway. When in doubt of whether progressive edema is likely, it is safest to intubate the trachea.
- One of the best monitors of fluid resuscitation in burn patients is urine output. A urine output of 0.5–1.0 mL/kg/hr in adults and 1.0–1.5 mL/kg/hr in children is considered an indicator of adequate organ perfusion.
- Dose requirements for all anesthetic agents are generally increased in burn patients with their hypermetabolic state and hyperdynamic circulation.
- Pharmacodynamic changes are common after burns and appear to account for many of the clinically relevant alterations in anesthetic drug pharmacology.
- Burn injury causes proliferation of extrajunctional acetylcholine receptors, leading to hypersensitivity to succinylcholine and resistance to non-depolarizing neuromuscular relaxants.
- Opioid doses titrated to response remain the mainstay of pain therapy in burned patients. Opioid side effects must be anticipated and managed.

# Further reading

1. Alvarado R, Chung KK, Cancio LC, et al. Burn resuscitation. *Burns* 2009;**35**:4–14.

2. Bak Z, Sjoberg F, Eriksson O. Hemodynamic changes during resuscitation after burns using the Parkland formula. *J Trauma* 2009;**66**:329–336.

3. Diver AJ. The evolution of burns fluid resuscitation. *Int J Surg* 2008;**6**:345–350.

4. Gallagher G, Rae CP, Kinsella J. Treatment of pain in severe burns. *Am J Clin Dermatol* 2000;**I**:329–335.

5. Latenser BA. Critical care of the burn patient: the first 48 hours. *Crit Care Med* 2009;**37**:2819–2826.

6. MacLennan N, Heimbach DM, Cullen BF. Anesthesia for major thermal injury. *Anesthesiology* 1998;**89**:749–770.

7. Mitra B, Fitzgerald M, Cameron P. Fluid resuscitation in major burns. *ANZ J Surg* 2006;**76**:35–38.

8. Norman AT, Judkins KC. Pain in the patient with burns. *Contin Educ Anaesth Crit Care Pain* 2004;**4**:57–61.

9. Orgill DP. Excision and skin grafting of thermal burns. *N Engl J Med* 2009;**360**:893–901.

10. Pham TN, Cancio LC, Gibran NS. American Burn Association practice guidelines burn shock resuscitation. *J Burn Care Res* 2008;**29**:257–266.

11. Warren J, Fromm RE, Orr RA, Rotello LC, Horst M, American College of Critical Care Medicine. Guidelines for the inter- and intrahospital transport of critically ill patients. *Crit Care Med* 2004;**32**:256–262.

**Chapter**

# 20

# Anesthetic management of the pediatric trauma patient

Ramesh Ramaiah and Sam Sharar

## Introduction

Despite improvements in education and injury prevention, trauma remains the number one cause of death among children over one year of age in the United States, accounting for approximately 15,000 deaths per year. The leading causes of traumatic injury in school-aged children are motor vehicle crashes and bicycle accidents. Among younger children, child abuse is the number one cause of injury in infants, and falls from height in toddlers. Injury patterns in pediatric patients are unique compared to adults due to their small size and anatomic immaturity. Head trauma is the most common isolated injury – 80% of hospitalized pediatric trauma victims have associated head injury, and traumatic head injury is the leading cause of death in pediatric trauma (70%). Thoracic injuries are the second leading cause of death. Due to the compliant chest wall (non-calcified rib cage) in young children, severe intrathoracic injury can occur without obvious external injuries or rib fractures. Depending on the healthcare system, anesthesiologists may be involved in the management of pediatric trauma at the injury scene, in the emergency room, in the operating room, or in the intensive care unit. Therefore, anesthesiologists should have a clear understanding of the pathophysiology of pediatric trauma, as well as associated age-dependent anatomical and physiological changes.

## Initial assessment and resuscitation

### Primary survey

The initial phase of patient assessment and resuscitation is focused on potential life-threatening injuries that compromise oxygenation and circulation. The principles of initial pediatric trauma care are to prevent hypoxia, recognize hypovolemia, restore circulating blood volume, and identify major neurologic injury. Rapid and prompt assessment of a child's airway, breathing, circulation, and neurologic disability (ABCDs) are crucial to successful management of pediatric trauma. Length-based weight-conversion devices such as the Broselow Pediatric Emergency Tape can assist in the acute management of injured children, as they provide rapid estimates of the child's weight, correct sizes for resuscitation equipment, and medication dosages (Figure 20.1).

**Airway and breathing**: As in all emergencies, airway control is the first priority in pediatric trauma care. The anatomy of the pediatric airway, however, differs from

*Essentials of Trauma Anesthesia*, ed. A. J. Varon and C. E. Smith. Published by Cambridge University Press.
© Cambridge University Press 2012.

## Harborview Medical Center – Basic Pediatric Equipment and Dosing Guide

| Broselow Color Zone | GRAY | | PINK | RED | PURPLE | YELLOW | WHITE | BLUE | ORANGE | GREEN | | |
|---|---|---|---|---|---|---|---|---|---|---|---|---|
| Approximate Weight (kg) | 3 | 5 | 6 | 8 | 10 | 13 | 16 | 20 | 26 | 32 | 40 | 45 |
| Approximate Age | Newborn | 2 mos | 4 mos | 8 mos | 1 yr | 2 yr | 4 yr | 5–6 yr | 7–8 yr | 9–10 yr | 12 yr | 13 yr |
| HR | 100–160 | 100–160 | 100–160 | 100–160 | 90–150 | 90–150 | 80–140 | 70–120 | 70–120 | 70–120 | 60–100 | 60–100 |
| RR | 30–60 | 30–60 | 30–60 | 30–60 | 24–40 | 24–40 | 22–34 | 18–30 | 18–30 | 18–30 | 12–24 | 12–20 |
| Minimum SBP | 40 | 50 | 60 | 60 | 70 | 70 | 80 | 80 | 80 | 90 | 90 | 90 |
| ETT [uncuffed /* cuffed >1 y/o] | 3.0 / 2.5 | 3.5 / 3.0 | 3.5 / 3.0 | 3.5 / 3.0 | 4.0 / 3.5 | 4.5 / 4.0 | 5.0 / 4.5 | 5.5 / 5.0 | 6.0 / 5.5 | 6.5 / 6.0 | 6.5 / 6.0 | 7.0 / 6.5 |
| NG / Foley | 5 Fr | 5 Fr | 5–8 Fr | 8 Fr | 8–10 Fr | 10 Fr | 10 Fr | 12 Fr | 14 Fr | 14 Fr | 14 Fr | 16 Fr |
| Chest Tube | 10–12 Fr | 10–12 Fr | 10–12 Fr | 10–12 Fr | 16–20 Fr | 20–24 Fr | 20–24 Fr | 24–32 Fr | 28–32 Fr | 32–36 Fr | 36–40 Fr | 36–40 Fr |
| Central Venous Line | 3.5–5 Fr UVC | 3 | 3–4 | 3–4 | 3–4 | 3–4 | 4 | 4 | 4–5 | 4–5 | 5+ | 5+ |
| Vent Settings–VT (mL) | 24–36 | 40–60 | 48–72 | 64–96 | 80–120 | 104–156 | 128–192 | 160–240 | 208–312 | 256–384 | 320–480 | 360–540 |
| Vent Settings–Rate (BPM) | 24–30 | 24–30 | 20–25 | 20–25 | 15–25 | 15–25 | 15–25 | 12–20 | 12–20 | 12–20 | 12–16 | 12–16 |
| C-Collar (Jerome Sizing) | P-0 | P-0 | P-0 | P-1 | P-1 | P-1 | P-2 | P-2 | P-2 | P-3 | use adult collar | |
| Fluid Bolus (mL) | 60 | 100 | 120 | 160 | 200 | 260 | 320 | 400 | 520 | 640 | 800 | 900 |
| Maintenance Fluids (mL/hr) | 12 | 20 | 28 | 35 | 40 | 45 | 55 | 65 | 70 | 75 | 100 | 115 |
| PRBC (mL) [unit = 350 mL] | 30–45** | 50–75** | 60–90 | 80–120 | 100–150 | 130–195 | 160–240 | 200–300 | 260–390 | 320–480 | 400–600 | 450–675 |
| FFP (mL) | 30–45 | 50–75 | 60–90 | 80–120 | 100–150 | 130–195 | 160–240 | 200–300 | 260–390 | 320–480 | 400–600 | 450–675 |
| Apheresis Platelets (mL) | 15–30 | 25–50 | 30–60 | 40–80 | 50–100 | 65–130 | 80–160 | 100–200 | 130–260 | 160–320 | 200–400 | 225–450 |
| Cryoprecipitate | 5–9 mL | 8–15 mL | 9–18 mL | 12–24 mL | 15–30 mL | 20–39 mL | 24–48 mL | 30–60 mL | 39–78 mL | 6 units | 6 units | 6 units |
| ** call blood bank (292–6525); consider Pedi-Pak | | PINK | RED | PURPLE | YELLOW | WHITE | BLUE | ORANGE | GREEN | | | |
| Acetaminophen PO/PR (mg) | 40 | 60 | 80 | 80–120 | 120 | 160 | 160–240 | 240 | 320 | 320–400 | 650 | 650 |
| Fentanyl IV (mcg) | 6–9 | 10–15 | 12–18 | 16–24 | 20–30 | 26–39 | 16–32 | 20–40 | 26–52 | 32–64 | 20–40 | 22–45 |
| Flumazenil IV (mg) | 0.03 | 0.05 | 0.06 | 0.08 | 0.1 | 0.13 | 0.16 | 0.2 | 0.2 | 0.2 | 0.2 | 0.2 |
| Glucose IV (mL of $D_{50}W$) | 6 ($D_{10}$) | 10 ($D_{10}$) | 3–6 | 4–8 | 5–10 | 6–13 | 8–16 | 10–20 | 13–26 | 16–32 | 20–40 | 22–45 |
| Loreazepam IV (mg) | 0.15–0.3 | 0.25–0.5 | 0.3–0.6 | 0.4–0.8 | 0.5–1 | 0.65–1.3 | 0.8–1.6 | 1–2 | 1.3–2.6 | 1.6–3.2 | 2–4 | 2–4 |
| Mannitol IV (gm) | 3 | 5 | 6 | 8 | 10 | 13 | 16 | 20 | 26 | 32 | 40 | 45 |
| Metoclopramide IV (mg) | 0.3 | 0.5 | 0.6 | 0.8 | 1 | 1.3 | 1.6 | 2 | 2.6 | 3.2 | 4 | 4.5 |
| Midazolam IV (mg) | 0.15–0.3 | 0.25–0.5 | 0.3–0.6 | 0.4–0.8 | 0.5–1 | 0.65–1.3 | 0.8–1.6 | 0.5–1 | 0.65–1.3 | 0.8–1.6 | 0.5–2 | 0.5–2 |
| Morphine IV (mg) | 0.15 | 0.25 | 0.3 | 0.4–0.8 | 0.5–1 | 0.65–1.3 | 0.8–1.6 | 1–2 | 1.3–2.6 | 1.6–3.2 | 2–4 | 2.2–4.5 |
| Naloxone IV (mg) | 0.03 | 0.05 | 0.06 | 0.08 | 0.1 | 0.13 | 0.16 | 0.2 | 0.26 | 0.32 | 0.4 | 0.45 |
| Oxycodone PO (mg) | 0.15–0.45 | 0.25–0.75 | 0.3–0.9 | 0.4–1.2 | 0.5–1.5 | 0.65–1.9 | 0.8–2.4 | 1–3 | 1.3–3.9 | 1.6–4.8 | 2–6 | 3–8 |
| Pancuronium/Vecuronium (mg) | 0.3 | 0.5 | 0.6 | 0.8 | 1 | 1.3 | 1.6 | 2 | 2.6 | 3.2 | 4 | 4.5 |
| Phenobarbital–IV Load (mg) | 60 | 100 | 120 | 160 | 200 | 260 | 320 | 400 | 520 | 640 | 800 | 900 |
| Phenytoin–IV Load (mg) | 45 | 75 | 90 | 120 | 150 | 195 | 240 | 300 | 390 | 480 | 600 | 675 |

**Figure 20.1.** The Broselow patient length-based system as modified for use at the Pediatric Level 1 Trauma Center at Harborview Medical Center (Seattle, WA), including estimated age-appropriate vital signs, recommended sizes of airway, ventilation, and other key medical equipment, and recommended doses of resuscitation fluid, blood products, and sedation/analgesia medications. Abbreviations. HR: heart rate, RR: respiratory rate, SBP: systolic blood pressure, ETT: endotracheal tube, NG: nasogastric tube, VT: tidal volume, PRBC: packed red blood cells, FFP: fresh frozen plasma.

that of the adult airway in several ways that can make airway management in this population challenging:

- Small oral cavity and relatively large tongue, adenoids, and tonsils predispose to airway obstruction, particularly in semiconscious or comatose children.
- Large occiput naturally flexes the neck in the supine position and leads to airway obstruction, as well as increasing the risk of injuring the unstable cervical spinal cord.
- Large mass of adenoid tissue can make nasotracheal intubation difficult or bloody.
- More cephalad (C2–C5) and anterior larynx can make visualization of the glottis difficult.
- U-shaped and floppy epiglottis may necessitate use of straight blade for direct laryngoscopy.
- Maximal anatomical airway narrowing is at the cricoid cartilage, as opposed to the glottis in adults, and this may limit endotracheal tube size.
- Narrow tracheal diameter and small distance between tracheal rings makes needle cricothyroidotomy difficult.
- Short trachea (e.g., 5 cm in infants) increases risk for right mainstem intubation.

In pediatric trauma patients, prevention of hypoxia is a high priority because of their propensity for rapid oxygen desaturation (due to low functional residual capacity and high oxygen consumption compared to adults), and their brisk bradycardic response to hypoxia. Children presenting with respiratory compromise should receive 100% oxygen and have pulse oximetry monitored continuously. If the child is unstable, airway management should consist of initial bag-valve-mask ventilation, followed by endotracheal intubation. Indications for endotracheal intubation in pediatric trauma patients include:

- Difficult bag-valve-mask ventilation or the anticipated need for prolonged assisted ventilation.
- Glasgow Coma Scale (GCS) (Table 20.1) score of less than 8, to protect the airway, prevent aspiration, and provide hyperventilation, if necessary.
- Respiratory failure secondary to chest trauma or other causes.
- Decompensated shock resistant to initial fluid resuscitation.
- Loss of upper airway protective reflexes.

Bag-valve-mask ventilation can be as effective as, and may be an alternative to, endotracheal intubation in the prehospital setting, depending on the training and experience of the prehospital providers. In the hospital emergency department setting, however, endotracheal intubation is the gold standard for airway management in severely injured children. In general, orotracheal intubation is preferred in children due to inherent risks associated with nasotracheal intubation, including adenoid bleeding and unintended intracranial tube placement in the settings of basilar skull or midface fractures. Careful attention must also be given to maintaining neutral position of the cervical spine during laryngoscopy and intubation, to prevent worsening of a spinal cord injury.

Although debated in the past, cuffed endotracheal tubes are now considered acceptable for children cared for in the operating room and intensive care unit locations. In addition, the 2010 International Consensus on Cardiopulmonary Resuscitation states that both cuffed and uncuffed endotracheal tubes are acceptable for infants and children undergoing emergency intubation. Cuffed tubes are potentially advantageous in circumstances of poor

**Table 20.1.** Modified Glasgow Coma Scale in children

| Sign | Evaluation | Score |
|---|---|---|
| Eye opening response (E) | Spontaneous | 4 |
| | Opens to voice | 3 |
| | Opens to pain | 2 |
| | None | 1 |
| Verbal response (V) | Appropriate words or social smile | 5 |
| | Cries but consolable | 4 |
| | Persistently irritable | 3 |
| | Restless, agitated (moans only) | 2 |
| | None | 1 |
| Best motor response (M) | Obeys commands | 6 |
| | Localizes pain | 5 |
| | Withdraws from pain | 4 |
| | Abnormal flexion | 3 |
| | Abnormal extension | 2 |
| | Flaccidity | 1 |

lung compliance such as high airway resistance or a large glottic air leak, provided appropriate precautions are taken regarding tube size, position, and cuff pressure. The presence of a cuff (to obliterate air leaks associated with positive pressure ventilation) may also obviate the need for reintubation with a larger uncuffed tube, thereby reducing the risks associated with laryngoscopy in children with head, neck, or face injuries. In addition to the endotracheal tube size recommendations based on patient height provided in Figure 20.1, the following formulas could be used for estimating appropriate tube size based on patient age:

- Uncuffed endotracheal tube size (mm ID) = (age in years + 16)/4
- Cuffed endotracheal tube size (mm ID) = (age in years + 12)/4

The short tracheal length in children creates a high risk for endobronchial intubation (right mainstem). The estimation of proper oral endotracheal tube depth in non-infant children is obtained by multiplying the internal diameter size of the tube by the factor "3," or by adding "10" to the child's age. In infants, the depth of tube insertion is based on their body weight, using the rule "1, 2, 3, and 4 kg equals 7, 8, 9, and 10 cm," respectively. Proper placement is confirmed by the presence of end-tidal carbon dioxide ($ETCO_2$), bilateral breath sounds, and chest X-ray.

**Circulation:** Recognizing hypovolemic shock in the setting of major pediatric trauma is essential for successful resuscitation. In children, the normal range of vital signs varies by age (Figure 20.1). Tachycardia is usually the earliest finding in hypovolemia, followed by altered mental status, respiratory compromise, delayed capillary refill, skin pallor, and hypothermia. Children have excellent cardiac reserve, such that blood pressure is typically well preserved in mild to moderate hypovolemia (i.e., < 30% blood loss). Thus, initial normal blood pressures may impart a false sense of security regarding circulating volume status. Hypotension and decreased urine output are more ominous signs of hypovolemic shock; however, they may not occur in children until more than 30% blood volume has been lost.

(A)

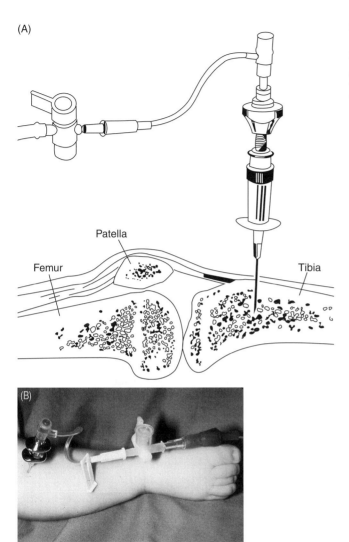

Patella

Femur

Tibia

**Figure 20.2.** Intraosseous needle placement diagram (A) and example in a small child (B). The intraosseous needle is most commonly placed in the proximal tibia 1–2 cm below the tibial tuberosity, but can also be placed in the distal femur or distal tibia.

Establishing vascular access can be challenging in all children, but particularly so in those with significant traumatic injuries that require more than one access site. Delays in securing intravenous (IV) access can be potentially detrimental to children because of their inherent small blood volume and risk for rapidly developing hypovolemic shock. If peripheral access cannot be obtained within three attempts or less than 90 seconds in young children, intraosseous access (Figure 20.2) should be considered. Other options for IV access include saphenous vein cutdown and central veins (internal jugular, subclavian, femoral). In patients with cervical immobilization it is difficult to place central lines above the diaphragm, thus femoral vein cannulation is an alternative option.

In the immediate post-injury phase, aggressive fluid resuscitation is vital in children, as hypoperfusion and hypoxia can induce anaerobic cellular metabolism resulting in the formation of inflammatory mediators that can have various deleterious systemic effects.

There are no evidence-based data to unequivocally support either crystalloid or colloid as the preferred resuscitative fluid in trauma. Initial fluid resuscitation in children should consist of warmed isotonic crystalloid solution (e.g., lactated Ringer's) as a bolus of 20 mL/kg. If there is no physiologic response or there is evidence of persistent volume loss, a second bolus of 20mL/kg should be administered. The goal of the initial crystalloid resuscitation is to rapidly achieve age-appropriate normal hemodynamic values and to restore adequate tissue perfusion. Children with evidence of hemorrhagic shock who fail to respond to initial crystalloid resuscitation efforts should also receive blood (10mL/kg) and undergo immediate surgical evaluation for possible operative interventions. The resuscitation practice of "permissive hypotension" (i.e., providing only enough volume to reach minimal accepted hemodynamic values) is advocated in selected adult trauma patients (e.g., penetrating trauma victims with no traumatic brain injury); however, its application to pediatric trauma is undefined and not typically practiced. Dextrose-containing fluids are avoided to minimize the risks of hyperglycemia, particularly in children with traumatic brain injury. However, dextrose-containing fluid may be administered to infants and younger children because this age group is more prone to hypoglycemia.

Children are more susceptible than adults to accidental hypothermia due to their higher surface area-to-volume ratio, resulting in vasoconstriction, hypoperfusion, acidosis, and coagulopathy. Preventive measures taken to avoid hypothermia include use of warmed IV fluids, warm blankets, convective air warmers, and warmed humidified ventilation. Increasing the temperature of the operating room to $> 24°C$ is a simple yet effective maneuver. If the child is refractory to these measures, peritoneal lavage with warm saline may be useful.

**Neurologic function**: Once airway, breathing, and circulation have been addressed, rapid assessment of neurologic function ("disability") should be performed. A quick, initial neurological evaluation can be made using the AVPU mnemonic (*Alert*, responsive to *Voice*, responsive to *Pain*, or *Unresponsive*). In most cases, a more formal assessment of neurologic function in children can be performed using the GCS modified by pediatric age-specific verbal responses (Table 20.1).

## Secondary survey

The secondary survey occurs after the primary survey is complete and the child is judged to be in a stable condition. The secondary survey includes a complete history and detailed head to toe examination to rapidly identify and begin to treat all non-life-threatening injuries. The mnemonic AMPLE can be helpful in quickly obtaining a relatively comprehensive history of the injury mechanism, as well as preexisting medical conditions:

A – Allergies (medications, including anesthetics)
M – Medications currently used (including steroid use)
P – Past illnesses and medical history (including recent viral illnesses)
L – Last meal or oral intake (assume full stomach unless otherwise confirmed)
E – Events/environment related to the injury scene

Because of age-related communication limitations with children, such history must often be obtained from family members, others present at the injury scene, or prehospital personnel with knowledge of the injury scene and medical care provided during transport to the hospital. Priorities for treatment and further diagnostic investigations (e.g., imaging and laboratory studies) can then be determined, including appropriate subspecialist consultation and decision for operating room intervention. If the child becomes unstable at any point during the secondary survey, a return to the primary survey and resuscitation is obligatory.

Patient examination during the secondary survey involves exposing the child by fully undressing to assess for any hidden injuries, but with special care taken to avoid hypothermia. Key portions of the physical examination in injured children include:

- Palpation of the skull and face for pain/deformities.
- Careful assessment of cervical spine for tenderness while maintaining cervical spine immobilization until it is "cleared" by a combination of physical exam and radiographic assessment; note that due to their more cartilaginous spine structure, young children have a higher incidence than adults of "spinal cord injury without radiographic abnormality" (SCIWORA), and may require computed tomography (CT) or magnetic resonance imaging (MRI) rather than plain film imaging studies in cases of high concern.
- Assessment for flail chest segments, chest wall tenderness, and crepitance, as well as auscultation for poorly transmitted or asymmetric breath sounds, and for heart murmurs.
- Abdominal examination for external signs of internal injury (e.g., "seatbelt sign"), distension, tenderness, open wounds, and presence of bowel sounds; note that crying children often "swallow" significant amounts of air that can lead to abdominal distension, which can limit the utility of the abdominal palpation exam and increase the risk of vomiting and aspiration.
- Rectal examination for sphincter tone (e.g., absence of tone in complete spinal cord injury), prostate position, and presence of blood in the stool.
- Perineal examination for hematoma or blood in the urethral meatus (e.g., urethral injury).
- Careful examination of all extremities for deformity, open wounds, distal pulses, and motor/sensory function.

After the history and physical examination, blood samples are typically collected for hemoglobin and electrolyte assessments, but may also include coagulation studies, type and cross-match, and arterial blood gas analysis in cases with severe injuries. In older children, the possible use of drugs or alcohol should be assessed by blood or urine toxicology, particularly if urgent surgical intervention and general anesthesia are planned. Hemoglobin levels sampled early in hypovolemic shock patients are not always a sensitive indicator of blood loss because hemodilution from crystalloid resuscitation may not yet have occurred.

The recommended radiological examination during initial assessment and stabilization of major blunt trauma in pediatric patients includes plain films of the chest, pelvis, and cervical spine. In stable patients with intra-abdominal injuries, the diagnostic test of choice is rapid abdominal CT scanning. Diagnostic peritoneal lavage (DPL) and focused assessment with sonography for trauma (FAST) can also be used for evaluation of intra-abdominal injuries, but require operators with special expertise and training in order to perform and interpret these exams properly in children. Other radiological examinations (e.g., extremity plain films) are performed based on the physical examination findings. Children with suspected child abuse injuries and who are less than two years of age generally require a more complete skeletal survey including radiographs of the skull, chest, abdomen, and long bones.

# Anesthetic management

Following the initial resuscitation, children may require urgent surgical intervention to control ongoing bleeding or treat traumatic brain injury. In addition, some acutely injured children who are otherwise stable may require procedural sedation in the emergency department for brief diagnostic or therapeutic procedures, or for radiological evaluation. Still other children may require more elective (non-emergent) surgical intervention for treatment of their traumatic injuries.

**Preoperative evaluation and preparation**: Because of the critical nature of certain traumatic injuries, preoperative evaluation may be limited in some children who require emergent surgery. In these cases the AMPLE mnemonic (see above) can provide a brief outline of the key preoperative data necessary to plan a safe, yet emergent anesthetic. For example, a deceleration mechanism of injury in a motor vehicle crash raises the likelihood of cervical spinal cord injury. Toddlers and school-aged children have relatively large heads perched atop a relatively cartilaginous cervical spinal column, such that with deceleration injuries they have an increased incidence of flexion-extension injury to the cervical spine at C2 and C3 levels. Spinal ligamentous injuries without obvious bony abnormalities occur more frequently in this age group compared to adults, and may result in a risk of SCIWORA. SCIWORA occurs in roughly half of the pediatric patients with spinal cord injury, and therefore requires careful attention to maintaining neutral cervical spine positioning during perioperative airway management (e.g., laryngoscopy), even if lateral plain films of the neck appear normal.

Except in the most urgent of surgical cases, a thorough anesthesia-oriented physical examination should be performed that focuses on the airway, breathing, and circulation, and also defines the extent of associated injuries and their impact on the conduct of anesthesia. For children who arrive in the operating room already intubated, proper endotracheal tube positioning must be confirmed and endobronchial intubation excluded. Premedication is avoided in the non-intubated patient who is hemodynamically unstable or if increased intracranial pressure is suspected. However, in stable children, a small dose of either anxiolytic (e.g., midazolam) or hypnotic drug that maintains consciousness (and protective airway reflexes) can be given to facilitate separation from parents and monitor placement prior to induction.

The operating room should be adequately staffed and equipped for children of all ages and sizes, including age-appropriate airway equipment and properly diluted medications with labels. To facilitate proper management of hypovolemic shock, IV and intraosseous access supplies, fluid and blood warmers, a rapid transfusion system, and pediatric-appropriate infusion pumps should also be available, as well as a defibrillator with appropriately sized paddles for both internal and external defibrillation. The ambient operating room temperature should be warmed, preferably to 26°C for infants and young children. Full monitoring capabilities should be available and include:

- Electrocardiography (ECG) – Bradycardia is more frequently seen in children compared to adults, and is usually indicative of hypoxia, ischemia, acidosis, cardiac contusion, or hypothermia.
- Blood pressure – Non-invasive blood pressure and an age-appropriate cuff should be selected. An arterial line is indicated in hemodynamically unstable children, those with anticipated large blood loss, and those with traumatic brain injury. The vessels used for arterial line placement will depend on the site of injury, and include the radial, femoral, dorsalis pedis, and axillary arteries.

- Pulse oximetry – In children in hypovolemic shock or hypothermia, pulse oximetry could be difficult to obtain and may require use of multiple probes in different sites.
- $ETCO_2$ – In smaller patients and those with hypovolemic shock, $ETCO_2$ may be less accurate, because of a relatively higher ratio of dead space to tidal volume than in adults.
- Central venous access – Central line placement can be challenging above the diaphragm in small children, particularly those with cervical immobilization, thus femoral line access is preferred. Central access may be useful for both volume administration and assessment of volume status, and may be requisite in patients without peripheral access (e.g., children with extensive cutaneous burn injuries).
- Temperature – Temperature monitoring is important in children to assess for both hypothermia and hyperthermia. The common sites for temperature monitoring include nasopharynx, esophagus, rectum, and bladder.
- Urine – Urine monitoring will provide a useful guide for volume resuscitation with the goal of maintaining urine output of at least 0.5–1 mL/kg/hr.
- Intracranial pressure (ICP) – ICP monitoring is indicated in head-injured children with GCS < 8 for proper hemodynamic and ventilation management in both the operating room and the intensive care unit.

## Induction and intubation

**Intubation technique**: As with adults, pediatric trauma patients should always be treated as having a "full stomach"; thus, rapid sequence induction (RSI) and intubation is indicated if the preoperative airway examination suggests no obvious impediment to direct laryngoscopy and oral endotracheal intubation. Accordingly, all equipment for RSI should be prepared – including multiple backup plans for airway management in the case of unanticipated difficulty – before administering induction agents and neuromuscular blocking drugs (NMBDs). Because of the possibility of SCIWORA and the fact that the cervical spine is often not fully cleared (i.e., both clinically and radiographically) prior to emergent surgery, careful attention to positioning and maintaining in-line cervical stabilization during airway management is crucial to avoid creating or worsening cervical cord injury. As mentioned above, airway management in pediatric patients is challenging because of the anatomical differences of the pediatric airway as compared to the adult airway. After preoxygenating the child as best as tolerated using 100% oxygen, RSI by classic or modified technique (i.e., gentle positive pressure as needed) is performed while cricoid pressure is provided. An appropriately sized endotracheal tube is placed and its position confirmed by observing $ETCO_2$ with repeated breaths, and by auscultation of bilateral breath sounds. Cricoid pressure should not be used in the presence of suspected tracheal or laryngeal injury.

**Induction agents**: Various induction agents may safely be used in injured children, with the final choice determined by clinical condition and provider familiarity. Etomidate 0.1–0.2 mg/kg IV is an ideal induction agent in trauma patients because of its rapid onset, hemodynamic stability, and its effect to decrease the cerebral metabolic rate of oxygen consumption (hence, decreased cerebral blood flow and ICP). For these reasons, etomidate is the preferred induction agent in trauma patients with traumatic brain injury and hypovolemia. There is unresolved controversy over the potential long-term effects of etomidate's known transient suppression of adrenocortical function; however, many providers believe its obvious short-term benefits outweigh its potential long-term risks. Ketamine 1–2 mg/kg is an alternative induction agent free from hemodynamic depression;

however, it is traditionally avoided in the presence of traumatic brain injury due to its potential to raise ICP. Other common induction agents (i.e., propofol) can also be used, but usually in smaller than standard induction doses due to risk of hypotension in patients with hypovolemia and shock.

**Neuromuscular blocking drugs**: NMBDs that facilitate direct laryngoscopy and endotracheal intubation are key to successful RSI. Succinylcholine at a dose of 1.5–2 mg/kg provides optimal intubating conditions in children within 60 seconds and a duration of 5–8 minutes. It is still considered the muscle relaxant of choice for injured children by many anesthesia providers unless specific contraindications to its use are present, including suspected muscular dystrophy, crush injury, hyperkalemia, burns, or acute upper motor injuries more than 24 hours old, and a family history of malignant hyperthermia. However, some providers argue against its use in young children due to a concern for undiagnosed myopathy and consequent development of hyperkalemia and adverse cardiac events. Succinylcholine can cause bradycardia in infants and young children due to their predominant parasympathetic tone, such that pretreatment with atropine is considered in this age group. Lastly, although succinylcholine can transiently elevate ICP, this effect has not been shown to adversely affect the outcome in patients with associated traumatic brain injury. Rocuronium is another NMBD frequently used for RSI and, as a non-depolarizing relaxant, is free of the potentially harmful side effects of succinylcholine. In doses of 1.0–1.5 mg/kg, rocuronium provides optimal intubating conditions in 60–90 seconds; however, its duration of action of more than 30 minutes must be considered in patients with a potential difficult airway in terms of both laryngoscopy and mask ventilation.

## Maintenance of anesthesia

No single anesthesia technique has been demonstrated to be superior in children undergoing either emergent or elective surgery for traumatic injury. A balanced general anesthesia technique using opioid and oxygen (with or without air, depending on hemodynamic stability and concurrent lung or thoracic injuries), NMBD, and judicious use of inhalational anesthetics such as sevoflurane and isoflurane is typical, and provides both intraoperative hemodynamic control and postoperative analgesia. Commonly used opioids in this setting include fentanyl (titrated boluses or bolus plus infusion), hydromorphone (titrated boluses), and remifentanil (continuous infusion plus long-acting opioid for postoperative analgesia). Nitrous oxide is avoided in injured children because of the risk for diffusion into unanticipated closed air spaces (e.g., pneumothorax, pneumocephalus). There is a tendency to maintain light levels of anesthesia in trauma patients with potential hemodynamic instability, which at times can lead to deterioration in clinical condition as a result of increased sympathetic activity. At the extreme, severely injured, hemodynamically unstable children may not tolerate IV or volatile anesthetics of any kind, in which case oxygen and NMBD alone may be necessary, preferably accompanied by a hemodynamically stable amnestic agent such as scopolamine. In such cases, assessment of the depth of anesthesia by end-tidal volatile agent monitoring or cerebral function monitoring may be helpful, but has not been demonstrated to be superior to any other technique. Intraoperative laboratory assessment of arterial blood gases, hemoglobin, electrolytes, coagulation parameters, and glucose should be obtained as indicated, and used as the basis for many intraoperative management decisions. As with adults, regional anesthesia in traumatized children is gaining popularity with the increased use of ultrasound guided block techniques, and should be used by those with appropriate expertise in children whenever possible to manage pain both during and after the surgical procedure.

# Intraoperative fluid management

Fluid management during emergent, post-injury surgery in children involves not only the usual challenge of estimating intraoperative blood loss, insensitive fluid losses, and pediatric-specific fluid replacement, but may also include the extension of prehospital and emergency department resuscitation efforts into the operating room, as surgeons work to control ongoing traumatic blood loss. In some cases, given the frequency of head injury in the pediatric population, one must balance the need for volume resuscitation with the avoidance of cerebral edema when concurrent traumatic brain injury is present. The general goals of intraoperative fluid management in these cases are to achieve age-appropriate hemodynamic vital signs, maintain adequate cerebral perfusion pressure (at least 50–60 mm Hg), ensure urine output (at least 0.5 mL/kg/hr), and maintain adequate circulating hemoglobin and coagulation factors.

When estimating the fluid requirements in the intraoperative period, the factors taken into consideration are preoperative fluid deficit (e.g., fasting time, preoperative injury-related blood loss), insensitive and third space fluid losses, and intraoperative blood loss. If there is a need to increase intravascular volume, isotonic crystalloids are used initially, but additional volume expansion can be achieved with colloids or blood products. Both colloids and blood products remain in the intravascular space for a longer period than crystalloids, and as a result may decrease the total volume infused and theoretically lessen tissue and cerebral edema. Hypertonic saline solution may be used in the initial resuscitation of selected adult patients with traumatic brain injury to reduce intracranial pressure and improve cerebral perfusion pressure; however, limited data are available to support this practice in children. Blood (packed red blood cells [RBCs] or whole blood) should be administered to hemodynamically unstable children or those with hemoglobin $< 7$ gm/dL, in volumes of 10 mL/kg, to ensure adequate tissue oxygen delivery. If time permits, type-specific blood is preferred over uncross-matched type O Rh-negative blood. In the acute setting with ongoing bleeding, however, there may not be any time available for type-specific blood. If the situation demands administration of at least one blood volume of O Rh-negative blood, subsequent use of type-specific blood may cause agglutination or hemolysis due to circulating antibodies from uncross-matched blood. Another sample should be sent to the blood bank to determine the optimal blood type component for further transfusions (patient's own blood type versus O negative). After such massive blood transfusion, platelet levels and coagulation factors should be assessed and replaced as indicated. Recent studies in severely injured adults have shown significant benefit of administering a high ratio of fresh frozen plasma (FFP) to RBCs, compared to the traditional approach where RBCs are given first and FFP later after coagulation factor testing; however, this practice has not been extensively studied in pediatric trauma. Hypocalcemia that develops following blood transfusion should be treated with calcium chloride 10 mg/kg or calcium gluconate 30 mg/kg and guided by serial laboratory testing.

Although hypovolemic shock is typically successfully treated with volume repletion alone, if hypotension persists even after adequate intravascular volume is ensured, the use of vasoactive agents may be indicated. Phenylephrine may be effective to increase blood pressure transiently; however its pure alpha-mediated vasoconstrictive properties may be undesirable in patients already experiencing inadequate tissue perfusion and oxygenation. Agents such as dopamine and dobutamine may be more effective in maintaining organ perfusion in this setting. However, epinephrine infusion may be indicated in critically ill patients because of its enhanced myocardial contractility and increased blood pressure (both alpha and beta adrenergic receptor effect).

## Postoperative care

Multiply injured or critically injured children who require emergent surgical treatment will most likely be transferred to the intensive care unit for continued care, including volume resuscitation, hemodynamic and ventilatory support, and adequate sedation/analgesia. Before transport, one should reassess the patient and ensure adequate oxygenation, ventilation, hemodynamics, and temperature. Cervical spine precautions (e.g., cervical collar immobilization and log-rolling) should be continued during transport and all postoperative phases in children whose spines are not yet cleared. Vital signs are monitored continuously during the transport, and age-appropriate drugs and equipment for resuscitation and airway management must be immediately available. On arrival in the unit, the provision of a comprehensive patient report, including injury mechanism, prehospital care, emergency department care, and intraoperative events should be provided to the critical care team, since the anesthesia provider is the key link to care continuity throughout these various phases of coordinated trauma care. This is particularly important in non-pediatric hospitals, where the majority of traumatized children are cared for, and where the critical care team may be less familiar with pediatric care issues compared to a children's hospital.

## Key points

- Trauma remains the leading cause of morbidity and mortality in children over one year of age. Early resuscitation efforts to prevent hypoxia and restore circulating blood volume are critical for the successful management of pediatric trauma.
- The majority of hospitalized pediatric trauma patients have associated traumatic brain injury, it being the leading cause of death in this age group.
- Anesthesiologists face several challenges in the management of pediatric trauma, including airway management, IV access, fluid management, and temperature regulation, all in the midst of challenging and often rapidly changing circumstances.
- The knowledge of age-dependent anatomical and physiological differences between children and adults is critical for successful acute and perioperative anesthetic care of pediatric trauma patients.

## Further reading

1. Lam WH, MacKersie A. Paediatric head injury: incidence, aetiology and management. *Paediatr Anaesth* 1999; 9:377–385.

2. Kleinman MD, de Caen AR, Chameides L, et al. Pediatric basic and advanced life support: 2010 international consensus on cardiopulmonary resuscitation and emergency cardiovascular care science with treatment recommendations. *Circulation* 2010;**122**:S466–S515.

3. Tobias JD, Ross AK. Intraosseous infusions: a review for the anesthesiologist with a focus on pediatric use. *Anesth Analg* 2010;**110**:391–401.

4. Roberts I, Alderson P, Bunn F, et al. Colloids versus crystalloids for fluid resuscitation in critically ill patients. *Cochrane Database Syst Rev* 2004;**4**:CD000567.

# Anesthetic management of the geriatric trauma patient

Sylvia Y. Dolinski and Olga Kaslow

The United States will soon experience record growth in the number of older individuals. The fastest growing segment of the population is the very old (more than 85 years of age). According to the US census bureau, the number of centenarians is expected to rise to more than 200,000 by the year 2030. In 2009, there were 33 million licensed drivers over the age of 65, which represents a 23% increase in 10 years.

There is a decline in all organ function each year with age. However, individual decline remains unpredictable, in part due to concomitant coexisting disease and associated organ dysfunction. The functional reserve (the difference between baseline functioning and function required in the face of trauma and serious illness) is narrowed, leading to rapid decompensation, multiple organ dysfunction, and ultimately death. There is a lack of definition as to what age is considered geriatric. There only seems to be a uniform definition of the very old – that being greater than 85 years of age.

## Etiology of trauma in elderly

Falls are the leading cause of trauma among the elderly. Each year, one in three adults over the age of 65 falls. The rate of falling increases with age. Those over 85 years have a four-fold increased incidence of falling compared with individuals aged 65 to 84 years. Traffic accidents, including pedestrian struck, also account for a large number of trauma victims. Burns, elder abuse, and neglect are not uncommon causes of injury.

The following age-related physiologic changes are important contributing factors to trauma:

- Visual loss
  - Cataract formation decreases the vision and increases requirements for bright light.
  - Impaired pupillary response affects the eye accommodation to light and darkness.
  - Decreased peripheral vision.
- Cognitive dysfunction
  - Memory decline; impairment in thought process.
  - High prevalence of depression and dementia.
- Unsteady balance and gait
  - Degenerative changes of visual, vestibular, and proprioreceptive sensory systems.
- Slowed reaction time
  - The time between perception of a hazard and avoidance behavior becomes longer.

*Essentials of Trauma Anesthesia*, ed. A. J. Varon and C. E. Smith. Published by Cambridge University Press.
© Cambridge University Press 2012.

- Syncope
  - The most common causes are cardiac dysfunction, cerebrovascular disease, and orthostatic hypotension.

# Age-related changes in physiology

## Cardiovascular function

Cardiovascular function declines with age, resulting in a decrease in cardiac reserve and predisposition to congestive heart failure. Arteriosclerosis is part of the normal aging process that results in loss of larger artery elastin and deposition of calcium, which results in an increase in vascular stiffening.

- Systolic hypertension results from two mechanisms:
  - The stiffened aorta increases the systolic pressure more than a compliant younger aorta that absorbs some of the pressure from the ejected blood volume.
  - The pressure pulse wave travels down the arterial tree faster and the subsequent reflected pulse pressure wave is propagated back toward the heart sooner. In a compliant younger patient, the reflected pulse pressure wave returns to the aortic root early in diastole, which helps augment diastolic blood pressure and coronary blood flow; whereas, in the elderly, the reflected pulse pressure returns at times before the heart has completed ejection. This leads to subsequent augmentation of systolic blood pressure, a decrease in diastolic pressure, and an increase in myocardial afterload.
- The development of higher myocardial wall stress in response to increased afterload leads to left ventricular hypertrophy.
- Augmentation of systolic pressure and left ventricular hypertrophy leads to prolonged myocardial contraction and concomitant impaired diastolic relaxation.
- Impairment of diastolic relaxation results in higher left ventricular end-diastolic pressure necessary to achieve the same stroke volume. In addition, the heart is dependent on atrial contribution to late ventricular filling.
- Fat and collagen deposition along the conduction system predisposes to slower resting heart rate or block; in addition, *adaptive* atrial enlargement to facilitate atrial contribution to stroke volume increases the propensity to atrial fibrillation.
- With age, an increase in cardiac output is dependent on stroke volume.
- Beta-adrenoreceptor responsiveness is blunted.

### Anesthetic concerns

- Acute blood loss is poorly tolerated by the elderly as cardiac output is unable to be improved by heart rate. Fluid boluses into a stiff heart with diastolic dysfunction and arrhythmias places the elderly trauma patient at risk for heart failure.
- Anesthetics cause withdrawal of sympathetic nerve activity upon which an impaired cardiovascular system may rely. This can exaggerate cardiovascular dysfunction.
- Anesthetics impair the heart and vasculature function *directly*, leading to negative inotropy and vasodilatation.
- The aging myocardium is less responsive to circulating catecholamines.

# Respiratory function

Respiratory function impairment leads to worsening in ventilation-perfusion mismatch. Structural alterations of the upper airway lead to increased aspiration risk. Bronchial duct ectasia and loss of elastic recoil of the lung are common in aged humans, leading to airspace enlargement and increased dead space.

- Chest wall compliance decreases with age due to increased fibrosis of thoracic musculature and calcification of costal cartilages. The chest wall becomes more barrel-shaped and the diaphragm flattens. Consequently, the work of breathing normally is elevated compared to a younger patient.
- Vital capacity is decreased, whereas functional residual capacity and closing capacity are increased.
- Pulmonary capillary blood volume and pulmonary membrane permeability diminish with age. Thickening of the alveolo-capillary membrane results in worsening of oxygen diffusing capacity.
- Lower baseline arterial oxygen saturation increases the risk of more rapid progression to hypoxemia.
- Response to hypoxemia and hypercarbia declines.

## Anesthetic concerns

- Increased risk for aspiration.
- Preoxygenation by only four maximal breaths prior to induction of anesthesia may not be sufficient in the elderly due to the decreased vital capacity and increase in residual volume.
- Abdominal or chest surgery compounded by narcotic requirements for pain control and the elderly's baseline increased work of breathing may lead to early respiratory failure.
- Opioids and benzodiazepines along with small residual amounts of inhalational anesthetics increase the upper airway resistance and amplify the reduced respiratory response to hypoxemia and hypercarbia. This may lead to upper airway obstruction, apnea, and hypoxemia.

# Renal function

Renal function declines yearly by a loss of nephrons.

- Glomerular filtration rate is reduced to 50% by the age of 80.
- Thirst response is diminished.
- The renin-angiotensin-aldosterone system's ability to adapt to fluid and pressure changes is reduced.
- Urine concentrating ability declines.

## Anesthetic concerns

- Urine output as a marker of renal perfusion is less reliable.
- Impaired excretion and conservation of water and electrolytes lead to predisposition to hyper- or hypovolemia, and hyper- or hypotension. Resuscitation with normal saline increases the predisposition to hyperchloremic metabolic acidosis.
- Postoperative renal failure susceptibility from hypovolemic and medication induced nephrotoxicity.

# Central nervous system function

Central nervous system function (CNS) is altered with age. Neuronal mass gradually diminishes and thermoregulation is impaired. Elderly patients may have pre-existing neurocognitive dysfunction which may predispose to postoperative neurological impairment and/or delirium.

## Anesthetic concerns

- Thermoregulation impairment rapidly leads to hypothermia. This predisposes to coagulopathy, impaired wound healing, prolonged drug action, increased oxygen consumption, arrhythmias, and myocardial ischemia. Ambient temperature should be increased before elderly patients enter the operating room until they are covered by surgical drapes.
- Postoperative delirium occurs in 5–50% of the elderly. It manifests as a transient and fluctuating disturbance of consciousness which tends to occur shortly after surgery. The prevalence approaches 80% among critically ill patients. Possible etiologies for postoperative delirium include alteration in cellular proteins by potent inhalational agents, central cholinergic insufficiency, preexisting subclinical dementia, infection, altered electrolytes, anemia, pain, and sleep deprivation (see Table 21.1).
- Postoperative delirium should not be confused with postoperative cognitive dysfunction – a more persistent change in cognitive performance of the elderly patient; the symptoms include mild changes in personality, emotional instability, and impaired memory and focus. The causes of postoperative cognitive decline are multifactorial; risk factors include age, years of formal education, duration of anesthetic, postoperative infection, and repeat operation. Postoperative cognitive impairment might be significant enough to lead to prolonged hospital stay and increased healthcare costs.

# Pharmacological changes

Pharmacological changes associated with aging relate to both the pharmacodynamics and pharmacokinetics of anesthetic drugs. There are alterations in the following:

- Lean body mass and total body water (decreased).
- Drug metabolism and excretion (decreased).
- Serum albumin (decreased).
- Sensitivity to drug effects (increased).
- Total body fat (increased).

## Anesthetic concerns

- Trauma-associated injuries and shock modify the response to anesthetics.
- Highly protein-bound drugs have an amplified effect because of a greater amount of free drug available.
- Water-soluble drugs have an exaggerated *initial* effect from a smaller volume of distribution.
- Fat-soluble drugs have a *prolonged* effect from a greater volume of distribution.
- Incidence of drug–drug interactions is greater due to the increased number of medications that the elderly take.

**Table 21.1.** Common causes of delirium in the elderly

| Preoperative variables | • Old age (70 or over)<br>• Chronic diseases, infection<br>• Malnutrition<br>• Hearing and visual impairment<br>• Psychiatric conditions:<br>  – dementia<br>  – prior stroke<br>  – organic brain disease<br>  – depression<br>  – history of delirium<br>• Metabolic causes:<br>  – dehydration, ↓ albumin, ↓ hematocrit<br>  – electrolyte disturbances<br>• Medications:<br>  – anticholinergic drugs<br>  – antidepressants and antipsychotics with anticholinergic activity (amitriptyline, doxapram, imipramine, nortriptyline)<br>  – reserpine<br>  – hydrochlorothiazide<br>  – propranolol<br>• Drug and alcohol abuse and withdrawal |
|---|---|
| Variables related to trauma, surgery, and anesthesia | • Head trauma<br>• Cerebral ischemia due to arterial hypoxemia or insufficient flow<br>• Shock: hypotension, hypoventilation, hypoxemia, anemia<br>• Anesthetic drugs:<br>  – ketamine<br>  – anticholinergic crossing blood-brain barrier (atropine and scopolamine)<br>  – opioids and benzodiazepines<br>  – metoclopromide<br>• Surgical procedures: thoracic, cardiac, and orthopedic<br>• Inadequate analgesia |
| Variables related to postoperative period and resuscitation | • Sleep disturbances, postoperative fatigue<br>• Language difficulty<br>• Immobility, physical restraints<br>• Cardiac, respiratory, renal, and liver failure<br>• Endocrine imbalance and electrolyte deficit:<br>  – abnormal serum glucose, albumin<br>  – abnormal electrolytes (Na, K, $PO_4$, Ca, Mg)<br>• Drug intoxication and withdrawal |

Therefore, dose requirement is markedly reduced:

- Minimum alveolar concentration (MAC) of volatile anesthetics declines by 30% compared to a young patient. Anesthetic induction and emergence are slowed.
- 50% reduction of intravenous induction agents and opioids.

- Benzodiazepines may delay recovery and their use should be minimized or avoided.
- Increased age is associated with slower onset for succinylcholine and vecuronium. The onset time for succinylcholine is prolonged up to two minutes. Duration of neuromuscular relaxants is significantly prolonged in geriatric patients because of the high plasma concentration and slow elimination, further aggravated by renal and hepatic insufficiency. However, the metabolism of atracurium and cis-atracurium remains unchanged.

## Preoperative evaluation

Triage of the elderly trauma patient is complex because usual hemodynamic criteria for trauma team activation are often not present. Thus, the severity and extent of injuries are frequently underestimated.

- Normal blood pressure may signify hypotension in a patient who has baseline hypertension.
- Geriatric patients may be too debilitated to provide any information about their preexisting comorbidities and advanced directives. Reliance on prior physical exam scars may provide insight to past surgical conditions.
- Knowledge of the trauma victim's medication list is of paramount importance, since these medications can significantly alter response to resuscitation and hospital course. The most common medications taken by geriatric patients are antihypertensives (including beta-blockers and vasodilators), oral hypoglycemic agents or insulin, statins, thyroid hormone, steroids, and anticoagulants (see Table 21.2).

## Intraoperative management

### Airway

In the elderly, cervical spine (C-spine) injury such as C1-C2 and odontoid fractures may occur in falls, even from the standing position, and therefore should always be suspected. Adequate preoxygenation, followed by rapid sequence induction with simultaneous in-line stabilization of the cervical spine, may be performed to anesthetize an injured geriatric patient (see Chapter 3). Etomidate and succinylcholine are the preferred agents in the trauma setting. Induction doses of etomidate should be decreased in the setting of hypovolemia and bleeding.

Airway management in the elderly might present a challenge for the anesthesiologist:

- Mask ventilation of edentulous patients can be difficult with ineffective mask seal; two-person bag-mask ventilation with an oral airway is often required.
- Pharyngeal tissues become loose with age and can easily obstruct the upper airway or limit its patency.
- Preexisting arthritis of temporomandibular joints and gradual deterioration of laryngeal structures interfere with mouth opening and visualization of the glottis. Osteoarthritis and degenerative changes at the C-spine and atlanto-occipital joint levels can limit mobility of the neck during direct laryngoscopy. Subluxation of the C-spine unrelated to the original injury may occur while attempting intubation.
- Protective airway reflexes diminish with aging, putting the elderly at higher risk of aspiration.

**Table 21.2.** Commonly used medications by the elderly and anesthesia considerations

| Medication | Anesthesia considerations |
| --- | --- |
| Beta-blockers | – Inhibit patient's physiologic response to hypovolemic shock by blunting tachycardia associated with trauma and hemorrhage<br>– May lead to erroneous assumptions about the patient's hemodynamic state |
| Calcium channel blockers | – Blunt the tachycardic response to hypovolemia |
| Vasodilators | – Aggravate hypotension |
| Anticoagulants (warfarin) | – Exacerbate bleeding<br>– Associated with traumatic intracranial hemorrhage<br>– Warrant the need for close monitoring and aggressive reversal of coagulopathy |
| Antiplatelet agents (clopidogrel) | – Exacerbate bleeding<br>– Increase the grade of intracranial hemorrhage<br>– Poor response to reversal of coagulopathy |
| Statins | – Increase risk of multiple organ failure post-trauma, possibly by affecting immune system |
| Diuretics | – Aggravate hypovolemia and hypotension |
| Angiotensin-converting enzyme (ACE) inhibitors and angiotensin-receptor blockers (ARBs) | – Aggravate hypotension |

# Breathing

Age-related physiologic alterations must be taken into consideration while providing ventilation and oxygenation to the geriatric trauma victim.

- Elderly people are prone to rapid oxygen desaturation, so adequate preoxygenation is important and takes longer.
- Osteoporosis makes the thoracic cage more fragile, rendering the older patient susceptible to rib fractures, pneumo- and hemothorax, flail chest, and pulmonary contusion. Pulmonary contusion is one of the most common complications of blunt thoracic injury, which might deteriorate over time especially with excessive fluid resuscitation (see Chapter 16).
- Both general anesthesia and supine position increase the incidence of atelectasis in the postoperative period. Combined with a less effective cough, the geriatric patient is placed at high risk for respiratory failure, greater likelihood for mechanical ventilation and ventilation-associated pneumonia, and longer intensive care unit stay.

# Circulation

Geriatric trauma patients are more likely to develop shock than their younger counterparts with similar injures. However, shock in the elderly might be difficult to recognize and patients may appear stable in the face of serious systemic hypoperfusion. Modest hypovolemia might go unnoticed in an old person. Skin turgor, feeling of thirst, and urinary output are not reliable signs or symptoms. In addition, elderly patients are prone to chronic volume depletion due to inadequate fluid intake and diuretic use. In a trauma setting, hemorrhage, immobility, and improper nutrition all lead to poor tissue perfusion and organ dysfunction, rapidly progressing to complete organ failure.

Recognition of early shock might be difficult since both the blood pressure and the heart rate response to blood loss are unreliable in advanced age. Blood pressure might not change and even remain elevated in the patient with a history of chronic hypertension, interfering with recognition of shock. Significant bleeding may be suspected based on subtle signs such as altered mentation, narrowed pulse pressure, and delayed capillary refill. However, heart rate response may be blunted by beta-blocker use.

The following issues should be taken into consideration when addressing circulation in the geriatric patient:

- Base deficit (less than −6 mEq/L) on admission arterial blood gas, elevated lactate more than 2 mmol/L, along with delayed rate of clearance suggest occult hypoperfusion and is associated with increased mortality.
- Significant reduction in coronary perfusion and subsequent myocardial infarction may occur even in the absence of coronary artery disease in elderly patients, therefore, revealing a strong association between hypovolemic and cardiogenic shock.
- Patients on warfarin or clopidogrel may sustain significant hemorrhage even in the presence of minor injury. Aggressive correction of coagulopathy with fresh frozen plasma (FFP) and platelets should be initiated early, and if it becomes severe, in addition to coagulopathy of shock and trauma, recombinant factor VII should be considered. Prothrombin complex concentrates and fibrinogen may also reverse the effect of warfarin.
- Both crystalloid and colloid solutions are suitable for volume replacement in a hypovolemic elderly patient; early administration of blood has been advocated in order to improve oxygen delivery.
- Obtaining adequate IV access in a bleeding geriatric patient may be difficult. It is imperative to place at least two large-gauge peripheral IVs. Central venous catheterization may be beneficial due to slow circulation time and for improved drug delivery; however, attempting central venous access during emergency surgery may be impractical and unsafe due to suboptimal sterile conditions and improper positioning, which increase the risk for complications like pneumothorax, infection, and neck hematoma.

## Intraoperative monitoring

Geriatric patients are more dependent on preload than their younger counterparts but at the same time they are more susceptible to fluid overload, especially the ones with history of cardiovascular and renal diseases. Early placement of invasive cardiovascular monitors such as central venous pressure and pulmonary artery (PA) catheters has been advocated in the elderly with hemodynamic instability, significant trauma, known chronic cardiovascular disease, or with a base deficit of more than −6 mEq/L, in order to guide volume replacement and improve oxygen delivery (see Chapter 9). However, no specific monitoring techniques have been shown to be superior for managing fluid resuscitation in the setting of emergency surgery for trauma.

## Temperature control

Elderly patients are especially susceptible to hypothermia; they have less fat stores and subcutaneous tissue for insulation and also exhibit decreased shivering and non-shivering thermogenesis (see Chapter 7). General anesthesia further alters their thermoregulatory response secondary to drug-induced vasodilation. Exposure to trauma, shock, and massive resuscitation exacerbate hypothermia and its complications – metabolic acidosis, coagulopathy, and platelet dysfunction.

Aggressive warming must be initiated in the operating room:

- Increase the room temperature.
- Apply radiant heat and/or convective warming.
- All IV fluids and blood products should be warmed.

# Anesthesia for the most common injuries in the elderly

## Orthopedic trauma

Orthopedic injuries in the geriatric population occur as a part of polytrauma or as an isolated extremity fracture (see also Chapter 18).

**Surgical considerations**. Expedited orthopedic surgery for fracture stabilization of the pelvis and long bones allows early mobilization and fewer complications due to prolonged bed rest. The timing for surgical repair and its effect on morbidity and mortality remain controversial. There seems to be little evidence that surgical treatment of open fractures within six hours after trauma decreases the risk of infection. This widely held "dogma" was spread prior to systemic antibiotic use and has been challenged within the past ten years. The medically fit elderly patient should undergo surgery as soon as possible, but patients with multiple comorbid diseases should be medically optimized. Surgery for closed fractures within 24 to 48 hours is currently advocated. Delaying the operation beyond 48 hours has been associated with prolonged hospitalization, increased morbidity (e.g., deep vein thrombosis, decubitus ulcer development), and increased mortality. Improved ambulation results in fewer respiratory complications as well.

**Anesthetic considerations**. The time period 24 to 48 hours after orthopedic trauma should be sufficient to conduct a thorough preoperative evaluation of the patient including investigation and treatment of the patient's medical conditions, diagnosis of all injuries, and pre-anesthetic optimization of volume status, hemodynamics, and respiratory parameters. Both general and regional anesthesia may be safely employed for orthopedic surgery in elderly patients.

Regional anesthesia has the least effect on cognition, particularly if no sedation is used during placement and surgery. Therefore, regional anesthesia is advocated for isolated orthopedic injuries (see Chapter 8). Its use preserves the patient's mental status and spontaneous breathing when no or minimal sedation is used. Smaller doses of local anesthetic, however, result in a higher level of sensory blockade with both spinal and thoracic epidurals. Unfortunately, no study to date has definitively shown that regional anesthesia decreases the incidence of postoperative delirium. This is most likely because the pathophysiology of delirium after anesthesia and surgery remains obscure and multifactorial (Table 21.1), and may include hypothetical mechanisms such as disordered neurotransmission, inflammation, and stress.

- Contraindications to regional anesthesia include a non-cooperative patient and those treated with anticoagulants and antiplatelet medications.
- The volume status of the patient with isolated orthopedic injury should be optimized before proceeding to regional anesthesia. The hydration status of geriatric patients is often underestimated due to poor oral intake, preexisting fluid deficit, and significant bleeding sealed in a muscular compartment in a case of closed fracture.

General anesthesia is advocated for patients with multiple orthopedic and multi-system injuries and for those with contraindications to regional anesthesia (see Chapter 7).

Intraoperative management of the patient's fluid status should be guided by both non-invasive and invasive monitoring; their choice should be based on the patient's preoperative cardiovascular status, known comorbidities, and the extent of trauma (see Chapters 9,10).

## Hip fractures

The most common orthopedic trauma among the elderly is an isolated hip fracture, which is typically due to a fall. The incidence of hip fractures doubles each decade after 50 years of age. Risk factors include osteoporosis and low bone density, female gender, history of smoking, low weight, and decreased physical activity. It is an important cause of mortality and functional dependence among geriatric patients. Hip fractures occur in three anatomic locations:

- Femoral neck fractures (intracapsular) are commonly seen in active geriatric patients, and are often associated with blood flow interruption to the femoral head with its subsequent necrosis.
- Intertrochanteric fractures (extracapsular) typically affect dependent females.
  The blood flow to the femoral neck is preserved due to the good vascularization of the fractured area.
- Subtrochanteric fractures are not very common, comprising only 5–10%.

**Surgical considerations.** Early reduction and fixation of the fractured hip is the current management strategy. This results in lower morbidity and mortality and shorter hospital stay among medically stable geriatric patients.

**Anesthetic considerations.** There are no data supporting advantage of certain anesthetic techniques for hip surgery in the elderly: general, spinal, and epidural anesthesia and peripheral nerve blocks have been employed with similar success. Spinal and epidural anesthesia along with the lumbar plexus block may be used in the modality of a single shot as well as a continuous infusion through the catheter, which provides adequate analgesia during surgery and in the postoperative period.

## Splenic trauma

Non-operative management has become standard care for hemodynamically stable splenic injuries. Age should not be a criterion to abandon non-operative management.

## Chest trauma and rib fractures

Elderly patients with more than four rib fractures have worse outcomes. It is likely that the increase in work of breathing is too great and predisposes the geriatric patient to respiratory failure (see Chapter 16). Early thoracic epidural or paravertebral catheter placement may improve respiratory function and pulmonary toilet and decrease the need for mechanical ventilation. It has been shown that epidural analgesia decreases mortality in the elderly.

## Cervical spine injuries

Often these are multi-level injuries and more often involve C1 and C2 levels (see Chapter 14).

## Closed head trauma

- People aged 75 and older account for the highest rates of traumatic brain injury-related hospitalization and death (see Chapter 13).
- Falls and concomitant anticoagulation use in apparently minor head trauma lead to neurosurgical intervention 20% of the time. Thus, even minimal head trauma in these patients should prompt use of head computed tomography.
- The ability of the brain to recover from trauma significantly declines with age; even mild injury can lead to a devastating outcome.

The patient may present with isolated head trauma or in association with C-spine, long-bone fractures, and other organ injuries that make the anesthetic management more challenging. Closed head trauma may be represented by a skull fracture, concussion and contusion of the brain, subdural and epidural hematomas, traumatic vascular dissection, or diffuse axonal injury.

Intracranial bleeding in the form of subdural or intracerebral hematoma is a common complication in the elderly due to a variety of factors:

- Increased vulnerability of cerebral vessels.
- Stretching of the bridging veins following trauma.
- Reduced brain mass.
- Anticoagulant and antiplatelet therapy.

Elderly patients seldom develop an epidural hematoma due to formation of firm adherence between dura matter and the skull. The classic signs and symptoms of elevated intracranial pressure (ICP), such as change in mental status, headache, and non-focal neurologic deficit, may not be obvious in geriatric patients because of their smaller brain mass.

- Patients with depressed skull fracture, or epidural, subdural, or intracerebral hematoma, require emergent surgical intervention.
- Reversal of anticoagulation drugs is necessary before proceeding with surgery. While vitamin K takes hours to become effective, plasma, platelets, and cryoprecipitate provide a rapid preoperative correction of the coagulopathy. Recombinant FVIIa, fibrinogen, and prothrombin complex concentrates may also be used to reverse warfarin coagulopathy.

**Anesthetic considerations**. The following issues must be considered in elderly patients who sustain traumatic brain injury:

- Premedication with benzodiazepines and opioids should be avoided in patients with suspected elevated ICP as it further alters the patient's sensorium and predisposes to hypoventilation and hypoxia.
- Expedited airway control with rapid sequence induction and manual in-line stabilization of the C-spine should be achieved in a smooth fashion to minimize hypoventilation, hypercarbia, and hypoxemia.
- The choice of induction agent should be based on the patient's hemodynamic status. Etomidate has an advantage over propofol and thiopental for its minimal hemodynamic consequences in a trauma patient. If there is no increased mass effect, ketamine may be indicated in the face of overt hypotension.
- The main anesthetic goal for the head-injured elderly patient is to maximize oxygen delivery to the brain and control ICP. Therefore, maintaining an adequate cerebral perfusion pressure is crucial to ensure sufficient oxygen supply to the brain, especially in the presence of high ICP.
- Mean arterial pressure should be maintained at the usual pre-trauma level of geriatric patients, many of whom have chronic hypertension.
- When there is hemodynamic instability, a PA catheter may help guide administration of fluids and vasopressors to optimize cerebral oxygen delivery.

## Outcomes of the geriatric trauma patient

Overall, the outcomes in the geriatric trauma patient are worse due to increased prevalence of chronic diseases and decreased physiological reserve.

- Elderly patients with blunt trauma have a two-fold increased rate of mortality.
- Triage is difficult to base on mechanism of injury, as low impact mechanisms can cause profound injury in the elderly.

Prevention of delirium and cognitive dysfunction should be initiated early. A multi-disciplinary approach is advocated and should include the following:

- Optimizing preexisting medical conditions and control of infection.
- Maintaining adequate oxygenation and cerebral perfusion.
- Correction of dehydration and electrolyte imbalance.
- Providing strong preoperative analgesia and emotional support.
- Early mobilization and nutrition.

## Key points

- The elderly are the largest growing segment of the population and are increasingly maintaining active lifestyles longer, putting them at risk for injury.
- Geriatric patients are more likely to present in occult shock.
- The combination of age-related decline in organ function, diminished physiologic reserve, and coexistence of one or more chronic diseases alters the ability of the elderly patient to compensate for the stress of trauma.
- It is not chronologic age that is important, but *physiologic* age in predicting survival in the geriatric patient population, especially in the very old.

# Further reading

1.  Deiner S, Silverstein JH, Abrams KJ. Management of trauma in the geriatric patient. *Curr Opin Anaesthesiol* 2004;**17**:165–170.

2.  Jaberi M. Geriatric trauma. In: Sieber F. *Geriatric Anesthesia*. New York, NY: McGraw Hill; 2007.

3.  Lewis MC, Abouelenin K, Paniagua M. Geriatric trauma: special considerations in the anesthetic management of the injured elderly patient. *Anesthesiol Clin* 2007;**25**:75–90.

4.  Silverstein J. Trauma in the elderly. In: Smith CE, ed. *Trauma Anesthesia*. New York, NY: Cambridge University Press; 2008.

5.  Web-based Injury Statistics Query and Reporting System by the Centers for Disease Control and Prevention. www.cdc. gov/ncipc/wisqars/. Accessed April 24, 2011.

6.  Williams J, Johnson C, Ashley S, et al. Geriatric trauma. In: Wilson W, Grande C, Hoyt D, eds. *Trauma*. Volume 1. New York, NY: Informa Healthcare; 2007.

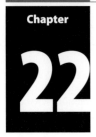

# Anesthetic management of the pregnant trauma patient

Nicholas Nedeff and Pertti Hakala

## Introduction

Traumatic injuries are the most common cause of maternal mortality in the United States. While only 6 to 8% of pregnancies are affected by trauma, these injuries are responsible for about 20% of maternal deaths. The most common cause of maternal death related to trauma is motor vehicle collision, accounting for roughly two-thirds of the deaths. Domestic violence and falls also account for a significant number of deaths. Further, it is estimated that drugs and alcohol are involved in 20% of maternal trauma.

Trauma in the pregnant patient results in several unique challenges. There are significant physiological and anatomical changes in the pregnant patient. These alterations impact clinical assessment, interpretation of diagnostic studies, patient management, and the type of injuries that may occur. With the exception of anesthesiologists, trauma team clinicians and staff typically have little training or experience in the care of the pregnant patient. Therefore, a multi-disciplinary approach involving the trauma surgeon, anesthesiologist, obstetrician, and other members of the trauma team, is important for optimal patient care. Perhaps the most unique challenge is simultaneously caring for two patients, fetus and mother. In doing so, it is critical to recall that the best strategy in caring for both patients is to optimize the treatment and resuscitation of the mother.

## Physiology and anatomy

The pregnant patient undergoes many anatomical and physiological changes through the course of pregnancy. It is of paramount importance to recognize such alterations in order to optimize the care of the mother and the fetus.

## Hematologic

- Blood volume progressively increases throughout pregnancy: a 25% increase is seen in the second trimester, and an increase of 40–50% by the third trimester. The increase in blood volume is likely a protective mechanism to compensate for blood loss during childbirth. This is one reason maternal heart rate and blood pressure may remain relatively unchanged from baseline despite blood loss of up to 1.5–2 L (30–35% blood volume).
- Hematocrit decreases. Well known as "the physiologic anemia of pregnancy," this alteration is due to a 40–50% increase in plasma volume with a 20–30% increase

*Essentials of Trauma Anesthesia*, ed. A. J. Varon and C. E. Smith. Published by Cambridge University Press.
© Cambridge University Press 2012.

in red blood cell volume. Thus, by 34 weeks gestation, the hematocrit is typically between 29% and 34%.

- Clotting factors increase significantly during pregnancy and create a hypercoagulable state with greater risk for thromboembolism. Factors VII, VIII, IX, and X and fibrinogen are increased. Patients are also at increased risk for developing disseminated intravascular coagulation (DIC) secondary to placental injury, such as placental abruption.
- White blood cell count is elevated during pregnancy and values of 12,000–15,000/mm$^3$ are not uncommon.

## Cardiovascular

- Cardiac output (CO) increases significantly. By the tenth week, CO can be increased by 1.0–1.5 L/min, and 30–50% by the third trimester. This is due to both an increase in plasma volume and a decrease in vascular resistance.
- Heart rate increases typically by 10–15%.
- Blood pressure decreases by approximately 20%. This is secondary to progesterone-induced decreases in systemic vascular resistance of about 35%.
- Pulmonary artery pressure (PAP) and central venous pressure (CVP) are usually decreased, but may be variable during pregnancy. Despite this, the response to volume is unchanged compared to the non-pregnant patient.
- Uterine blood flow increases throughout pregnancy and, at term, can be up to 20% of CO. A decrease in uterine blood flow to compensate for acute maternal hemorrhage may occur. Therefore, fetal distress may signal maternal hypovolemia earlier than tachycardia and hypotension.
- Electrocardiogram changes can manifest in a number of ways. The normal position of the heart is altered due to the enlarging uterus and can be reflected as left axis deviation. Q waves, flattened or inverted T waves in leads 2, 3, and AVF, and non-specific ST changes may also be observed. In addition, ectopy is more frequently seen in pregnant patients.
- Supine hypotension syndrome is hypotension caused by the gravid uterus compressing the inferior vena cava and reducing CO by up to 30% when the patient is supine. This syndrome is typically seen beyond 20 weeks gestation and is usually corrected by changing the patient's position, most commonly, to the left lateral decubitus position.

## Pulmonary

- Functional residual capacity (FRC) decreases by 20–25%. This is due to both weight gain and the presence of a gravid uterus, leading to an elevation in the diaphragm by up to 4 cm, or two costal spaces.
- Oxygen consumption increases by 20% or more at term. Increased oxygen consumption coupled with decreased FRC predisposes pregnant patients to develop hypoxia more rapidly during periods of apnea. In spite of adequate preoxygenation, these patients typically develop arterial desaturation within three minutes after cessation of ventilation. This phenomenon can occur as quickly as one minute, as compared to the non-pregnant patient who can typically tolerate five to seven minutes of apnea before the oxygen saturation measured by pulse oximetry (SpO$_2$) starts to decline.

- Tidal volume and respiratory rate are both increased and result in an increase in minute ventilation of up to 40%, with increased tidal volumes being a major causative factor. This leads to a mild respiratory alkalosis, with a mildly elevated maternal arterial oxygen tension ($PaO_2$) and a decrease in arterial carbon dioxide tension ($PaCO_2$) by up to 10–12 mmHg. Notably, although a $PaCO_2$ of 35–40 mmHg in the non-pregnant patient is considered normal, in the pregnant patient such levels may reflect hypoventilation and an early sign of respiratory failure.
- Vital capacity is relatively unchanged as decreases in FRC are offset by increases in inspiratory reserve capacity.

## Gastrointestinal

- Gastroesophageal sphincter tone and gastric emptying are decreased due to increased progesterone levels. Most pregnant patients by the second or third trimester have gastroesophageal reflux to some extent. These changes increase the risk of aspiration and pneumonitis.
- Although the position of the liver and spleen are relatively unchanged, the intestines are displaced into the upper abdomen and, in some instances, may be partially shielded from injury by the uterus. However, unlike in non-pregnant patients, intestinal injuries may occur from trauma to the upper abdomen.

## Renal and genitourinary

- Renal blood flow and glomerular filtration rate increase and lead to natriuresis.
- Patients are more prone to urinary tract infections due to ureteral dilatation and ureteral reflux.
- Blood urea nitrogen (BUN) and creatinine are decreased; values half that of normal non-pregnant values are typical. As a result, normal values in the non-pregnant patient may be an indication of significant renal dysfunction in the pregnant patient.
- Physiologically, uterine blood flow increases greatly throughout pregnancy. The increase is roughly ten-fold, from about 60 mL/min to up to 600 mL/min. Because of this, the gravid uterus can be a significant source of hemorrhage.
- Anatomically, by week 12, the uterus changes from being considered an intra-pelvic organ to an intra-abdominal organ. The uterus continues to grow with the vertex typically reaching the level of the umbilicus by week 20, and to its maximal height, typically around the costal margin, sometime between the 34th and 36th weeks. Fundal height decreases in the last two weeks of gestation as the fetus descends.
- Early in pregnancy the uterus is not only small, but also relatively thick-walled. As pregnancy progresses, the uterus increases in size and becomes more thin-walled.
- Placental blood flow is not autoregulated; hypovolemia and anemia will lead to decreased fetal blood flow often manifesting as a sign of fetal distress even though maternal vital signs may appear relatively normal. The placenta has very little elasticity, which puts the patient at risk of placental separation or abruption secondary to shear forces exerted on the uteroplacental interface.
- Early in pregnancy, the fetus is protected from trauma due to the relatively large amount of amniotic fluid surrounding it. However, as the pregnancy progresses, this cushion becomes increasingly smaller. Also, in the event of trauma, amniotic fluid may lead to amniotic fluid embolism or DIC.

## Musculoskeletal

- During pregnancy, the sacroiliac joint space increases and the pubic symphysis widens. Thus, the interpretation of pelvic X-rays when diagnosing pelvic fracture may become more difficult.

## Endocrine

- The pituitary gland increases in size by 30–50% during pregnancy. The anterior pituitary gland becomes more prone to necrosis, secondary to shock, and may result in pituitary insufficiency.
- Pregnant patients have altered glycemic regulation, which can result in gestational diabetes.

A summary of the physiologic changes of pregnancy is provided in Table 22.1.

## **Mechanisms of injury**

Pregnant patients have similar mechanisms of trauma as non-pregnant patients. However, the incidence of certain types of trauma, and the injury patterns suffered, may differ. In addition to maternal injuries, fetal injuries and the possibility of fetal loss must also be considered.

## Blunt trauma

- In pregnant patients, blunt trauma is the most common trauma mechanism. Motor vehicle collision is the most common type of blunt trauma and accounts for over half of all injuries in the pregnant patient. They also account for the majority of fetal deaths. The incidence and severity of maternal injuries, premature labor, fetal injuries, and fetal loss are significantly lower in restrained as opposed to unrestrained patients. Seatbelts with both shoulder and lap restraints offer greater maternal and fetal protection as compared to a lap belt alone.
- The incidence of trauma due to falls is increased in pregnant women. Falls occur more frequently late in pregnancy, as the gravid uterus becomes more prominent and balance is altered due to a change in center of gravity. Falls are also among the leading causes of fetal death.
- Domestic violence is also increased among pregnant patients compared to non-pregnant patients. It is estimated that domestic violence accounts for 5 to 15% of trauma among pregnant women. It is more common in the second and third trimester of pregnancy and often involves the abdomen.

## Penetrating trauma

- Penetrating injuries, such as stab wounds and gunshot wounds, account for a small percentage of trauma among pregnant women. Although gunshot wounds are uncommon, there is a significant risk of fetal death.
- Early in pregnancy, the fetus is relatively well protected from penetrating injuries due to the thick muscular uterine wall and amniotic fluid. In the case of firearms, the uterus

**Table 22.1.** Summary of the physiologic changes of pregnancy

| Hematologic | |
|---|---|
| Blood volume | Increase |
| Plasma volume | Increase |
| Red blood cell volume | Increase |
| White blood cell volume | Increase |
| Coagulation factors | Increase |
| Hematocrit | Decrease |
| **Cardiovascular** | |
| Cardiac output | Increase |
| Heart rate | Increase |
| Blood pressure | Decrease |
| Systemic vascular resistance | Decrease |
| Central venous pressure | Decrease |
| Pulmonary artery pressure | Decrease |
| **Pulmonary** | |
| Minute ventilation | Increase |
| Tidal volume | Increase |
| Respiratory rate | Increase |
| Oxygen consumption | Increase |
| $PaO_2$ | Increase |
| Functional residual capacity | Decrease |
| $PaCO_2$ | Decrease |
| **Gastrointestinal** | |
| Gastroesophageal sphincter tone | Decrease |
| Gastric emptying | Decrease |
| **Renal and genitourinary** | |
| Renal blood flow | Increase |
| Glomerular filtration rate | Increase |
| Uterine blood flow | Increase |
| BUN | Decrease |
| Creatinine | Decrease |

Abbreviations: BUN = blood urea nitrogen; $PaCO_2$ = arterial carbon dioxide tension; $PaO_2$ = arterial oxygen tension.

and amniotic fluid have the ability to absorb energy from projectiles and reduce the likelihood and extent of fetal injury.

- As pregnancy progresses, the uterus takes up more space in the lower abdomen and partially shields the intestines and other organs from injury. However, the uterus becomes more susceptible to penetrating injuries with its now thinner walls. In addition, with the relative decrease in amniotic fluid, the chances of penetrating trauma resulting in significant injury increase as pregnancy progresses.

## Burns

- Burns are relatively uncommon among pregnant patients, and are managed much the same way as in non-pregnant patients (see Chapter 19). The airway, the extent and severity of the burn, and fluid resuscitation are key components in managing these patients.
- Supplemental oxygen should be used and the threshold for tracheal intubation should be low as oxygenation and ventilation may be impaired and because of the risk of carbon monoxide poisoning. The latter is especially worrisome in pregnancy as fetal blood has a higher affinity for carbon monoxide; the fetus is thus more prone to acidosis and hypoxemia and elimination may take longer than from maternal blood. Just as in the non-pregnant patient, significant airway edema can develop rapidly leading to airway compromise; securing the airway may become more difficult.
- Assessing the extent and severity of the burn is important in predicting outcome. Patients with less than 30% burn surface area have lower morbidity and mortality rates. The rule of nines is used, just as in non-pregnant patients, to estimate surface area of burn and guide fluid therapy (see Chapter 19).

## Assessment and management

The possibility of pregnancy should be considered in all female trauma patients of child-bearing age. Prompt recognition is important so that necessary team members can be notified and any additional equipment needed to care for the patient can be secured. Furthermore, recognition will allow for more accurate interpretation of the signs, symptoms, and diagnostic studies when evaluating the patient.

Management priorities for optimizing care in the pregnant trauma patient are to assess and resuscitate the mother, followed by the secondary survey which includes fetal assessment. While pregnancy is an important consideration, it should not interfere with performing necessary tests and procedures (e.g., radiographic studies) or managing the patient's injuries.

## Initial management

Initial management of the pregnant patient should focus on the ABCs of resuscitation, just as in the non-pregnant patient. However, while conducting the initial assessment, it is important to keep in mind the changes that occur with pregnancy, as they impact the management of these patients.

# Airway

There are several important factors amongst pregnant patients that make the incidence of failed intubation greater, thus complicating airway management. The airway is often edematous at the level of the cords and above. This may make conventional laryngoscopy technically more difficult and require the use of a smaller tracheal tube. In anticipation, having a smaller endotracheal tube (i.e., size 6.0 or 6.5) and surgical backup readily available are recommended. The increase in breast size may hinder insertion of a standard laryngoscope. In such instances, the use of a short handle laryngoscope may be advantageous.

Trauma patients are already considered at high risk for aspiration and this risk is compounded in pregnancy due to the decrease in gastric emptying and lower esophageal sphincter tone. For these reasons, rapid sequence induction and intubation is recommended for securing the airway (see Chapters 3 and 7). Alternatively, when difficult intubation or ventilation is anticipated, an awake oral fiberoptic intubation may be indicated. Manual in-line immobilization is done if there is suspicion of cervical spine injury.

Adequate preoxygenation and the ability to rapidly secure the airway are imperative as pregnant patients can become hypoxic with short periods of apnea. If an awake technique is chosen, it is important to limit the amount of sedation and consider the effects of any prehospital medications that may have been given in order to prevent oversedation and loss of the airway.

# Breathing

Ensuring adequate oxygenation and ventilation is essential because pregnant patients are more prone to hypoxia and hypoventilation due to increased oxygen requirements and decreased oxygen reserves. Supplemental oxygen should always be used in parturients during the initial assessment to reduce the likelihood of hypoxia. Maternal hypoxia is poorly tolerated by the fetus and often manifests as fetal decelerations or bradycardia. Hypercarbia and acidosis also lead rapidly to fetal distress.

# Circulation

Aggressive fluid and blood resuscitation of the mother to restore intravascular volume and correction of severe anemia are indispensable for improved outcome. Fetal distress is often an early sign of inadequate resuscitation, as significant blood loss is fairly well tolerated by the mother and vital signs may be minimally altered from baseline values. The use of vasopressors to maintain blood pressure should be minimized as they may further decrease fetal blood supply, despite improvement in maternal values.

In patients who are more than 20 weeks gestational age, use of left uterine displacement may prevent or minimize the "supine hypotension syndrome" that results from compression of the inferior vena cava by the enlarged uterus. If the patient is on a backboard, left uterine displacement can be achieved by tilting the entire backboard approximately 15°, which is commonly achieved by placing a wedge or blankets under the backboard.

# Fetal evaluation

After the airway, ventilation, control of hemorrhage, protection of the spine, restoration and maintenance of vital signs, and prompt treatment of other life-threatening conditions have been addressed, the focus can shift to the fetus.

An initial step in fetal evaluation is the confirmation of fetal heart tones. Another critical step is estimating gestational age, which can occasionally be elicited through the patient's history. After the primary survey is completed, evaluation of uterine size should be done to help confirm or determine gestational age. This can be done by ultrasound examination (ideal) or by physical exam (measurement of fundal height). Whether or not the fetus is viable is an important endpoint for decisions regarding patient management. The fetus is generally considered viable at greater than 23 weeks gestation. This is an important distinction, as emergent Caesarean section (C-section) may be performed in cases of fetal distress not resolved with conservative management.

Advanced Trauma Life Support (ATLS) guidelines recommend that continuous fetal monitoring be initiated during the secondary survey in patients with more than 20 weeks gestation. The length of time for fetal monitoring varies based on maternal vital signs and severity of trauma. Continuous monitoring is performed throughout the period of maternal hemodynamic instability. If the mother is stable, monitoring is recommended for a minimum of 4–6 hours for minor trauma and a minimum of 24 hours for severe trauma. The potential benefit of monitoring fetal heart rate is that signs of fetal distress can be earlier indicators of significant maternal hemorrhage than tachycardia and hypotension (the normal fetal heart rate is 120–160 bpm).

The secondary survey should encompass the same components as for a non-pregnant patient. In addition, a complete pelvic and perineal exam should be performed, ideally, by an obstetrician.

## Obstetric issues

There are a number of conditions unique to pregnant patients that require treatment. These range from isoimmunization to fetal loss. Presenting signs and symptoms of many of these entities include abdominal pain and tenderness, vaginal bleeding, maternal instability, and fetal distress.

- Amniotic fluid embolism has a high mortality rate and the management focus is early recognition and aggressive supportive therapy.
- Maternal isoimmmunization occurs in up to 30% of the cases and can be screened using the Kleihauer-Betke test. Rh-negative patients should receive Rh immune globulin within 72 hours of the injury.
- Pre-term labor should be initially managed with fluids and tocolytics. C-section may be indicated when the fetus is viable, in distress, and initial therapies fail.
- Uterine rupture requires aggressive fluid and blood resuscitation, operative management to control bleeding, and delivery of the fetus. In some cases hysterectomy may be required.
- Premature rupture of membranes may lead to pre-term labor, infection, sepsis, fetal distress, and demise.
- Placental abruption has an incidence of 1–5% in minor trauma, and 20–50% in major trauma. It is also associated with a high fetal mortality, with some estimates as high as 60%.
- Fetal concerns include direct fetal injury, umbilical cord rupture, and fetal loss. In these cases emergency C-section may be beneficial if the fetus is viable.

## Imaging studies

A number of non-invasive imaging techniques are used for patient assessment. Focused assessment with sonography for trauma (FAST) is routinely used to evaluate the abdomen and can be safely used for fetal assessment as well.

Radiation exposure should be avoided whenever possible. The greatest risk to the fetus is during the first trimester, particularly within the first eight weeks, as this encompasses the period of organogenesis. Radiation exposure remains a concern throughout pregnancy, as there may be many harmful effects, such as increased risk of lymphoma. Radiation exposure of 5 to 10 rad or greater can lead to a developmental disorder. While necessary tests should not be withheld, it is important to use clinical judgment regarding necessity of tests rather than ordering them by protocol. In addition, measures should be instituted to avoid unnecessary exposure, such as using a lead shield to cover the abdomen, reducing exposure time by limiting repeat films, and using fluoroscopy judiciously.

- Radiation dose from radiographs is fairly low with values of 0.005 rad for chest and 0.5 rad for pelvis.
- Computed tomography (CT) delivers a significantly larger radiation dose, with abdominal CT approaching 5 rad and whole body reaching up to 9 rad.
- Fluoroscopy exposes the patient to more radiation than CT and its use should therefore be limited as much as possible.
- Magnetic resonance imaging does not expose patients to radiation and offers an alternative imaging method.
- For patients with equivocal FAST exams, peritoneal lavage should be considered as an alternative to CT, particularly in the first trimester, as the uterus is still intrapelvic and the fetus is most sensitive to the effects of radiation.

## Operative management

Pregnant trauma patients may require surgical intervention for definitive treatment of injuries. Common surgeries include exploratory laparotomy, orthopedic procedures for pelvic or limb repair, and gynecologic or obstetric procedures such as C-section.

### Anesthetic considerations

Proper backup equipment and personnel should be on hand for induction and intubation in the event there is difficulty or failure to intubate the trachea. Adequate venous access, at least two large intravenous catheters, is crucial to allow aggressive resuscitation. Volatile agents should be kept below minimum alveolar concentration (MAC) of 2.0 for surgery, and below 1.0 MAC for C-section. Oxygen concentration should not be less than 50% in order to maximize fetal oxygen delivery. Review of maternal medications prior to surgery is important. For example, magnesium potentiates the effects of neuromuscular relaxants. Orogastric tubes are preferred to nasogastric tubes, for gastric decompression, as the nasal mucosal surfaces are friable and edematous; similarly, oral versus nasal temperature probes are preferred.

### Monitoring

For all pregnant patients undergoing surgery, the presence of fetal heart tones should be confirmed before and after surgery. After 20 weeks gestation, continuous intraoperative fetal monitoring is recommended. An exception is when fetal heart rate monitoring is not possible due to surgical site interference. Monitoring requires a dedicated person familiar with the fetal monitor, typically a labor and delivery nurse. An obstetrician needs to be notified any time these patients go to the operating room, as they need to be immediately available should emergency C-section be required.

Numerous anesthetic agents reduce or abolish normal fetal heart rate variability without affecting fetal well-being. Although heart rate variability is lost as a marker for fetal well-being, fetal heart rate and uterine contractions can still be determined.

## Emergent C-section

There are several reasons for performing an emergent C-section in the pregnant trauma patient. Indications for emergent C-section include:

- Fetal distress in a stable mother with a viable fetus.
- Perimortem mother with viable fetus. In this situation, the timing of delivery is crucial as delivery within five minutes of maternal cardiac arrest has a 70% newborn survival rate, compared to delivery after six minutes, which is associated with less than 15% survival. Some authors refer to this as the "four-minute" rule. During such time, it is important to continue effective chest compressions and resuscitation to the parturient.
- Maternal cardiac arrest. Regardless of fetal viability, this is done to improve the quality of maternal resuscitation.
- In some cases C-section is performed during surgery due to persistent fetal distress or maternal cardiac arrest.

Because the need for emergent C-section can occur at any time, appropriate obstetric and pediatric/neonatal personnel and equipment must be immediately available.

## Cardiopulmonary resuscitation (CPR)

Pregnancy does not change the manner in which CPR is performed, or the manner in which vasopressors or defibrillation are used during cardiac arrest resuscitation. The airway should be secured to ensure oxygenation and ventilation, which are typically difficult via face mask ventilation in pregnant women. The patient should remain in left lateral tilt. Emergent C-section should be performed if the patient does not respond to initial CPR efforts. In a non-viable pregnancy ($< 24$ weeks), the focus should be on saving the mother. Delivery of the fetus improves resuscitative efforts by improving the quality of chest compressions, decreasing metabolic demands, and increasing venous return. If the fetus is viable, then the focus is on saving both the mother and child.

## Key points

- Pregnancy must be suspected and evaluated in all female trauma patients of reproductive age.
- The best strategy in caring for a mother and her fetus is to optimize treatment and resuscitation of the mother.
- Significant blood loss of up to 1.5–2 L (30–35% blood volume) may occur with little change in maternal vital signs.

- Fetal distress is often an earlier indicator of significant maternal hemorrhage than tachycardia and hypotension.
- The chances of a difficult or failed intubation and aspiration are much higher in pregnancy. Therefore, backup equipment and personnel should be in place prior to intubation attempts.
- Necessary tests and treatments should not be withheld because of pregnancy, as benefits outweigh the risks. When possible, measures should be taken to protect the fetus.
- Patients > 20 weeks gestation should be positioned with a left lateral tilt to avoid the supine hypotension syndrome.
- Fetal monitoring should be considered for pregnant patients with ≥ 20 weeks gestation.
- Obstetricians and pediatricians should be immediately available for emergency delivery in cases where the fetus is viable.
- Anesthesiologists can play a crucial role in patient outcome, as they are often more experienced than surgeons with caring for pregnant patients, and are more experienced than obstetricians with caring for hemodynamically unstable patients.

## Further reading

1. American College of Surgeons, Committee on Trauma. *Advance Trauma Life Support for Doctors: ATLS® Student Course Manual.* Chicago, IL: American College of Surgeons; 2008.

2. Chestnut, DH. *Chestnut's Obstetric Anesthesia: Principles and Practice*, 4th edition. Philadelphia, PA: Mosby; 2009.

3. Grossman NB. Blunt trauma in pregnancy. *Am Fam Phys* 2004;**70**:1303–1310.

4. Hull S, Bennett S. The pregnant trauma patient: assessment and anesthetic management. *Int Anesthesiol Clin* 2007;**45**:1–18.

5. McAuley DJ. Trauma in pregnancy: anatomical and physiological considerations. *Trauma* 2004;**6**:293–300.

6. Tsuei BJ. Assessment of the pregnant trauma patient. *Injury Int J Care Injured* 2006;**37**:367–373.

# Index